SOURCES OF CONSCIOUSNESS

The Biophysical and Computational Basis of Thought

Advanced Series in Neuroscience – Vol. 5

SOURCES OF CONSCIOUSNESS

The Biophysical and Computational Basis of Thought

H S Green & **T Triffet**
University of Adelaide *University of Arizona*

World Scientific
Singapore • New Jersey • London • Hong Kong

Published by

World Scientific Publishing Co. Pte. Ltd.

P O Box 128, Farrer Road, Singapore 912805

USA office: Suite 1B, 1060 Main Street, River Edge, NJ 07661

UK office: 57 Shelton Street, Covent Garden, London WC2H 9HE

British Library Cataloguing-in-Publication Data
A catalogue record for this book is available from the British Library.

SOURCES OF CONSCIOUSNESS
The Biophysical and Computational Basis of Thought

ISBN 981-02-2921-6

This book is printed on acid-free paper.

Printed in Singapore by Uto-Print

Foreword

The primary purpose of this book is to offer certain insights to the understanding of human consciousness gained by the authors from theoretical and experimental research in the neurosciences over the last two decades.

Because of the explosive growth of such knowledge during this period, and the vast literature that now exists documenting the achievements of investigators worldwide, our presentation of background material is necessarily selective rather than comprehensive. In general, we have chosen to summarize only those topics, and within these only those treatments, that seem to us essential for our purposes, and for arriving eventually at a satisfactory explanation of the higher brain processes–the properties of mind. No attempt is made, for example, to treat every important contribution of the last twenty years to the neurosciences, cognitive science, artificial intelligence, or neural network theory and practice; in no sense is the book a survey of all, or even one, of these disciplines. Instead, only those concepts are included from these fields that we judge to be most important for understanding the conclusions presented in the final chapter.

Some of these concepts are, of course, our own from earlier publications and in a sense provide a unifying theme for the work, which might be described as 'mathematical neurophysics'. As it happens, hardly any of the scientists involved in developments in the above disciplines have been mathematical physicists, and thus have not approached the field in quite this way. As a result, several aspects of brain structure and function which we consider to be important for the understanding of consciousness have been somewhat neglected, *e.g.*, coupled ion-electric field effects at the neural membrane, the existence of small unit circuits of neurons containing internal feedback loops and their interconnection to form much larger networks, the role and information content of global waves of electrical potential directed through specific cortical regions, and especially the influence of quantum mechanical events on observable processes. Analyses of these aspects were required for our research to progress in a natural manner and should, we believe, constitute useful additions to the study of the neurosciences.

Bearing in mind this inherent bias as well as the preceding restrictions, investigators from other disciplines and readers approaching the subject for the first time should find the book to be a concise and accurate summary of the topics needed to dig deeper in other areas, with plenty of embedded pointers to more detailed treatments. An additional resource will be found in the collection of computer programs listed in the Appendices, from which many of the results presented have been derived. They are described and listed in a form that may easily be run and developed on most personal computers; some of them are also available on the World Wide Web of the Internet where they may be downloaded from the World Scientific home page (http://www.wspc.com.sg).

But most importantly, the theory of consciousness presented in conclusion — supported as it is by an actual model built on the laws that constitute the solid foundations of the mathematical, physical and chemical sciences — should prove useful to seasoned investigators willing to believe there is no 'devil in the details'.

Contents

Chapter 1

Introduction

1.1 The Emergence of Life

As we know it, consciousness is invariably associated with life. The simplest known building block of life is the individual cell, but this is already so complex that it is very difficult to be sure how it evolved from lifeless matter, or to devise a laboratory procedure which could produce a similar result. It seems probable, however, that the first cells were evolved in saline lakes or seas, since even today the extracellular environment of most cells is a fluid with a chemical composition similar to that of sea water.

An essential feature of any cell is the membrane that defines its boundary and preserves its integrity by creating a selectively permeable barrier separating the cell from its environment. Originally this may have been formed by chance by the closure of bilipid sheets formed in saline pools around polymeric chains incorporating fragments of nucleotides[1]. Energy to support the continuing chemical processes within would most naturally be derived from the sun, as it still is in the photosynthesis that takes place in most forms of vegetation. However, further evolution of the membrane was required to allow the substances needed for metabolic and reproductive processes to pass into the intracellular cytoplasm, as well as to resist the passage of others which would interfere with these processes - in particular calcium and sodium at the high concentrations found in sea water.

Since an essential characteristic of life is the ability to reproduce itself, a fundamental step in the evolution of a living cell was the synthesis of the DNA (deoxyribonucleic acid) that carries the genetic material needed for reproduction. But, although reasonable processes have been suggested for the formation of the nucleotides adenine, guanine, thymine and cytosine – the fundamental components of both DNA and RNA (ribonucleic acid) – in the oxygen-poor reducing atmosphere proposed for the early earth, and though certain evidence supports catalytic RNA as the precursor of DNA, how RNA itself first formed is still unknown. Only the most elementary steps required for such a synthesis have as yet been accomplished, but the principles involved are now well understood.

The simplest naturally occurring forms of cellular life are the procaryotes, including bacteria and certain types of algae, which have no well defined nucleus; but in more highly evolved cells, known as eukaryotes, a nucleus containing DNA does exist and is separated from the cytoplasm by a separate membrane within the cell. At an early evolutionary stage cells reproduced by the subdivision of a single cell found the advantages of cooperation in symbiosis, and multicellular life forms like amoeba emerged[2]. From this time onward the development of life is relatively easy to follow in the light of the geological record and the theories of natural selection and evolution developed by Darwin and his successors. It has become clear that terrestrial life has been very largely determined by natural selection operating within environmental constraints; but even so a very wide variety of different life forms has emerged, making it virtually certain that other forms are life are possible.

The distinguished mathematician and mathematical physicist Johann von Neumann was the first to develop a realistic proposal to bypass the lengthy processes of evolution by creating artificial forms of life[3]. In recent years there has been renewed interest in von Neumann's concept of artificial life[4], that is, of machines which might display many of the characteristics of living creatures. Since reproduction is one essential characteristic of life, the problem he emphasized was to determine the conditions under which an automaton, given access to the necessary materials, could fabricate an exact copy of itself.

This problem can be reduced to the construction of a computer capable of executing a program which includes instructions for its own construction and the copying of its program. Programs of this type have been relatively easy to implement on a computer; but the ability to reproduce is by no means the only attribute of animal species. In order to move and interact effectively with the environment all animals have evolved some degree of *motivation* and *intelligence*, and the development of control programs required to emulate motivated and intelligent behaviour poses a separate set of problems.

In the past, motivation and intelligence have been somewhat vaguely defined concepts, often used to distinguish animate from inanimate matter, and therefore associated exclusively with the nervous system of waking animals. The modern trend, however, is to make concepts like information and memory more precise and to quantify them where possible. One of our aims in this volume will be to discover properties of the nervous system underlying motivated and intelligent behaviour, and to relate them to information and memory. Later (in Chapters 5 and 6 of this volume) we shall make a study of some simple animals and inanimate systems that display motivation and intelligence, in what could be considered an acceptable sense of these words.

Motivation may be regarded as responsible for a type of behaviour best described as *goal fixation*. This behaviour is displayed by many insects and other simple animals, as well as the primates, in pursuit of the fundamental requirements of reproduction and nourishment. In the higher animals motivated behaviour of this type is believed to be related to activity in the brain stem and the limbic system, the most primitive parts of the brain, and has a clear relation to the processes of natural selection. In the higher animals, and especially in humans, goal fixation may also be motivated by the endeavour to satisfy intellectual and artistic needs not so directly related to survival, but in which the limbic system is undoubtedly involved. It is not difficult to simulate goal fixation in inanimate systems, as we shall show in Chapter 6, and the conclusion will be reached that though it is a common attribute of consciousness, it is not necessarily associated with consciousness.

Intelligence is also a common attribute of consciousness. Elsewhere[5] we have attempted a definition of intelligence in terms of

(1) sensitivity - the ability to respond to external stimuli

(2) impressibility - the ability to form of memories of experiences

(3) activity - the ability to perform tasks without supervision
(4) plasticity - the ability to adapt, or learn, as a result of experience
(5) foresight - the ability to anticipate future developments, and, incidentally, to make mistakes!

Artificial intelligence should exhibit most, if not all, of these properties; and, in fact, it is not too difficult to model intelligent behaviour, especially by computer simulation and the use of non-linear analysis. In recent years there has been a rapid development of different kinds of computers and computer programs, including computer viruses that are able to reproduce themselves, and some that have in addition all the characteristics of intelligence that have been identified above. It is already possible to construct artificial neural networks which perform complex parallel processing, and artificial brain components such as synapses[6] that exhibit the same sort of behaviour as their biological counterparts. The intelligence exhibited by intelligent materials, often exploiting non-linear characteristics of matter, is reproducible by mathematical and computer modelling. Today there is a rapid growth of areas of science concerned with narrowing the gap between artificial and animal intelligence[7–11], and little reason to believe that this separation can never be eliminated. It now seems possible that in the development of intelligent materials a condition which could be recognized as consciousness might appear. Again we are led to the view that intelligence may be, but is not necessarily associated with consciousness.

So far, however, neither the theories nor the implementations of real and artificial life have succeeded in elucidating the precise conditions under which consciousness, as distinct from intelligence, may be expected to emerge; evidently some important element is lacking. Consciousness confers the great advantage of choice to the individual, and thus is highly relevant to many factors affecting the survival and multiplication of a species. Its development is strongly favoured by natural selection in any highly competitive environment, and consequently would be enhanced in the course of evolution, though the genetic factors that influence intelligence and consciousness have not yet been determined, probably because they themselves have not been fully understood. The reproductive capacity of some species, including man, has clearly been more influential in the process of natural selection than either intelligence or consciousness; and in recent times the surface of the earth and its atmosphere have been transformed by their activities, not always in an optimal manner even from the point of view of continued survival.

In their operation machines have failed to mimic the action of the conscious brain, most conspicuously in the ability to make self-interested decisions, the outcome of which cannot be predicted even in principle. What is lacking in attempts to create artificial consciousness is precisely the sort of integral uncertainty that most physicists associate with quantal phenomena, which suggests that the development of quantum processes in this context could play a vital part in what might be regarded as the crucial step in the evolution of animate species.

1.2 The Nature of Consciousness

One of the first requirements for the discussion of consciousness is an acceptable definition. Early ideas on this subject were formulated by Descartes who, in his famous syllogism *Cogito, ergo sum*, identified his capacity for thought as a precondition for his own existence, and developed a theory of the relation between mind and brain that has been a fertile source of metaphysical and philosophical enquiry ever since. Much of this discussion has been based on an unquestioning acceptance of what we shall call a *deterministic* interpretation of the laws of nature. At first this interpretation was an apparently inevitable consequence of Newton's laws of motion, which in principle permit the detailed prediction of all future events from sufficiently accurate data concerning the present or past. One of the most successful applications of Newton's laws was to the prediction of the motions of the planets and other heavenly bodies. However, there was no evidence to suggest that the same laws should not apply to animate matter. It followed that the sense of freedom of action enjoyed by human beings must be illusory, inasmuch as their own future behaviour was as completely determined as the motions of the planets.

The essence of the resulting dilemma was that although, as Descartes recognized, consciousness is the source of all certain knowledge of the external world, it can have no role in a universe completely subject to deterministic laws: even though it exists, it makes no difference to the course of events.

It was not until the twentieth century that imperfections were discovered in the applicability of Newton's laws to natural phenomena, leading first to the formulation of the theory of relativity and later to the development of quantum mechanics. The theory of relativity was consistent with a deterministic interpretation of the laws of nature and would seem to have little relevance to the subject under discussion; in any event, it is safe to say that the discovery of quantum mechanics has led to the most immediate challenge to determinism. Although the first applications of quantum mechanics were to sub-microscopic phenomena, it implied that predictions based on the deterministic Newtonian laws must always have limited validity. Quite recently a number of books have appeared[12–15], in general agreement with our thesis that quantum mechanics has an important bearing on the question of consciousness, though at odds with one another and with our own point of view in some other respects.

The reader should be aware that, from the time of its inception, the interpretation of quantum mechanics has been an extremely controversial subject, although there is no room for argument about the correspondence between its consequences and observation. Some theoretical physicists have been unable to accept that the Newtonian concept of a universe whose past and future development was completely predictable from its creation could be wrong. In Chapter 7 we shall discuss in more detail the deterministic theories: the theory of hidden variables[16,17], the theory of the universal wave function[18,19] and the theory of many worlds[20,21]. These differ from one another in essential respects, but they seem to be attempts to restore some of the features of classical mechanics. We shall find that although they reproduce the observable consequences of quantum mechanics, they also require a multiplicity of phenomena that are unobservable, and are therefore products of the imagination! Our own view is that imagination is often an invaluable stimulus to creative activity, and in principle there should be no objection to the invention of unobserved phenomena to explain what is observed, but only provided that this is consistent with all the facts *and* simplifies the explanation. It is particularly valuable where it has the power to predict observable phenomena that would otherwise be inexplicable. But the deterministic theories are now sufficiently old to allow us to conclude that they are unlikely to fulfill these criteria.

We are therefore among the advocates of an interpretation of quantum mechanics close to what has come to be known as the Copenhagen interpretation[22,23]. This is that most of the observations made of phenomena at the atomic and molecular level are fundamentally unpredictable. Quantum mechanics allows the calculation of the probabilities that a measurement made on a microscopic system will have certain values, and these probabilities are experimentally verified. However, it also allows a numerical value to be attached to the uncertainty, or indeterminacy, in the measured value of any microscopic observable, and this has likewise been confirmed by experiment. It is therefore very well established by now that most events originating at the microscopic level are not determined, in the sense that they cannot be predicted with certainty. It is also well known that at least some microscopic events, subject to the laws of quantum mechanics, have macroscopic consequences; this is true particularly of the events by which atomic events are detected. Such events are also fundamentally unpredictable.

The important question here is whether there are events of this kind, which are easily detected but are not predictable on the basis of macroscopic laws, in the animal brain. In the course of this book we shall show that there are. The action of a cell in the brain is controlled by the flux of ions through channels in its membrane, and these channels are so small and narrow that they can contain only a few ions at a particular time. The individual ions are undoubtedly subject to the laws of quantum mechanics. Admittedly, there are many channels, and if the flux of ions through different channels were uncorrelated, it would still be possible to predict the action of a cell with reasonable certainty. But in the living animal the ionic flux is well known, in many instances, to be crucially affected by variations in the potential in the electrolytic fluid in contact with the cell, so that the quantal events are strongly correlated.

Later we shall provide a theoretical and quantitative basis for the important conclusion that the electrical activity of the cortex is not completely subject to deterministic laws but is affected by the indeterminism of events at the microscopic level. It will be shown that some of the electrical activity is the result of the *selective* amplification of electric fluctuations originating at the sub-microscopic level, and these are certainly subject to the laws of quantum mechanics. From this it will follow that quantum mechanical indeterminacy is indeed relevant to the nature of consciousness.

Our view of quantum mechanics, and its importance for the workings of the brain, leads naturally to a pragmatic definition of consciousness in terms of awareness and volition. Awareness implies the attention given to elements of short-term memory, including sensory impressions, and the likelihood that these will be transferred to working or long term memory. Volition implies the direction given to a train of thought or the decision making that guides the performance of a sequence of voluntary motor actions; in such processes a search of memory is usually implied. In some processes, of course, awareness and volition are both active at the same time.

There are various reasons, other than those we have already mentioned, for concluding that quantum sensitivity with its attendant uncertainty enter the operation of the human brain on the lowest functional level. The experimental findings that support this conclusion include the background of random firings that persists in the resting brain[24], the possible response of a retinal photoreceptor to a single photon of visual light [25–27], and recent evidence that chaotic processes[28] – notoriously sensitive to initial conditions – appear in many types of cortical activity, such as those accompanying recall from long term memory, creative associative reasoning, voluntary activity, and the arousal of consciousness. The relevance of quantum mechanics to the phenomenon of consciousness was anticipated by a number of distinguished physicists and neurophysiologists [29–31].

It is important to observe that awareness and volition are not exclusively subjective notions. As we shall discuss in more detail later, they are closely related to fluctuations in potential within the animal cortex that can be observed experimentally in the extracellular fluid by electroencephalography and similar techniques. The fluctuations in potential have components with characteristic frequencies, and though these are known to be closely correlated with cellular activity, it is not generally possible to distinguish between cause and effect. We shall see later that there is a considerable amount of experimental evidence pointing to a close correspondence between conscious activities and certain types of rhythmic electrical activity in the cortex. Of course there is also electrical activity associated with the various unconscious functions essential to animal life, most of which persists in sleep and other states of unconsciousness; but this kind of activity is not difficult to distinguish observationally from that which we associate with consciousness.

This brief introduction to the theory of consciousness leaves many important questions to be discussed. The detailed considerations supporting the theory are drawn from the physical sciences, from the neurosciences, and from computing science. From the physically based theory of electrolytes comes an understanding of the non-linear processes responsible for the amplification and propagation of electrical impulses in the nervous system, and their selective transmission across the neural membrane. From the neurosciences comes an understanding of the organization of the nervous system, including the animal cortex with its delicate balance of excitatory and inhibitory cells, each of which is associated with a particular cell functionally dedicated to input, transmission or output. From computer science comes an understanding of the mode of operation of the biological neural networks of the nervous system and the cortex, and its description in terms of information processing.

In the following Chapters we shall discuss in some detail the relevant material from these sciences in both mathematical and non-mathematical terms. Useful background material will be summarized in the next few Sections.

1.3 Schrödinger's Cat and Wigner's Friend

Following the general acceptance by the Copenhagen school's interpretation of quantum mechanics, it was evident that a revision of the classical theories of measurement and observation would also be required. This was attempted by Dirac and von Neumann in two very influential text-books [32,33] that first appeared not long after the discovery of quantum mechanics. In subsequent years their theories of measurement were to become an even more potent source of confusion than the issue of determinism.

The original formulation of quantum mechanics by Born, Jordan and Heisenberg [34,35] in 1925 and 1926, was in terms of matrices and is known as matrix mechanics. The formulation in terms of wave functions by Schrödinger came about a year later and is known as wave mechanics. In their application to sub-microscopic phenomena the two formulations were seen to yield identical results, and they soon came to be regarded as equivalent. However, there is in fact an important difference between them. Whereas the matrices of matrix mechanics are constructed entirely from quantities that are, in principle, observable, the wave functions of wave mechanics usually incorporate factors that have no observational significance. In spite of this, both Dirac and von Neumann took it as axiomatic that *the state of any isolated system in nature may be represented by a wave function.* Consequently, the wave function was interpreted as a *state vector*, in a particular representation. According to von Neumann's theory, when a measurement is made on a microscopic system, its wave function or state vector is changed in a way that depends both on what is measured and the result of the measurement. This has given rise to an endemic belief that, because it cannot be predicted, *the outcome of a measurement must remain not merely uncertain, but indeterminate and therefore undecided, until it enters into consciousness.* If this were true, it would undoubtedly establish a very direct connection between the concepts of quantum mechanics and consciousness. But in fact the acceptance of the statement italicized above has a variety of paradoxical, if not incredible, consequences[36,37]. We shall give two examples.

Schrödinger[38] was the first to invent a vivid illustration of the strange implications of the above interpretation of von Neumann's theory of measurement; some of the details are contained in a letter reproduced by the authors[39]. A cat is confined to a box that also contains a lethal device, which may be activated by the decay of a radioactive nucleus. On the basis of quantum mechanics, the time of decay of the nucleus cannot be predicted with certainty, but it is possible to compute the probability that it will decay within any interval of time. If and when the nucleus decays, the lethal device will function and the cat will die. The system consisting of the nucleus, the lethal device and the cat can be regarded as the apparatus of an experiment to measure the time of decay of the nucleus. According to Schrödinger's application of von Neumann's theory, the system at any time may be represented by a state vector with two components, one corresponding to the possibility that the nucleus has not decayed and the cat is still alive, and the other to the possibility that the nucleus has decayed and the cat is dead. The result of the experiment, depending on the state of the cat, is undecided, and the cat is neither dead nor alive, until the fact enters the consciousness of the experimenter. On the other hand, the result of the experiment is certainly not indeterminate for the cat, assuming that it is still alive.

Subsequently Wigner invented a more elaborate paradox, known as the paradox of Wigner's friend[40]. Like Schrödinger's cat paradox, this paradox deals with the possibility that a microscopic event will have a macroscopic effect. But this example concerns the possibility that a flash of light may be emitted by a microscopic object. It is supposed that, if it is emitted during a particular interval of time, the flash will be noticed by one of Wigner's friends. As we have already noted, the retina of the eye is in fact sensitive to radiation consisting of a very small number of photons. After some time, Wigner asks his friend whether he has observed the flash, and receives the answer "Yes" or "No". Before the answer is given, the system consisting of the object and the friend is represented by a wave function with two components, one corresponding to the possibility that the flash has been emitted and noticed, and the other to the possibility that it has not. When the friend's answer enters Wigner's consciousness, the wave function changes rapidly to another from which one or other of the two components is missing. On the other hand, he is able to verify that his friend already knew whether he had seen the flash before the answer was given! From this Wigner seems to have concluded that, by some non-linear process, the conscious mind is able to change the state of the external system; and that, therefore, the action of the brain is subject to laws essentially different from those of ordinary matter.

It should be emphasised that Schrödinger's account of the cat paradox, and the account just given of the paradox of Wigner's friend are not consequences of the orthodox Copenhagen interpretation of quantum mechanics. It is known that Born, Jordan, Heisenberg and Bohr all held the common-sense view that the fate of Schrödinger's cat was decided if and when the lethal device was activated, and that the emission of a photon by an atom becomes virtually certain if and when the photon is detected by any means. In the penultimate Chapter of this book we present a version of quantum mechanics consistent with the Copenhagen interpretation based on information theory and with a common sense interpretation of the paradoxes. There we shall find no reason to dissent from the view that the brain is governed by the same fundamental laws as ordinary matter; these are marvellous enough!

There is some consensus in the literature that there is a serious difficulty if the concept of a wave function or state vector is extended to macroscopic measuring devices and observers. This difficulty, from our point of view, stems from the fact that measurement and observation both involve irreversible processes, which cannot be adequately described in terms of such concepts. Quantal theories of irreversible processes[41–43] all make use of a generalization of the theory of the *statistical matrix* (the statistical operator, in von Neumann's terminology or the density matrix in Dirac's). The statistical matrix has elements that are probabilities and can be measured; therefore, unlike the wave function or state vector, it has a meaning for systems that are in interaction, or have interacted with their environment. In Section 7.1 we shall state and prove a theorem to the effect that there is no system in nature (with the dubious exception of the entire universe) that can be represented by a single wave function, so that the use of the statistical matrix is necessary.

This still leaves a role for consciousness in discovering, *after* a macroscopic event, which of the various unpredictable possibilities was realized. We shall find it important to recognize that the processes of measurement and observation require the transfer of information, as defined in the quantal mechanics by Brillouin[44], again using the theory of the statistical matrix. In Section 3.4, we shall illustrate this, on the basis of quantal information theory, by constructing a quantum-mechanical model of the action of individual cells and of a miniature neural network in the brain[45]. The model reproduces most of the essential features of the physiological brain, including action potentials that can be initiated by events at the quantum mechanical level in the extracellular environment. Subsequently we have developed both classical and quantum-mechanical models of more extended neural networks of the animal cortex that also function in much the same way as their biological counterparts.

The relevance of a quantum mechanical model of cortical action to Schrödinger's cat paradox and the paradox of Wigner's friend becomes apparent when it is noted that the information content of the cat's brain or the friend's brain is neither indeterminate nor subjective, but is stored in their long-term memories, which can be accessed by an appropriate stimulus. For the complete resolution of the paradoxes, the theory of quantal measurement, which is concerned with the information gained concerning a microscopic system by the operation of a macroscopic measuring device, has to be extended to provide a theory of observation, concerned with the transfer of the information to the brain of an intelligent observer.

The brain has a number of special qualities that are relevant to a theory of observation. It is obvious that not all macroscopic objects are well adapted to the detection of events at the microscopic level, since it may be very difficult to determine from them, by inspection or otherwise, whether interaction with a microscopic system has actually occurred. Most efficient detectors of microscopic events are in a metastable state, so that the interaction, however small, is sufficient to induce a large transfer of information which is easily detected at the macroscopic level. But, as will become clear in following Chapters, the cortex of an intelligent observer may also be classified in this way, so that there is no essential difference, in that respect, between an efficient inanimate measuring device and the conscious observer who takes note of the measurement. In this sense, the measuring device has at least one essential attribute of an artificial consciousness.

The common sense view is that the conscious act of observation, as distinct from the process of detection of a microscopic system, has little or no effect on what is observed. On the other hand, what is consciously observed does affect the nervous system of the observer, especially those parts concerned with the formation and retention of memory. The animal cortex retains not only a memory, but a sequential memory of *information actually gained* in the process of observation. In indeterministic quantum mechanics, this information is quite distinct from *information that may be gained.*

The term 'information', as used here and elsewhere in this volume, has much the same meaning as in ordinary language. But since the ordinary usage is somewhat vague and variable, information is here given the more exact, indeed quantitative, meaning proposed by Shannon[46] in the classical context and, as already mentioned, by Brillouin[44] in the context of quantum mechanics. These definitions, in terms of probability and the statistical matrix, will appear in Sections 4.2 and 7.3, but it is important to note at the outset that information theory usually deals with the objective information associated with a specified system that may, at least in principle, be gained by observation. It is a calculated quantity that differs from the subjective information that is available at any time to a particular observer. When information is gained by an observer, the subjective information to be gained naturally decreases by the same amount. But if the system is or includes the nervous system of the observer, the subjective information available to the observer is certainly represented in the information associated with the system.

The nervous system, and the animal cortex in particular, has some remarkable properties not found in other systems in a metastable state. These include the selective ability not only to gain information, which is a function of awareness, but also the ability to create information, which is a function of volition. It is the outcome of these functions of the animal cortex that cannot be predicted in advance and lies within the domain of quantum mechanics. But they are functions that are not difficult to reproduce in inanimate matter, at least in a rudimentary form. The nervous system is distinguished from other known systems by the complexity of its organization, by its elaborate provisions for the continuous acquisition of information through the senses, the purposeful initiation of motor activity, and above all by the development of the sequential memory that supports the continuous processing of information.

1.4 Real and Artificial Neural Nets

The basic function of the nervous system of an animal is to transfer information between different cells and different parts of the body. This transfer is accomplished by physical processes, especially by the movement of ions and related electrical activity; and it will be found useful to make a distinction between the information conveyed by ionic currents and that associated with the random motion of ions and molecules of the nervous system which have little effect on the processing of information.

Even plants have a rudimentary nervous system consisting of cells that communicate information by ionic currents. At just what point in the process of evolution consciousness first appeared remains largely a matter of definition; but if, as we have suggested, it is associated with quantum-mechanical choice and decision-making, it could well be regarded as a potential property of all matter. As Teilhard de Chardin has pointed out[47], the mere existence of conscious life implies the potential for its existence in inanimate matter.

In particular, evolving slowly in a constantly changing environment, constrained by available energy, forced to add layer to existing layer, function to existing function to satisfy ever expanding information requirements, the control program of the animal brain has been driven relentlessly toward complexity and nonlinearity[30]. As a result its principles are obscured by illogical indirections and its operations by seeming discontinuities inaccessible to linear analysis.

Simply to tense a muscle, for example, an elaborate sequence of neural activations and inhibitions is often required for the signal to propagate through the brain structures involved[48]; and the prevailing balance of excitatory and inhibitory synaptic activation is sufficient to ensure that in some circumstances extremely small increments of potential can cause massive organizational changes in information. And yet, the mental processes that most distinguish the higher animals – awareness, including self awareness, the ability to remember, to plan ahead, to think and act creatively – have arisen from these very characteristics and depend on them critically[15]. For this reason if the objective were merely to create an artificial nervous system with functional capabilities similar to humans, the best approach might be to reproduce these biological capabilities at the highest level, and in the most direct possible way[49].

If, however, we wish to understand the underlying functions in the accepted manner of the sciences they must be investigated from the lowest level, by building hierarchies of basic mechanisms consistent with the body of physical, chemical and neurobiological science[50]. Since this is our objective in the present volume, at the most fundamental level we shall consider the dynamics of ions and their interaction with the electric field at the membrane of a neuron, and focus attention sharply on the characteristics of the *graded* and *action* potentials produced within the cell[51]. The internal electric potential of such a cell is normally of the order of 50-100 mV (millivolts) below that of the extracellular fluid. Graded potentials are fluctuations of a few mV in the internal potential within the cell, in the course of which the cell is said to be *potentiated.* Under conditions that we shall study in detail in subsequent chapters they may develop into firings, or action potentials, during which the internal potential rises briefly to a level that may exceed the potential outside the cell. As these potentials and associated potential waves in the extracellular fluid constitute the primary means by which information is transferred throughout the nervous system, their properties may be expected to strongly influence, if not fully determine, all higher processes.

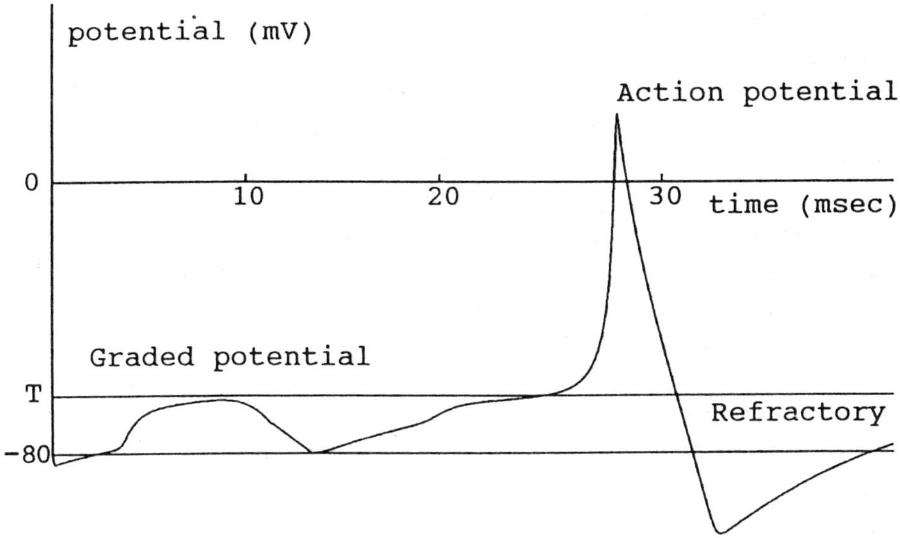

Fig. 1.1: Time variation of the electrical potential (mV) in the axon hillock of a typical neuron subjected, first, to a current pulse that does not cause this potential to exceed the threshold T (-65 mV) of the neuron, but produces a graded potential; and next, to a slightly larger pulse that causes the potential to exceed T and produce an action potential, followed by an insensitive refractory state.

In the vertebrates, a typical neuron consists of a *soma*, or cell body, an *axon*, or fibre that transmits potentials to the *synapses* where it communicates with other neurons, and *dendrites* which receive information from other neurons. The action of a cell is determined chiefly by the value of the potential at the *hillock* near where the axon leaves the body of the cell, and an action potential is possible only if this potential exceeds a certain threshold value. This is illustrated by the typical potential within a firing neuron, shown in Figure 1.1. The information that the neuron can transfer depends on the frequency of its firing peaks. In the following Chapter we shall discuss the way in which this affects the formation of working memory and its consolidation as a result of the prolonged potentiation called *long-term potentiation.* However, neither of these essential functions can be performed unless, as in other threshold problems associated with systems in a metastable state, the potential accumulated at the the axon hillock of the cell body fails to exceed some definite value.

The course of higher processes is also dependent on the passage of information bearing signals across synaptic junctions (Figure 1.2). At the synaptic *cleft*, the axon of the *presynaptic* neuron is separated from another, *postsynaptic* neuron by a thin layer of electrolytic fluid. As we shall see in more detail in the following Chapter, the transmission of a potential from one neuron to another is conditioned by the release of one of a variety of neurotransmitter substances from the presynaptic axon terminal and quantum chemical effects at surface of the postsynaptic cell. The neurotransmitters depend for their efficacy on a release of calcium which occurs when they interact with receptor molecules embedded in the postsynaptic membrane. Current research suggests, for example, that the release of the neurotransmitter glutamate and its subsequent interaction with the receptor molecule NMDA underlies the long-term potentiation which occurs specifically in the *amygdala*, responsible for the formation of emotional responses and memories[52], and that the neurotransmitter serotonin released by fibers, emanating from the raphe nuclei and terminating in widely distributed patterns throughout the brain, provides fine-tuning for many of the basic bodily and psychological functions, such as sleeping and eating cycles, cardiovascular and respiratory activity, mood changes, and aggressive behavior.[53].

The influence on conscious behaviour of information transmitted by various chemical substances diffusing locally from stimulated neurons should not be underestimated. Indeed, evidence is accumulating that emotional responses controlled by mid-brain structures depend on recruiting groups of neurons in just this way[48,54], and there can be little doubt that the positive or negative reinforcement of trial behaviors by the release of such substances in the brain constitutes an important component of learning[55].

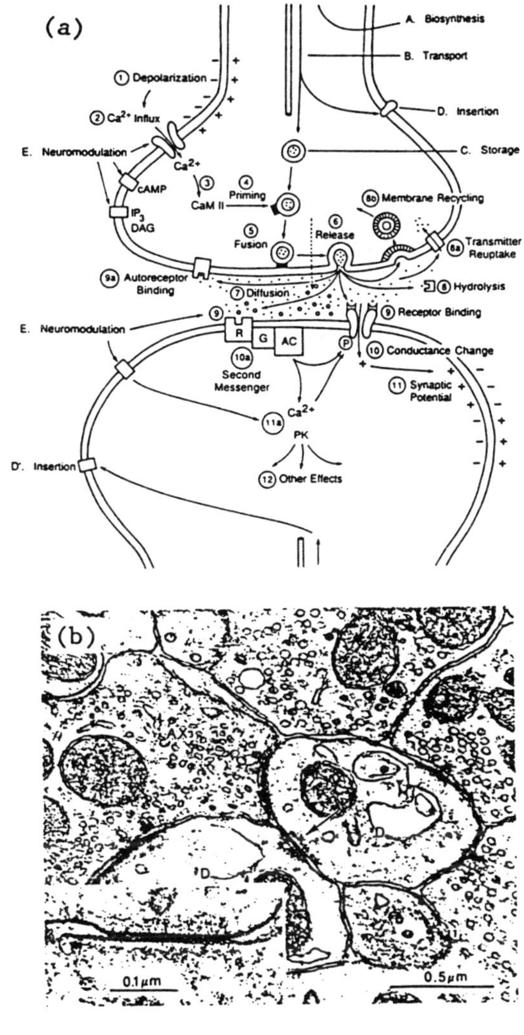

Fig. 1.2 (a) Biochemical mechanisms of a chemical synapse: long-term steps in the synthesis, transport and storage of neurotransmitters and neuromodulators, and the insertion of membrane channel proteins and receptors; and (b) large scale micrograph of a chemical synapse (AX-D) and an electrical synapse (D-D, with enlargement at arrow) in the cortex of a cat.

But the release of these neurochemicals depends in turn on receipt of the stimulating signal. Similarly, in the last analysis all higher processes, such as left and right brain coordination[56], feature extraction and related action cascades[57], and the comparative sensory feedback cycles essential to self-awareness[58], must be initiated and sustained by electrical signals that manipulate neural membrane potentials near threshold - so near, in fact, that quantum probabilities defined by net potentials must be assigned to the outcome for every neuron involved. Fortunately, the methods of mathematical physics make it possible to deal with the collective behavior of such systems without dependence on details at this level, as we have done in Chapter 7.

However, the larger scale features of neural connectivity, the circuitry networks that constitute the primary pathways for information exchange in the brain, must be taken into account. Consequently, we have chosen to model functions of the allocortex, cerebellum and cerebrum with linked sets of characteristic 'unit circuits', small groups of interconnected neurons containing one or more feedback loops, which have been observed in microanatomical studies and suggested to be the basic building blocks of these structures[59,60].

As shown in Chapter 6, many of the features of artificially intelligent behavior, such as pattern recognition and adaptive learning, can be generated in this way without recourse to back-propagation of error, location of minima in energy surfaces, or other computation-intensive neural network techniques[61]. The controlling transfer functions become those of the unit circuits, and these functions allow each unit to perform a sequence of internal 'computations' in response to specific stimuli. Repetition of the stimulus will adjust the connection and interconnection weights and cause the output of the unit to reach a steady state which, in conjunction with that of the others, will result in a unique network output. Inhibitory feedback loops within each unit circuit, together with the more extended feedback loops associated with them, make the required corrections automatically.

Following the remarkable advances initiated by Golgi and Ramon y Cajal in the last century and continued by Lorente de No[62,63] and others more recently[64–66], much information has been gathered concerning the types of neurons in the cerebral cortex and their synaptic connections, and regions responsible for the processing of specific sensory information or specific motor functions have been identified. For example, the important role of the cerebellum in the control of motor activity has been elaborated by Eccles[48] and considerable insight has been obtained concerning the role of the allocortex, including the hippocampus, in the sequential ordering of sensory data[67,68]. Additionally, Shepherd[69], Szentagothai[59] and Ito[60] have provided excellent descriptions of the details of synaptic organization revealed by these studies.

In spite of the apparent complexity of its organization, it has become apparent that many parts of the cortex may be subdivided laterally into interconnecting columns or zones, based on the primary pyramidal or Purkinje cells which they contain, and vertically into layers which contain cells of distinctive types. The cerebellum is subdivided into zones consisting of a network of these columnar units, the cerebrum into segregates or areas with specific sensory or motor activities, and the cells in each column have been found to be dynamically as well as spatially related. Hence, the structure defined by the columns, zones and areas must be taken into account in partitioning the cortex into semi-autonomous functional units.

Great interest attaches to the exact nature of the fundamental unit circuits, their detailed connections and functional characteristics, several examples of which are featured in Chapter 6. Additionally, their interconnections within a column or zone with others nearby and with afferents from other brain structures, occur in well-defined bands rich in neural dendrites and heavily penetrated by lateral axonal processes, most of which are unmyelinated. In the cerebrum the most prominent of these, the outer and inner lines of Baillarger, appear in layers 4 and 5, but similar banding is seen in all six layers[68–70], and these bands may function in certain respects as wave guides for the integrated electromagnetic field changes observed in alpha, beta and other types of brain waves, including event-related potentials[71,72].

There has been detailed study of the electrical activity manifested by the cortex, and especially of the way in which cells process information by the integration of graded potentials of a few mV in their dendrites and transmit the result to synapses with other cells by action potentials of more than 50 mV in their axons. It is also recognized that this internal activity of a cell is correlated with potential spikes, also of a few mV, in the extracellular fluid; but the method of generation of periodic potentials of similar amplitude, such as the theta-rhythm in the hippocampus and the alpha-rhythm in the cerebrum, is not well understood.

Such activity in the extracellular fluid has been regarded by some as a mere by-product of intracellular processes, in spite of evidence that electromagnetic radiation[73] and electroconvulsive therapy[74] can affect the nervous system. Morever, the work of Lorente de No, Marrazzi and Lorente de No, Adey, Rall, and Rall and Shepherd[75–79] has pointed to a role for extracellular potentials of up to 10 mV in the transmission of information between cells. There are other instances[80,81] where experimental evidence for the importance of such transmission has appeared; but until recently, even where there is obviously a direct relation between extracellular activity and animal behaviour, the distinction between cause and effect has been difficult to establish. Understanding of the influence of the extracellular on the internal electrical activity of the cortex has undoubtedly been retarded by many questions that have long remained unanswered. However, today there are important advances from improved experimental techniques that promise new insights, especially in the light of physically based theoretical interpretation and mathematical models.

On the experimental side, much of the new information is derived from developments in electroencephalography. The analysis of fluctuations in the extracellular potential over extended regions of the cortex, and especially the frontal regions, has revealed definite patterns of theta-activity (in the 4-9 Hz waveband) accompanying the conscious activity associated with tasks such as mental arithmetic or tracing a maze[82]. Even where the fluctuations are not clearly identified with a particular wave band, they have been found to be chaotic rather than random, and to conceal a series of underlying frequencies. The models presented in this volume have been developed largely for the purpose of investigating the effects of such extracellular fluctuations on the animal cortex, which must be taken into account if the application of quantum mechanics is to be understood.

The models of cortical action to be developed in subsequent chapters are naturally related to those developed by the authors in a series of papers extending over a number of years (see ref. [83], and earlier references contained therein), but as will be seen from their specifications, represent an advance in several respects. Quite apart from the inclusion of quantal and extracellular field effects, the approach differs most from the neural network models developed by various other authors such as Hinton and Anderson[84], Hopfield and Tank[85], and Rumelhart, McClelland et al.[9] by their strict observance of neuroanatomical structure and the degree of fidelity to neurophysiological fact.

It will be noted that the more important apparent difficulties in the concept of extracellular communication between neurons are now resolved. For example, one of these concerned the possibility that too many neurons could respond indiscriminately to an extracellular signal, since the latter lacks the specificity of a synaptic transmission. But it is shown that an extracellular potential is transmitted by the membrane only if it has one of certain characteristic frequencies dependent on the geometry of the membrane; and the frequencies corresponding to the pertinent geometries are obtained explicitly. Many neurons may still satisfy the conditions for the transmission of such a potential, but this is an essential condition for the generation of extracellular fields with prescribed frequencies. Each neuron which responds with a graded or action potential to a particular frequency contributes to the component of the extracellular field with that frequency, and thereby helps to sustain periodic potentials such as the alpha and theta-rhythms.

There are many other implications of the inward transmission of periodic potentials from the extracellular fluid which are consistent with present experimental knowledge. There is, for instance, an increasing amount of evidence that the activity of wide variety of cells in the cortex is synchronized to extracellular potentials[86,87]. From this it follows that, because of the interrelations of excitatory and inhibitory cells, the response of the neural network to potentials in the extracellular field is not indiscriminate. On the contrary, these potentials produce a moving pattern of facilitation essential to the proper functioning of the neural system in the region affected.

A further problem which is resolved by the intervention of periodic extracellular potentials concerns the synchronization of potentials in different units of a system of neurons. This is a fundamental requirement of parallel processing, the importance of which becomes fully apparent in any attempt to model an extended neural network. Without such synchronization the activity rapidly becomes incoherent and disorganized. Cotterill[88] has proposed a method of synchronization based on the refractory period exhibited by cells after an action potential, but this proposal meets with serious difficulties where the refractory periods vary from cell to cell or begin at different times, as they do in a biological context. The alternative of synchronization by an extracellular wave presents no such difficulty.

There is, however, another less obvious problem, concerning the capacity of a system of cells to respond in a consistent way to a particular stimulus, even where the synaptic and extracellular components of this stimulus are the same. This problem arises because cells may be found at various levels below threshold and therefore will require different degrees of excitation on different occasions to fire. The resolution of the problem requires an understanding of the mode of formation and distribution of memory in the cortex. In earlier work[89] we have considered the well known experiments of Kandel[90] on learning and habituation in *Aplysia Californica* (a giant sea-snail) from the point of view of ionic theory, and concluded that calcium currents were implicated in this type of learning.

But it is clear that something additional to the proper distribution of calcium is required for the formation of long-term memory, and this probably remains true even if the role of neurotransmitters in regulating concentrations of calcium is taken into account. Nevertheless, calcium currents could still initiate the formation of lasting memory[91], and there is now good evidence to this effect in the phenomena of long-term potentiation[92–96] and synaptic plasticity[97–100] of cells in the hippocampal formation and elsewhere.

We have accepted the suggestion of several of these authors that long-term potentiation and synaptic plasticity are essential to the development of memory. This can also be regarded as a more explicit form of Hebb's rule [101]. The model assumes that the 'weight' associated with a synapse, which determines its effect on the transmitted potential, may increase with use, but only under certain conditions, specified in detail in Chapter 6. When such a process of sensitization is complete, a system of cells will reliably perform what, by obvious analogy with computational models, may be considered a 'program'[102].

A relatively wide variety of programs may be performed by the same small group of cells, and this we believe to be promising for the construction of artificial systems of acceptable size within the bounds of current technology.

1.5 The Brain as a Turing Machine

Because of its remarkable capacity to process information, the animal brain has often been compared with an electronic computer. In its extreme form, the idea was that the only significant differences between animate and inanimate 'machines' are in the amount of available memory and the degree of complexity of their circuits. Since, even today, the memory of computers is insignificant in comparison with the number of neurons in the human brain, and the circuitry is also simple in comparison, it is not possible to decide whether such a analogy is appropriate on empirical grounds, and it is important to have in mind a clear idea of what a computer is or might become. It may then be possible to answer the question: is the animal brain a form of computer?

The first general formulation of the action of a classical computer was made by Turing[103] in an attempt to determine the limits of numerical computation. He found that for any computer there must be certain uncomputable results, analogous to Gödel's unprovable propositions[104] within any logical system. But, more importantly from our point of view, he described in mathematical terms what may be called a *Turing machine.* The precise specifications of the machine itself were unimportant; it could be thought of as a 'black box' with a finite number of internal states. The machine requires a 'tape' for its operation, which is not part of the machine, but consists of a sequence of segments. On each segment there is a symbol that can be read and possibly changed by the machine, and without serious restriction these symbols may be supposed to be binary digits, 0's or 1's. The machine performs a completely predictable sequence of operations in time. In each operation, the machine scans a particular segment of the tape, and, depending on its internal state *and* on whether the symbol on the segment is a 0 or a 1, does three things:

(1) changes its own internal state;
(2) either changes the symbol or leaves it unchanged; and
(3) selects the segment of the tape that is to be scanned in the next

operation; this may be the same segment, or one of the two neighbouring segments of the tape. The sequence of operations is terminated if a particular sequence of symbols is read from the tape.

From this description it will be seen that a Turing machine with a given initial internal state performs a computation with data represented by the initial sequence of symbols on the tape, and with results represented by the final sequence of symbols on the tape. The tape is obviously quite analogous to the devices used to load a program into a computer and to monitor the result. It provides the information required for the operation of the machine, and the binary digits are the 'bits' of information. In principle, any computation can be performed by the machine with input and output of information from and to the tape, and any automatic computer can be perceived to operate in the way described. The question then naturally arises: does the brain consist of or contain a machine that operates in the same way? To justify an affirmative answer to this question, it is necessary to find an analogue of the 'tape', and identify processes within the brain that correspond to the three actions specified above as necessary for the operation of a Turing machine. A simple analogue of the tape can be suggested in the sequence of sensory impressions presented to the brain by its external environment. Considering its capacity to form memory, there is no doubt that the state of the brain may be changed by sensory impressions, though there may be some doubt that it is necessarily changed. There is also no doubt that in some circumstances it is able, through motor actions, to alter the nature of these sensory impressions, and also to select the sensory impressions that will be experienced next, though it is a matter of experience that this is not always possible. It is therefore reasonable to conclude that the action of the brain is similar to that of a Turing machine, but only under certain conditions. This conclusion has the corollary that, subject to the same conditions, *it should be possible to construct a robot that would function in much the same way as a human being.*

The last point was made very cogently by Turing, in another well known paper [105]. He proposed an *imitation* game, in which a player is required to distinguish between an unseen person and an unseen computer on the basis of their spontaneous answers to a series of questions. It does indeed seem quite plausible that, in the future, it will be possible to program a computer to answer all questions, not always truthfully or consistently, but sufficiently well to convince the questioner that the computer was really a human being. Turing then argued, in effect, that if there was no detectable difference between the behaviour of a robot and that of an animate being, the latter should be thought of as a kind of robot.

Whether by intention or not, most attempts to model the neuronal activity of the brain have been strongly suggestive of the action of a classical Turing machine. In one of the earliest models, due to McCulloch and Pitts[106], individual neurons were represented, in effect, as elements of a computer, providing a predetermined output in response to any given input. The further development of such models could be interpreted as providing Turing's 'black box' with an internal structure of interconnected units, each of which had the essential properties of a Turing machine. Conceptually, the interconnection of any number of Turing machines is still a Turing machine, and its action is in theory replicated by Turing's *universal* machine, whose specification includes those of all others. However, the more recent developments have tended to support Turing's contention that a computer could be devised to emulate at least the computational action of the brain, not only in the actual performance of a particular task, but in the internal mechanisms underlying the performance.

Today it is clear that, in spite of the enormous capacity and complexity of the brain, there are many tasks of a routine nature that can be performed more rapidly and reliably by a computer. Although it is still possible to point to various types of activity where the performance of the animate brain is much superior, their number is steadily diminishing. Since these have been the subject of a great deal of research, it is worth considering some of them. There are 'expert' programs that encapsulate the accumulated knowledge of specialists in various professions. Computer programs have been written that excel in solving a wide variety of problems, such as restoring the initial configuration of a Rubik cube, or showing that any map needs only four colours to distinguish territories with a common border. Also, programs for playing games like chess (though not, at present, the oriental game of Go) are now approaching or surpassing the limits of human capability. Progress has also been made in the programming of computers for pattern recognition[107], though over a period of time most programs have made use of iterative procedures that do not closely resemble and are obviously not as efficient as corresponding processes in the brain. The performance of such programs can often be greatly enhanced by a more faithful modelling of the brain, which in important respects has reached a peak of efficiency through processes of natural selection operating over a geological span of time. Some programs based on this principle will be discussed and are available to the reader, as listings in the Appendices, and as described in the Foreword to this volume.

There have been important attempts to simulate actions of the brain which rely on a representation of cortical circuits that is intensively computational, as will appear in more detail in Chapter 6. This was perhaps inevitable as long as most computers were sequential and designed primarily for computation. However it has become increasingly clear that the internal architecture of the brain differs from that of such computers in several important respects. To begin with, the brain is a parallel, as distinct from a sequential processor: it is able to execute a multitude of functions simultaneously. There is no difficulty in simulating parallel processing on a modest scale in a sequential computer, but a parallel processor can do it more efficiently, and today parallel processing is becoming an increasingly common feature of machines designed for computation on a large scale. But also the brain has a remarkable capacity for self-organization and association of data derived from different sources in memory. Again, as Kohonen has shown[11], these processes can be simulated in detail on a conventional computer, but again elaborate calculations are required to do what appears to be commonplace in the brain. Still another distinctive feature of the brain is its capacity for learning by experience, assisted by simple feedback mechanisms that are partly built into the nervous system and partly derived through the senses. In comparison, most simulations of feedback by computational methods[108] appear to be rather slow and inefficient.

It is important to notice that consciousness plays no essential part in the mental processes that we have considered so far, which have been, or in principle can be, simulated. In most instances such processes are more 'naturally' accomplished, in the sense that physical and chemical processes, rather than computation, are involved. But, more importantly, they are normally carried out by unconscious or autonomous activity with at most occasional conscious intervention. Like breathing and the circulation of the blood, they are essential to the welfare of the animal and it would be highly detrimental if they did not proceed automatically and without conscious effort. Even the learning of refined motor activity, a great deal of which occurs in early childhood, is instinctive in this sense. In the following pages, we shall note and acknowledge the importance of unconscious processes, but shall study them in detail only where they have a significant bearing on consciousness.

How, then, should a participant in Turing's imitation game frame questions to distinguish between a conscious human being and an unconscious computer? If our earlier conclusions are correct, we should try to elicit manifestations of the unpredictable consequences of quantum mechanics. Unpredictability in the form of inconsistency and random decision-making is easily simulated; but the result of many years of unpredictable but strongly correlated decision making, leading to the formation of a system of values, artistic, aesthetic and cultural preferences, and what we recognize as personality, is not.

This does not imply that a computer, or more generally, an inanimate system, can never be conscious. In recent years the development of computers with all the attributes of consciousness has become very much more likely as a consequence of advances in technology, and also as a result of the appearance of the concept of *quantal computing.* This arose from some early work by Benioff[109] and Feynman[110], and has been developed by Deutsch and Josza[111–113], who observed that a device with quantal input and output was, at least potentially, a very much more powerful computer than the classical Turing machine. The concept is not without problems, arising especially from the difficulty of making observations at the quantal level. We have already referred to the controversies surrounding the interpretation of quantum mechanics, which have arisen mainly because of a lack of understanding of the theory of measurement in quantum mechanics. In Chapters 7 and 8 we shall discuss this subject in some detail, since it has implications ranging from the essential properties of a quantal Turing machine to the nature of consciousness.

The ability of a quantal Turing machine for the parallel processing of a virtually unlimited amount of information in a single operation is of course not easy to realize, and not without cost. The input to the 'machine' must be by a microscopic system, that serves as a segment of a 'tape'. For the purpose of detection, the microscopic system must have at least one observable in an almost pure state. The 'scanning' or observation and modification of this state must be made by a suitably prepared 'machine', consisting of a macroscopic system in a metastable state. The creation of this state requires energy, and, in the scanning process, the macroscopic system reverts to a stable state, so that at least some of the energy is degraded. The machine must have provision for the formation of memory of the scanning process and for subsequent access to this memory. As we shall see in the course of this book, *the animate brain satisfies all of these quite exacting requirements with remarkable efficacy,* and it is not surprising that no artificial machine with comparable functions has yet been created, even though the specifications are known.

It is an inescapable feature of the quantal computer that its output cannot be predicted with certainty. This it shares in common with all other systems exhibiting quantal phenomena. The uncertainty of the outcome is a matter of experience which has to be accepted even by those who, like Deutsch[111], subscribe to deterministic interpretations of quantum mechanics, such as the 'many worlds' interpretation. While such unreliability would be considered an undesirable feature of a classical computer, it is just this feature that distinguishes the conscious brain.

In recent years there has been rapid parallel development of theory and technology tending to narrow the gap between inanimate and animate matter. During the decade of the 80's great progress was made both in computer architectures and neurobiological modelling. Connectionist theories, especially the seminal development by Hopfield[114], and the concurrent emergence of a number of practical machines featuring parallel rather than sequential processing of data streams[115,116], initiated a symbiotic process that continues to accelerate development in each field separately.

Accompanying neural network developments by Grossberg[7,8], Rumelhart and McClelland[9,10], Kohonen[11] and many others[117–120] have demonstrated the effectiveness of these for dealing with image manipulation, associative recall and other important capabilities of living creatures.

Currently, generic neural network IC chips are being developed by a number of engineering scientists and machines to take advantage of their enhanced performance are being designed[121,122]. Additionally, research on appropriate operating systems for hybrid computing system architectures combining neural network and expert system technologies is underway[123]. It is not unreasonable to think that the next few years will see a new family of computers featuring these developments in the marketplace, as well as a number of new advances in the simulation of first-order cognitive functions.

However, it is unlikely that systems of this kind will be able to emulate higher cognitive processes, such as unpredictable decision making, associative learning, willed behaviour and conscious awareness, for several reasons. Perhaps the most intractable of these is the fact that the functional units of biological brains are electrochemical rather than purely electrical in character, and as noted earlier, there is compelling evidence that the emotional reward system essential to learning is dominantly chemical[124–126].

For this reason if no other true emulation must in all likelihood await the development of more realistic computing systems, possibly systems based on chemically-mediated transistors subject to quantal effects[127–128]. While imperfect simulation of these effects is possible on existing systems[129–132], a new type of machine incorporating 'electrochemical transistors' at the IC level may be required for fully adequate treatment.

In Chapter 6 we summarize some results of preliminary experiments designed to develop such a device, which can be regarded as an artificial neuron in the same sense that the transistorized electrical connections in all current simulated neural networks may be so regarded. The device is different from these, however, in that its operation depends on its chemical as well as its electrical properties, and thus exhibits both refractory and long-term potentiation behavior - thereby offering the possibility of constructing artificial networks with properties more closely resembling those of true neurobiological networks, and on which the functional characteristics of the latter critically depend.

Anticipating the availability of computing systems incorporating such networks, our final Chapters are devoted to a discussion of quantum effects it may then be possible to simulate with greater fidelity, and of the reliance that may be placed on related measurements. Quantum particle and field concepts are recast in purely algebraic terms without dependence on wave functions, and combined with information theory to model nervous system activity. This development, the mathematical physical foundations of which are presented in full, supports the quantal theory of consciousness we offer in conclusion.

Though initially we have chosen to model brain processes quantum mechanically, we have done so in such a way as to facilitate formal transitions to the classical limit[133]. The great majority of observable functions may be described in this limit, but such a formulation offers the necessary vantage point from which some of the brain's more complex nonlinear operations, recognized as properties of 'the mind', may eventually be understood.

But, to summarize the conclusions reached earlier in this Chapter, there is a residual uncertainty associated with quantum mechanics that limits all definite knowledge, and what can be definitely known concerning any material system is summarized in the elements of its statistical matrix. There are various deterministic theories which try to extrapolate this information, for instance by attributing physical reality to Schrödinger's wave function; but the resulting paradoxes strongly suggest that the success of these theories is limited to the calculation of the conditional probabilities that form the elements of the statistical matrix. There are important implications for the functioning of individual cells in the brain. As we shall see in Chapter 7, quantum probabilities are associated with periodic components of the electric potential[134] in the electrolytic fluid forming the cellular environment, as they are with other types of electromagnetic and material waves. Since the transfer of information in the brain depends fundamentally on changes in potential, we shall give due emphasis to the effects of fluctuations in the extracellular potential in the development of models of cortical activity throughout subsequent chapters.

Chapter 2

The Mammalian Nervous System

2.1 Structure and Function

If awareness and volition are the correlates of consciousness, there seems no reason to suppose they are restricted to the human species. Though varying greatly in size and capabilities, the mammals as a class are rather closely related in the evolutionary process, and this is most evident in the similarity in structure of many parts of their nervous systems. In some respects, in particular in the limbic system that is concerned with the expression of emotions, the nervous system of humans appears to have remained at a very primitive level. But humans are especially distinguished from other mammals in the development of structures adapted to the understanding of language.

In the process of natural selection, the communication of information by speech and more recently by writing, has conferred advantages that more than offset manifest inferiority in several other directions. It represents a critically important step in the evolutionary process, mainly because it allows detailed information to be passed on not only from individual to individual but from generation to generation.

In this Chapter we shall review what is known about the mammalian nervous system, and the human nervous system in particular, from the point of view of structure and function. We shall take it for granted that the brain is the centre of awareness of the nervous system, but sensory information is transmitted by nervous action to the brain from all parts of the body. The spinal cord displayed on the cover of this volume is responsible for the transmission of activity to and from the trunk and limbs[135]. The ventral (front) part consists mainly of a tract of afferent, or outwardly directed, fibres which are the axons of neurons that transmit motor action initiated in the brain. The dorsal (rear) part consists mainly of a tract of efferent, or inwardly directed, fibres which are the axons of neurons that transmit motor feedback as well as the sensations of touch, pressure and pain, to the brain.

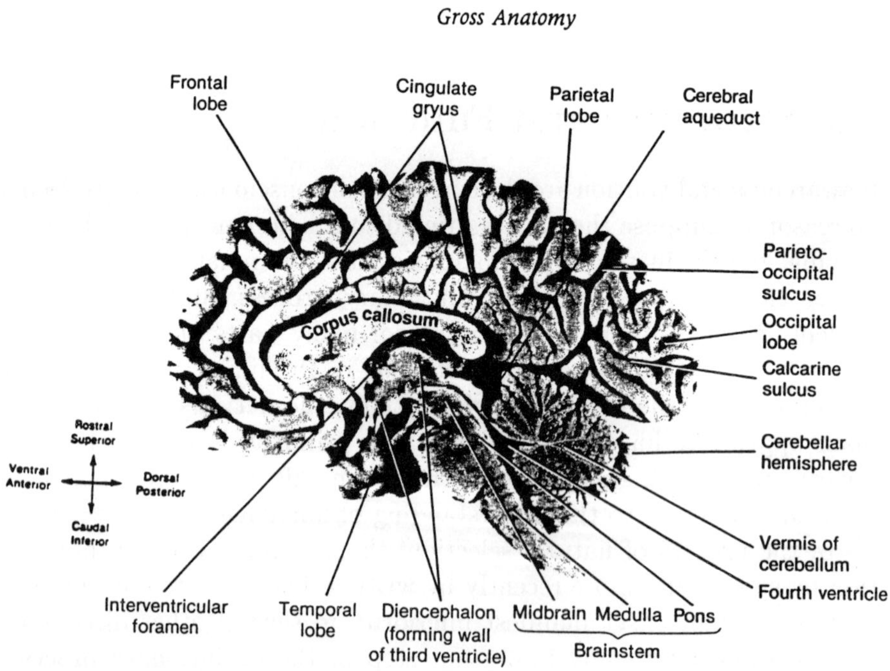

Fig. 2.1 Major regions of the human cerebrum, midbrain, cerebellum and brainstem shown in mid-plane cross-section; directional terms used in text are inset.

Generally speaking, the afferent fibres receive cortical input through various nuclei and tracts in the lower ventral portion of the brain, the anatomical structure of which is illustrated in Figure 2.1. The most important groups of fibres in the lower part of the brain are the medullary reticulospinal tract and the pontine reticulospinal tract and the pyramidal tract originating from cells of this name in the cortex. At their other ends, these fibres serve to activate limb nerves and the motor neurons that in turn innervate muscles in all parts of the body. The activity of the efferent fibres of the spinal cord is transmitted to the cortex by way of analogous tracts. In particular, a pyramidal tract and ganglia in the lower rear, or dorsal, part of the brain communicate directly with specific centres in the cortex.

The cortex consists of the outer surface layers of the brain proper. Its principal subdivisions, which as we shall see, have quite different functions, are the allocortex or thalamic/hippocampal formation, the cerebral cortex or cerebrum, and the cerebellar cortex or cerebellum. The allocortex forms part of the limbic system, occupying regions around the cavity known as the lateral ventricle found on each side of the cortex; the cerebrum covers most of the actual surface of the brain; and the cerebellum occupies a compact region of the hindbrain just below the cerebral cortex, as shown in the Figure.The interior of the brain is occupied to a large extent by tracts of fibres and various nuclei or ganglia. The fibres are simply axonal extensions of neurons carrying information in the form of electrical impulses between different parts of the nervous system, and the nuclei are dense clusters of neurons whose principal function is to pass this information from one centre to another. The position of these internal structures is often described in terms of the forebrain, the midbrain and the hindbrain or their subdivisions.

The thalamus, in particular, is a collection of important nuclei in the diencephalon, which is a medial subdivision of the forebrain. These nuclei relay a great deal of the motor and associated sensory activity of the brain. The hypothalamus is another collection of nuclei in the lower part of the same subdivision, but forms part of the limbic system. The midbrain or mesencephalon includes near the back the collicular nuclei, responsible for the relay of visual and auditory activity. The hindbrain extends down to join the spinal cord. The anterior subdivision of the hindbrain, called the metencephalon, contains the pons, including the pontine nuclei and those of the inferior olive. Below the pons, the oblong medulla adjoins the spinal cord, and contains the nuclei that relay most bodily somatosensory information.

It is not always possible to make a clear distinction between sensory and motor functions, since feedback plays an important role in most of the motor functions of the nervous system. As Wiesdanger and Miles have emphasized[136], the feedback is accomplished to an important extent by neural servomechanisms in which the performance of a movement is continuously monitored and compared with the desired performance; discrepancies between actual and desired movements elicit activity (often by a long loop from the muscle, skin or joint back to the motor cortex) to automatically compensate for the error.

The cerebellum is specialized for learning muscular activities that require fine control, and there are a variety of pathways carrying excitatory impulses between it and the motor association cortex. These include the afferent paths from the large pyramidal cells through the inferior olive to the climbing fibres, or through the pontine nuclei to the mossy fibres, and the efferent paths from the inhibitory Purkinje cells of the cerebellum via the dentate nucleus and the thalamus to both large and small pyramids of the cortex. However, all sensory processing functions – seeing, hearing, smelling, tasting, touching, balancing – as well as those responsible for emotions and memories reside in other regions of the cortex.

Visual input, for example, is from cells in the retina of the eye, with a variety of specialized functions adapted to sense intensity, colour, shape and motion in the field of vision. Two independent pathways to the cortex exist, one through the lateral geniculate part of the thalamus, another by way of the colliculus in the lower part of the brain; but they are probably not redundant, serving instead to distinguish between types of information provided by different specialized cells of the retina.

As a rule, sensory input from the left side of the body is processed in the right hemisphere, and *vice versa*. Thus, visual input coming from the right eye is transmitted via a synaptic relay in the lateral geniculate body to areas of the left side of the cortex, and similarly input coming from the left eye is transmitted to the corresponding areas on the other side. Auditory functions are organized in a similar way.

The input is from a specialized transduction mechanism in the cochlea of the inner ear. This in effect performs a frequency analysis, and the resulting impulses are transmitted through several synaptic relays[64] to the contralateral primary auditory area of the cortex.

The limbic system and the hypothalamus are found near the upper surface of the lateral ventricle, and are responsible for control of the emotions [137]. The septal nuclei and the associated hypothalamus are responsible for pleasurable emotions, the amygdala for disagreeable emotions. The hypothalamus connects to the septum and the septum to the mediodorsal thalamus and beyond. The amygdala connects with both the hypothalamus and the mediodorsal thalamus.

The hippocampus, shown in Figure 2.2, connects to both the hypothalamus and the septum. This structure located on the lower surface of the lateral ventricle plays an important part in the formation of long-term memory [138]. The (parietal and temporal) sensory association cortex is connected via the cingulate gyrus and the parahippocampus to the hippocampus, the hippocampus via the mediodorsal thalamus nucleus to the frontal convex cortex, and this to the sensory association areas. Another route is from the sensory association cortex to the frontal convex cortex, then to the anterior thalamic nucleus to the cingulate gyrus. The approach to the hippocampus via the entorhinal cortex is known as the perforant pathway; the commisural pathway connects the corresponding contralateral areas of the hippocampus by way of the septum and the lower side of the corpus callosum, which is in the middle of the brain and connects the two hemispheres.

The corpus callosum serves to coordinate information processing between the separate hemispheres of the cortex. Surgical procedures affecting this body of fibres have shown that in most respects the two sides of the cortex are able to function independently, though specialized in some respects. The effect of interrupting the normal flow of information between them may give the impression of creating two different personalities in the same individual.

It is worth noting that, quite different from the visual system, the olfactory system — together with the septum, amygdala, hippocampus, limbic and thalamic structures — forms part of the allocortex from which the human cortex evolved. Sensory input to the receptors for smell is directly converted by chemotransduction to nerve impulses

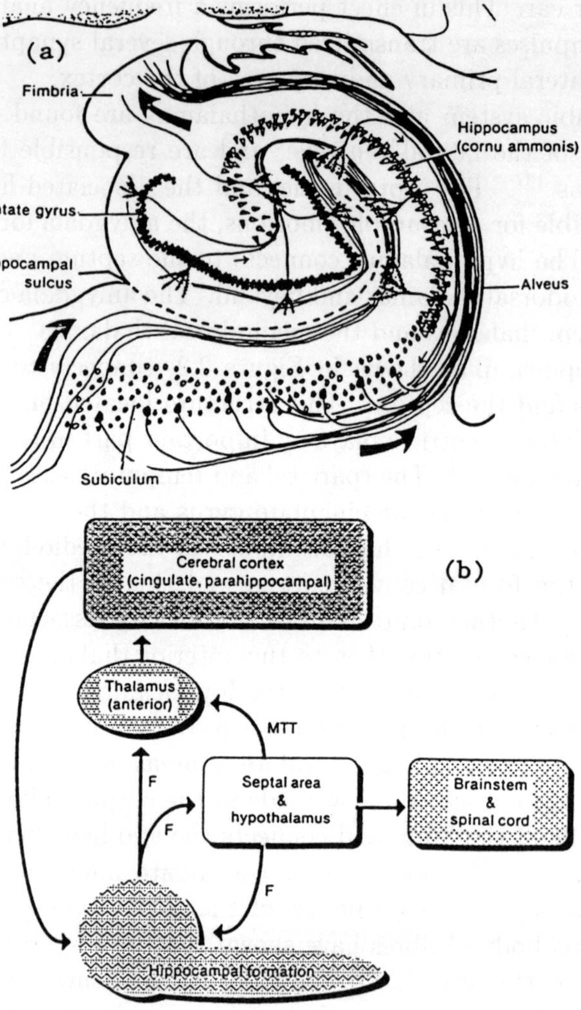

Fig. 2.2 (a) Diagram of the structure of the hippocampal formation showing the arrangement of different types of neurons, and indicating the primary input coming from the subiculum. The latter receives its principal input from the septal area and the hypothalamus, as shown in (b): a schematic of the participation of this formation in the limbic system.

that are transmitted to the olfactory bulb and thence directly and by way of the lateral olfactory tract to the cortex. As it is one of the more primitive parts of the brain, the system is not as well developed in humans as in many of the lower vertebrates; but, interestingly, its neural activity has been demonstrated to be exceptionally well correlated with variations in the extracellular field[139].

Later we shall find it necessary to give considerable attention to the environment of the neuronal network; but for the present we note that, apart from neurons, most of the remaining space in cortical regions is occupied by glial cells which, though they do not form part of the network, do interact with it through the extracellular fluid. This forms a continuous thin conductive, chemically active layer surrounding all of the actual neurons. From our point of view, the glial cells and extracellular fluid constitute integral parts of the nervous system; their influences will be analyzed and modelled in subsequent sections.

2.2 Cortical Organization

In this section our emphasis will be on the processes responsible for the acquisition, processing and utilization of information. Natural selection, operating over hundreds of millions of years, has developed these processes into a system of matchless efficiency.

The acquisition of information depends on the transmission from specialized sensory receptors, distributed over the entire body, through various nuclei and ganglia to the cortex. The utilization of information, by the physical movement of parts of the body, depends on the transmission of motor action from the cortex to groups of muscles. But the processing of this information, linking perception to action, involves the formation of memory, retrieval from memory, association, evaluation and various other operations. In the higher mammals, and especially in humans, these functions have been developed intensively in the brain, many concentrated in specific regions of the six neural layers that form the cortex.

For this reason we shall now concentrate attention on the organization of the cortex, stressing function and location rather than anatomical detail, which is easily found elsewhere[140], though important cellular and synaptic information is summarized in the following section. Those parts of the nervous system concerned with sensory input, memory formation, emotional influence, and motor output will be discussed separately. The less tangible processes associated with conscious and subconscious thought will be treated briefly, but in the main reserved for later chapters.

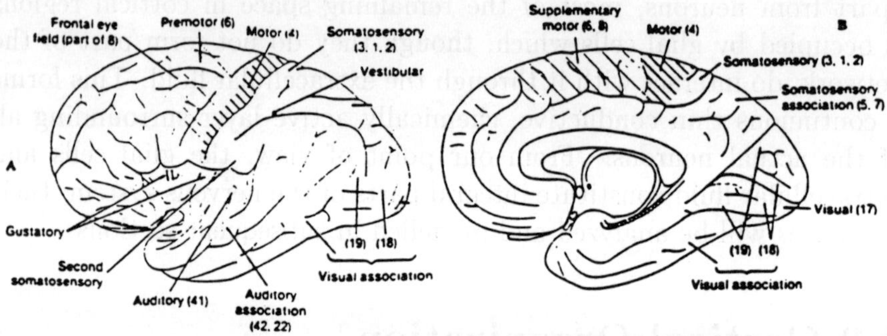

Fig. 2.3 External and cross-sectional diagrams illustrating important functional regions identified in the cortex, with Brodman numbers shown in parentheses.

Figure 2.3 shows the general locations of the areas of the human cortex responsible for some of the basic functions, but a more accurate way of specifying such regions is by the use of the Brodman numbers[141], shown schematically in Figure 2.4. There are areas corresponding to those featured in the following discussion in higher animals other than man, but in most instances they are quite undeveloped and barely recognizable. We consider first the organization of regions dedicated to sensory functions other than those of language and music.

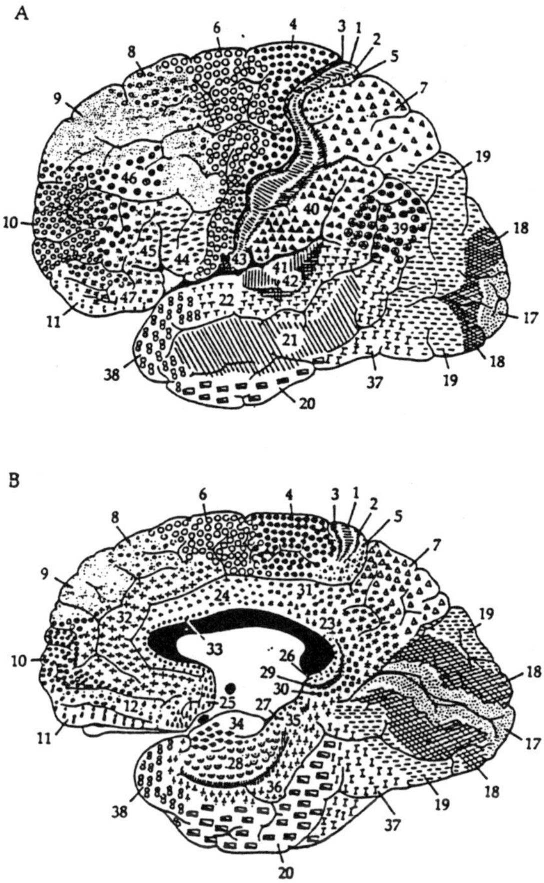

Fig. 2.4 Brodman's anatomically defined regions of the human cortex, with their numerical labels, displayed in external and cross-sectional views.

Most inputs to opposed hemispheres are processed symmetrically and coordinated continuously through the corpus callosum and septum. Visual perception occurs primarily in the striate and occipital areas (Brodman areas 17, 18 and 19) and adjacent temporal and parietal areas, while the perception of sound occurs mainly in the primary auditory area (Brodman area 41) of the superior temporal gyrus. The obvious difference between seeing and noticing, hearing and listening, is reflected in the way visual and auditory information is passed on and processed in other areas of the cortex. Actually, fixing attention to acquire information is so fundamental to the development of human knowledge that we shall be led to regard it as an essential part of conscious experience.

In nearly all individuals the recognition and production of speech is concentrated in the left parietal and temporal areas[142]. Brodman area 39 is concerned with the reading and understanding of written material from visual input, and area 40 with listening to and understanding audible speech. These are parts of the Wernicke area, located in or near the fissure of Sylvius, and one of the earliest such areas identified. Speech is also processed in the secondary auditory area, the planum temporale, Brodman area 42. The posterior speech centre of Wernicke is for the understanding of speech, the anterior speech centre of Broca with the production of speech– a motor function. The Wernicke area actually includes Brodman areas 39 and 40, the posterior parts of 21 and 22, and part of 37, while the Broca area includes Brodman areas 44 and 45.

The corresponding right parietal areas are normally concerned with relationships, especially the awareness of spatial relations such as pattern recognition and the position of the body in space. Musical appreciation which requires awareness of the relations of sounds, though not necessarily of rhythm or pitch, also resides in the right parietal areas; and speech, which is mainly controlled by the corresponding left parietal area, can be affected by the lack of this facility. It is also noteworthy that in a relatively small number of persons, usually left-handed, the normal functions of the left and right parietal and temporal areas are at least partly interchanged.

The hippocampus, already shown in Figure 2.2 of the previous Section, is situated in the wall of the lower temporal horn of the lateral ventricle, Brodman areas 35 and 36, adjacent to the entorhinal cortex, Brodman area 28, which is also part of the allocortex. It lies in close proximity to the septum, forms a part of the well-known Circuit of Papez, is connected directly or indirectly with most parts of the brain, and has been proved to play an essential role in the formation of long-term memory[143]. An individual suffering damage or interruption of blood supply to the hippocampus will have a clear memory of experiences up to a few days before the event occurred, but almost none of all subsequent events, and even those for some hours preceding the disability.

The primary motor cortex, Brodman area 4, controls movement in all parts of the body and occupies the precentral gyrus, a band extending to both right and left immediately in front of the central fissure. Consecutive segments of this band from top to side are dedicated to the movement of the toes, foot, leg, thigh, body, shoulder, arm, forearm, hand, fingers, thumb, neck, head, face, tongue and throat respectively.

Rapid feedback is essential in this part of the nervous system. It is therefore hardly surprising that the processing of somatosensory sensations such as hot and cold, pressure and pain, is the responsibility of segments of the postcentral gyrus immediately adjacent to the corresponding motor segments on the other side of the central fissure. Also of special interest is the fact that the cingulate band-like area occupying a gyrus just above the central upper lip of the cavity known as the lateral ventricle, Brodman areas 23, 24 and 25, is regarded as part of the limbic system and therefore directly responsive to emotional states.

The supplementary motor area, Brodman area 6 immediately in front of the motor area, also plays an important part in the initiation of motor activity.[144] There are several routes from this area via the motor association cortex and the cerebellum through the basal ganglia and back through the thalamus to the motor cortex[145,15]. Additionally, there exists an indirect route from the motor cortex via the pars intermedia of the cerebellum, as well as various others involved in the transmission of motor activity to the muscles. As one example, afferent spinal nerves have a ventral root but there is also direct feedback via dorsal roots from the skin, muscles and joints.

Of special significance for present purposes is the association cortex spread over the frontal and adjacent parietotemporal areas of the cerebrum, Brodman areas 9 through 12. It is responsible for the analysis and elaboration of sensory functions, the integration of information derived from different senses, and the planning of motor activity. Impairment by disease, accident or surgery results in behaviour that can be described as thoughtless, lacking in perception or motivation. Clearly, therefore, though other parts of the cerebrum such as the motor cortex ultimately become involved in any overt action, key properties that we regard as distinguishing mind from brain, including the initiation of thought and very likely consciousness itself, critically depend on the proper functioning of this region. For this reason these functions are emphasized in the modelling development of Chapter 6.

2.3 The Cellular Environment

The neurons that are responsible for the direct transmission of information, should not be regarded as the only functional part of the nervous system. In the animal cortex, the neurons come into close proximity with one another only at synapses, and over most of their area they are surrounded by glial cells which are only indirectly concerned in the transmission of information. Neurons and glial cells are separated by the thin layer of electrolyte that we refer to as the extracellular fluid. This layer has an ionic composition much nearer to that of sea water, with a greater concentration of sodium and calcium than is found in the intracellular fluid.

The neurons and their processes – dendrites and axons – occupy less than half of the cortical space and the glial cells most of the remainder. The external surfaces of the membranes of adjacent glial cells and neurons within the cortex are almost parallel and the layer of extracellular fluid that separates them is typically 100 - 150 Å thick. Although this separation is small, it is sufficient under normal conditions to preclude the direct transmission of significant potentials between neighbouring cells. Because of the large electrical conductance of the electrolyte, changes of potential at the surface of a cell are attenuated exponentially with distance from the membrane, and become negligible at distances greater than about 50 Å. However the large conductivity is a consequence of the rapid diffusion of ions, and in such a confined space a flux of ions across the membrane of a particular cell can affect the ionic composition of electrolyte in the adjacent extracellular space to a significant extent. Other cells in the neighbourhood may well be affected by this change in ionic composition, and it is therefore possible for any cell to interact indirectly with other cells through the extracellular fluid.

The extracellular fluid is generally uniform in character, but there are variations depending on the cellular environment. We first consider the fluid separating neurons from glial cells. There are in fact several types of glial cells, some called oligodendroglia providing the insulating layer of myelinated axons, others devoted to sealing the blood-brain barrier; but here we are mainly concerned with the neuroglia constituting a significant part of the grey matter of the cortex. Since their only direct interaction is with the extracellular fluid, the function of these cells long remained a mystery, but is now beginning to be apparent[147]. Although they cannot generate an action potential, the neuroglia are in other respects very much like neurons. The membranes of typical glial cells are always permeable to potassium ions, and from time to time there is an influx of calcium and sodium very similar to that which accompanies the small graded potentials observed in neurons. The resulting transfer of ions across the membranes have an important effect in the regulation of the concentration of potassium and therefore of the potential throughout the extracellular space. Moreover, the possibility of diffusion of ions across the membrane depends critically on variations in the potential difference between the intracellular and extracellular fluids, so that there is certainly the possibility for neighbouring cells to interact indirectly through the extracellular fluid, provided there is an ionic current across the membrane of at least one of them.

In fact it has been known for a long time that the axonal fibres of neurons, which do not normally form synapses with one another but in some regions run parallel in bundles, may interact through the extracellular medium. Evidence was cited by Marazzi and Lorente de No[76] to the effect that (i) impulses (action potentials) travelling in a fibre or group of fibres may act as liminal stimuli and set up new impulses in neighbouring fibres; (ii) the passage of impulses along a fibre or group of fibres may modify the electrical excitability of the neighbouring fibres, and that there could be (iii) modification of activity attributable to the interaction of neighbouring fibres: synchronization of spontaneous rhythmic firing; modification of the speed of conduction of impulses.

As shown in Figure 2.5, axons transmitting impulses over long distances are insulated with white myelinated wrappings that dominate the appearance of the deeper layers of the brain. To enhance the capability of axons to carry potentials without attenuation, the myelination is interrupted at what are known as the nodes of Ranvier, to allow the influx of calcium and sodium, and the efflux of potassium during the passage of an action potential. The axons of most motor neurons are of this type and terminate at synaptic boutons where, typically, the arrival of a potential results in the contraction of a muscle.

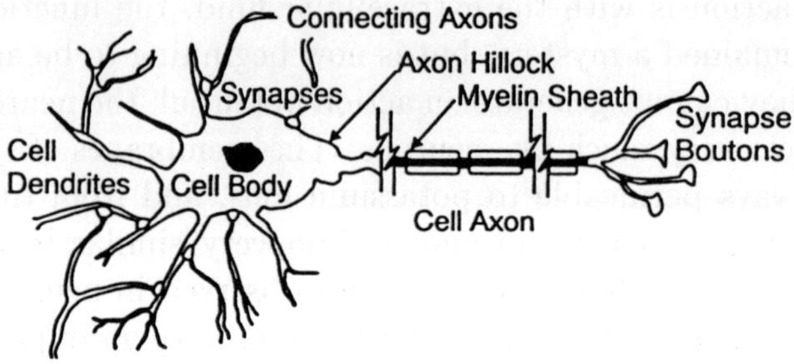

Fig. 2.5 Simplified diagram of a neuron with the principal large-scale features labeled. The insulating myelin sheath of the axon, and the synaptic boutons are a feature of motor neurons, but the cell body with its receiving dendrites, and the axon itself, are common to most types of neurons.

In contrast with these axons, many fibres in the more superficial layers of the cortex are relatively short and unmyelinated, causing them to appear largely filled with grey neural matter. However, the surface layer of the cortex provides a prominent avenue for fibres transmitting impulses between various parts of the brain. As will be seen by reference to Figure 2.6 shown in the next Section, there are at least three additional well-defined avenues below the surface separating layers in which different types of cell bodies are concentrated. The electrolyte near the surfaces of the fibres running through these channels can carry transient ionic currents, accompanied by transient potentials in their immediate neighbourhood. Such effects obviously contribute to the ambient extracellular field, and although they might appear to be merely incidental to the neuronal activity, we shall later refer in some detail to a substantial body of evidence that proves they are important conveyors of information within the cortex.

As a rule, the axonal and dendritic processes extending from the cell bodies, or somas, of neurons are surrounded by extracellular fluid which is remarkably uniform in ionic composition. But wherever an axonal fibre of one neuron closely approaches the membrane of another to form a synapse, the composition of the fluid in the resulting synaptic cleft may be somewhat different due to the presence of various neurotransmitter molecules and related imbalances of calcium. This is clearly a special arrangement designed to enhance the transmission of potentials from one neuron to another, which we shall also discuss in more detail, but here note that it too has its effect on the extracellular field.

The variations in the electrical potential and current in the extracellular fluid can be monitored experimentally in the living animal by means of probes introduced directly into the brain, but are most easily recorded from surface layers by non-intrusive methods based on the use of the electroencephalogram (EEG) and magnetoencephalogram (MEG).

Though the existence of fluctuations of potential on the scalp had been known since the nineteenth century, the invention of the EEG is credited to Berger[148], who was also the first to investigate the various types of activity displayed, and to recognize their importance in monitoring ambient mental processes. The EEG is able record an attenuated form of the activity in the surface layers of the cortex from any number of locations in contact with the scalp. Fluctuations of the order of 10 μV are observed there, corresponding to fluctuations of a few mV in the adjacent extracellular fluid. Even these are, of course, small compared with the action potentials of the order of 100 mV generated within the active neurons of the neural network proper. However, they give a very interesting independent insight into the activity of the cortex. For the most part the EEG potentials are not associated in any obvious way with particular cells, but represent a spontaneous cooperative activity of the cells in the neighbourhood. The operation of the MEG, on the other hand, depends on the detection of the very small magnetic fields (of the order of 10 pT) generated by ionic currents in the cortex. It is even possible to detect the bipolar currents associated with action potentials in this way.

It was some time before the information obtained from the EEG was even partially understood. This information is in fact of two kinds, derived from the slow changes of potential, and the more rapid fluctuations, respectively. The latter will be discussed later, in Section 3.2. The present discussion is therefore limited to the slow potential changes which reflect the mass action of the cells, including glial cells, in the surface layers of the brain. The slow potential changes, called DC potentials because of their uniformly positive or negative character, are to a large extent the manifestation of the relative concentration of potassium ions, which naturally varies as the result of nervous activity, though not always in the most obvious manner. There is usually, for instance[149], a positive shift in the transition from wakefulness to sleep, which is reversed on arousal. There are also some very interesting shifts of potential, both positive and negative, during the performance of various kinds of tasks, indicating readiness for motor action, or the expectation of success or failure. The shift is normally negative in anticipation or hope of success, and positive in anticipation or fear of failure. There is, therefore, a correlation between DC potentials and conscious activity, especially the activity of participating cells in the surface layers of the brain.

The DC potential may be regarded as the result of averaging a fluctuating EEG potential over a period of the order of a second. It often appears to change abruptly by up to 10 μV but rarely maintains a steady value. Since it is an average value, the interpretation of the DC potential requires an understanding of the relation between the average value of the superficial extracellular field and the activity of the cells, including glial cells, near the surface of the brain. Ellis[150] has made calculations on the basis of statistical mechanics showing that the average extracellular potential is directly related to the average intracellular potential, from which it may be inferred that changes in one must be accompanied by changes *of the opposite sign* in the other. Changes in the DC potential therefore reflect changes in the average potential within a large number of neighbouring cells, either as a result of excitation or potentiation, leading to negative shifts, or as a result of inhibition or refractoriness, leading to positive shifts. The larger the shift in the DC potential, the greater the number of participating cells, so that shifts of the order of 10 μV over a short period of time imply a high degree of synchronization of cellular activity.

On the other hand, there is a great deal of evidence that some of the more rapidly varying potentials detected by the EEG are not simply by-products of the activity within the cells, but an integral and indispensable part of the overall activity of the cortex.

There is no doubt that the activity of individual cells of the nervous system is easily affected by external changes of both electric and magnetic fields, especially those which are variable with a definite frequency. The effect of an electric field has for a long time been the basis of electroconvulsive therapy[74]. More recently, an analogous but less pervasive therapy has been developed based on the stimulation of parts of the cortex by means of a magnetic coil[151]. Especially significant is the evidence from EEG and MEG observations that much of the cellular activity of the nervous system is synchronous with rhythmic and other fluctuations of potential in the extracellular field[152]. In the hippocampal formation such activity is synchronous with the theta-rhythm, having frequencies in the 4-10 Hz band; the alpha-rhythm, with frequencies in the 8-12 Hz band, is observed in most parts of the cerebral cortex during relaxed mental states; the beta-rhythm, exhibiting frequencies above 14 Hz, is associated with more excited states; and a variety of other rhythmic variations of potential with higher and lower frequencies can be observed under special conditions.

However, EEG records often exhibit fluctuations that do not obviously correspond to any definite frequency. For example, the fundamental alpha-rhythm is easily disturbed when attention is given to any sensory stimulus; its characteristic frequency rapidly gives way to aperiodic fluctuations, then gradually reappears when the stimulus is removed. The evoked potentials of such a disturbance seem to emerge in the frontal and parietal association regions, then spread rapidly to other areas widely distributed over the cortex.

The incidence of periodic components of the extracellular potentials in the cortex is not restricted to the obviously rhythmic potentials; and in view of the close relationship between extracellular and intracellular activity, it is not easy to determine whether one controls the other. Experiments can demonstrate no more than the synchronization of the two types of activity, and it is left to a physically based theory to disentangle cause and effect. The conclusion reached in Section 4.5 is that the transmission of potentials across the cellular membrane is not, as a rule, exclusively in one direction or the other. There are apparent exceptions to this rule, particularly at synapses, where there are special provisions, involving neurotransmitter molecules and receptors, to ensure that transmission is initiated from the axoplasm of one cell and then from the extracellular fluid to another. However, even at synapses there may be inward *and* outward transfer of certain types of ions across both the presynaptic and postsynaptic membranes.

It has been known, since the work of Katz and Miledi[153] that, especially at synapses, an influx of calcium from the extracellular fluid is the normal precursor of an action potential. Moreover, Adey[154] has summarized a great deal of evidence from various sources to show that external fields with particular frequencies and amplitudes have an important effect on cellular activity. The amplitude of the external potential may be quite small, and in view of the attenuation of all potentials in the extracellular fluid, the amplitude at the membrane must be smaller still. It may be inferred that even very small extracellular potentials with suitable frequencies may have significant effects on the nervous system of an animal. We shall return to this subject in Section 3.2, where the significance of the rhythmic potentials will be discussed in more detail.

2.4 Neurons and Their Properties

Neuron Types

Though intimately linked to their environment and continuously influenced by its electrochemical state, neurons are undoubtedly the principal information processing elements, and the networks formed by their interconnections the primary transmission pathways of the brain. For this reason, inspired by the late 19th Century work of Ramon y Cajal[63], scientists of four successive generations have studied them in detail, documenting their microanatomical structure and electrophysiological functions in an extensive and definitive literature[155,156].

However, the human brain contains more than 10 billion neurons of many different types, and at least 10 trillion interconnections that form a wide variety of circuits. As a result its complexity is far from fully understood; but thanks to the pioneering investigations referenced above, and the dedicated research of many others[157–159], certain common features have emerged which enable some simplifying generalizations to be made.

The simplifications having to do with circuits will be reserved for discussion in Chapter 4; but as regards the neurons themselves it is possible to state, for example, that all those of mammalian nervous systems appear to be specializations of a single type, nearly always with three distinct treelike parts, appearing in Figure 2.5 of the previous Section: receptive dendritic 'branches', a cell body or soma forming an upper 'trunk', and a transmitting axon stemming from the lower trunk and 'root'.

The dendrites receive incoming potential pulses that flow through their many branches into the soma, which contains the nucleus and various neurochemical production components of the cell; and the axon, which contains a cytoskeletal support and molecular transmission structure, transmits action potentials originating in the region where it joins the soma to its bulblike bouton tips, the presynaptic portions of junctions with other neurons described in following Sections.

Nevertheless, these three basic substructures can vary so much that the resulting neurons appear quite different and have, in fact, been assigned different names, as illustrated for the cerebellar region of the cortex in Figure 2.6(a).

The highly specialized organization of the cerebellum is simpler, or at least easier to understand than that of most other cortical regions[60]; but the types of neurons present, though specialized to perform the 'calculations' required for fine control of bodily muscles, can be considered representative of those found elsewhere. The Purkinje cells (P), for example, whose inhibitory outputs represent the end result of such calculations, closely resemble the excitatory pyramidal cells of various sizes shown in Figure 2.6(b) that are found throughout the cerebrum – as are the granule (Gr), Golgi (Gl), basket (B) and stellate cells (S), a few of whose cell bodies and processes are revealed in Layers I, II, IV and VI. The Weigert stained section of a similar region of the neocortex is included to highlight the lateral communication channels discussed in the preceding Section, which also contain many unmyelinated axons paralleling those partly or completely insulated.

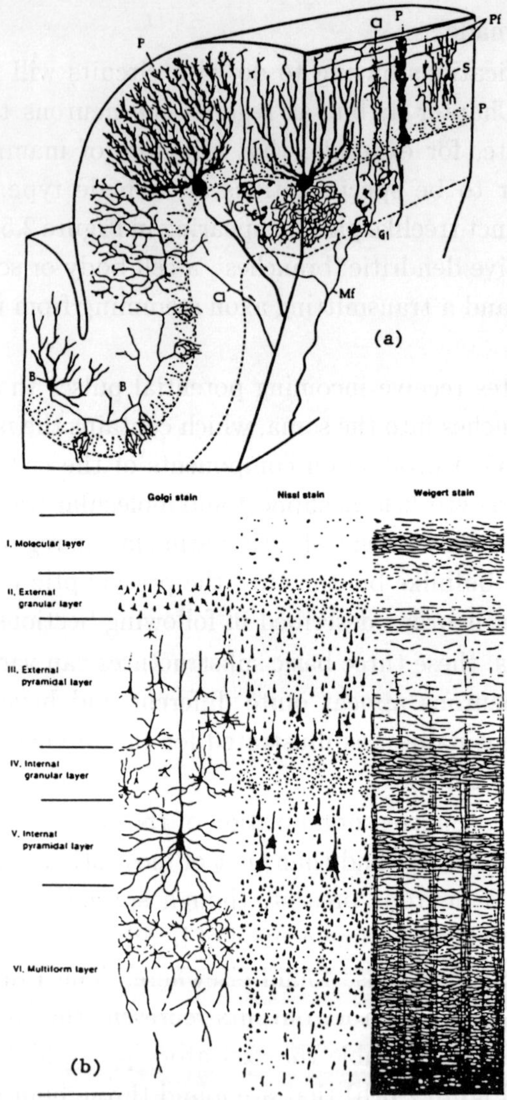

Figure 2.6 (a) Illustration of the layered structure of the cerebellum with the connecting parallel fibres (Pf), and the climbing fibres (Cl) and mossy fibres (Mf) that provide input. (b) Cross-section of the neocortex, stained by three different methods to reveal only: certain types of neurons with their processes, cell bodies, and connecting fibres.

The Neural Membrane

Since the membrane of a neuron not only encloses the reproductive nucleus and the molecular machinery required to assemble transmitter and other associated chemical substances, but also mediates its ionic interactions with the extracellular fluid in such a way that electrical potentials can be produced and sustained, it has been a focal point of biosciences research for many years[160–161].

This work has established that, though consisting essentially of opposed bilipid layers, the membrane is also penetrated by a wide variety of complex protein molecules that regulate the flow of ions of various sizes – principally sodium, potassium and calcium throughout its body and processes – and, additionally, of neurotransmitter molecules keyed to interact with specific receptor molecules and so lead to an influx of ions at the postsynaptic membrane and also at junctions, such as are illustrated in Figure 2.7.

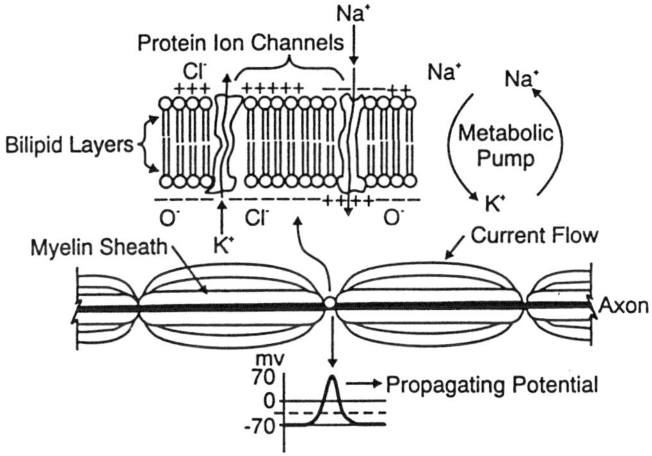

Fig. 2.7 Diagram of a segment of a myelinated axon of a neuron, illustrating the mechanism of propagation of an action potential by drift-current induced exchange of sodium and potassium ions through channels in proteins embedded in the bilipid layers of the membrane, and reversed after the passage of each such potential by metabolic pumping.

The ability of the membrane to generate and transport graded and action potentials is, perhaps, the most fundamental of its properties. A potential difference of about 100 mV between its inner surface, exposed to the cell cytoplasm, and its outer surface, exposed to the extracellular fluid, must be maintained; and this is accomplished by an ionic pumping mechanism of ancient origin[162].

The ionic composition of the extracellular fluid in most animals betrays the origin of life in sea water. However, the oceans are among the end products of a cycle of energy and entropy transfer driven by the Sun on the earth's surface; and as most of the natural processes in this cycle are irreversible and tend to increase the total amount of entropy, the sea is not a favourable environment for much of the essential activity of life. The concentrations of sodium, calcium, magnesium and chloride in solution are too high. It is hardly coincidental that an very important part of the chemical activity of a cell results in the expulsion of sodium and calcium ions, which are replaced by potassium ions in the electrolytic fluid enclosed by the cellular membrane. Typical ionic concentrations found within the cytoplasm are:

$C_{\mathrm{K}} = 135$ mM; $C_{\mathrm{Na}} = 5$ mM; $C_{\mathrm{Ca}} = 10^{-6}$ mM; $C_{\mathrm{Cl}} = 52$ mM.

It can be seen from these values that there is not enough chloride to secure the electrical neutrality of the electrolytic fluid within the cell. Nevertheless, the electrolyte must be almost neutral except very near membrane surfaces, and the balance of the negative charge is on a variety of protein that is relatively immobile, so that its contribution to the electrical activity of the cell is negligible.

The reduced levels of sodium and calcium are achieved by the action of enzymes within the structure of the cellular membrane; these are large molecules known as ATPases (adenosine triphosphatases), extending between the internal and external surfaces of the membrane. They continually recycle ATP (adenosine triphosphate) in a process that accounts for a considerable fraction of the metabolic activity of the cell. There are three types[163]:

(1) Na,K-ATPase; which, as its name implies, exchanges intracellular sodium for extracellular potassium. There is of course a limit to the reduction of the internal sodium concentration which can be achieved by this pumping action. Eventually the sodium must be returned to the cell, but this occurs by a different mechanism, discussed below, and

through other channels.

(2) H,K-ATPase; which exchanges intracellular hydrogen for extracellular potassium without a net transfer of charge. As in any electrolyte, the hydrogen ions are invariably bound to positive ions, but are readily available to participate in chemical reactions.

(3) Ca^{2+}-ATPase; which transfers calcium from the intracellular to the extracellular electrolytic fluid.

Sodium, potassium and calcium are not the only ions or molecules actively transported across the membrane, but these are most important for the electrical activity of the cell with which we are primarily concerned. As one consequence of the ionic pumping mechanism, the electrical potential gradient noted above is maintained; at the normal potential difference of approximately 100 mV there is approximate electrochemical equilibrium of the potassium inside and outside the cell. But because of the difference in potential between its surfaces, the membrane is polarized, with an excess of negative charge on its internal surface.

Thus, metabolic pumping plays an essential part in creating, restoring and maintaining a potential difference across the cell membrane which, in turn, provides a readily available source of electrochemical energy. Part of this energy is released in the transmission of signals from one part of a neuron to another by means of transient fluctuations of the potential difference across its membrane, resulting in the influx of calcium and sodium ions and efflux of potassium ions that temporarily undoes the work of the ionic pumps. These produce not only the small graded potentials in the dendrites and upper soma, but the large action potential spikes in the lower soma, which momentarily depolarize the membrane and move down the axon sustained by a similar mechanism at uninsulated nodes.

The mechanisms and characteristics of potential pulses and synaptic transfers are discussed in the next Section, but because of their special importance to the theme of this book, the former are treated in detail in the following Chapter.

2.5 Synapses and Neurotransmitters

Synapse Types

In a micrograph showing a cluster of neurons and glial cells, most of the external surface of a neuron is found to be adjacent to glial cells. There are, however, places where the membrane of the neuron is adjacent to that of another neuron, and in such places the thin layer of extracellular fluid separating two neurons can be identified with one of several different types of chemical synapse (Figure 2.8). The synaptic cleft provides the means by which one of the neurons communicates directly with the other, and most such synapses have special features designed to permit or enhance the transmission of information in one direction or the other[164].

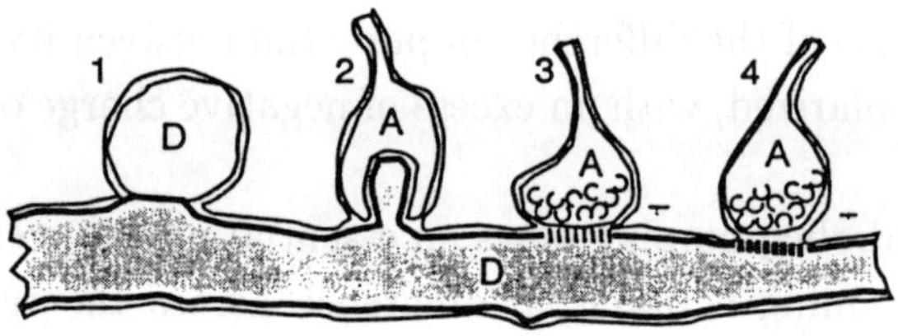

Fig. 2.8 An illustration of several common types of synaptic connections: (1) a tight electrical dendro-dendritic junction (D-D), (2) an axo-dendritic junction on a dendritic spine, (3) an asymmetric excitatory axo-dendritic junction and (4) a symmetric inhibitory axo-dendritic junction (A-D).

Axo-dendritic synapses clearly transmit information from the axon of one neuron to the dendrite of another; similarly, axo-somatic synapses transmit information from the axon of one neuron directly to the soma of another. The possibility of dendro-dendritic synapses is also sometimes encountered, some of which have been identified as tight electrical junctions, such as that labelled (1) in the Figure. Synapses usually occur at axon terminals, but are not necessarily located there.

It is also necessary to distinguish between two types of synapses, sometimes referred to as asymmetric and symmetric. At asymmetric synapses, a potential in the axon of one neuron tends to excite a potential in another, but at a symmetric synapse a potential in the axon of one neuron tends to inhibit a potential in the other. It follows that asymmetric synapses are formed by the axons of excitatory cells, but symmetric synapses are formed by the axons of inhibitory cells. The axons of inhibitory cells are seldom very long, and many are classified as local interneurons, though some have axons which reach out to more distant cells in the same group or neighbouring groups. It is often possible to recognize a symmetric synapse in a micrograph, by the presence of a layer of material in the extracellular fluid, midway between the membrane surfaces of the two neurons.

It is not surprising that a firing neuron, which raises the external potassium level, should tend to inhibit the firing of another in its immediate neighbourhood, but clearly some special mechanism is required to facilitate the transmission of the excitatory potential at an asymmetric synapse. Eccles was among the first to grapple with this problem, and has related that he was led to a solution by a dream[165], in which he visualized a stream of particles across the synaptic cleft from the presynaptic neuron to the other. At first he concluded that these particles were ions, making an electrical connection between the two neurons. Somewhat later he was convinced by colleagues that this interpretation of his dream was wrong, that the particles must have been molecules of some chemical substance, such as acetylcholine (ACh); but thus the neurotransmitter or chemical messenger theory of synaptic transmission was born.

Synaptic Transmission

The theory of synaptic transmission that subsequently evolved is remarkable not least for its complexity. There was no doubt that transmission is initiated by the influx of calcium to the presyanptic neuron that accompanies the arrival or passage of a graded or an action potential. There was also no doubt that the consequent activation of the postsynaptic neuron required the participation of the neurotransmitter at the postsynaptic membrane surface. However, according to Dale's principle[166], the type of neurotransmitter was always determined by the presynaptic cell. Therefore, in intermediate processes the neurotransmitter must be released at the presynaptic membrane and be transferred in some way to the postsynaptic membrane. The release from the presynaptic membrane into the synaptic cleft is from *vesicles.*

Vesicles are small bodies with a surface composed of the same lipid material as the cell membrane, and are routinely involved in the transport of large molecules in the intracellular space. They spend part of their time in random (Brownian) motion in the intracellular fluid, but when they come into contact with a cell membrane they tend to attach themselves and partly fuse with the membrane. While connected to the membrane in this way they are able to interchange material with their extracellular environment in a process known as exocytosis. Eventually they are detached from the membrane after a process called endocytosis, and drift into the intracellular fluid. It is known that the vesicles in the synaptic neighbourhood may contain quite high concentrations of neurotransmitter substances.

According to the theory described by Llinás[167], *immediately following* the arrival or passage of a potential, vesicles containing a neurotransmitter substance, such as ACh, attach themselves to certain sites in the presynaptic membrane and release the neurotransmitter into the synaptic cleft. The process is described in more detail by Jahn and Südhof [168] as follows: "Neurons transmit information by releasing neurotransmitters from presynaptic nerve endings. In the resting stage, transmitters are stored in synaptic vesicles. When an action potential arrives in the nerve terminal, the membrane depolarizes and voltage-gated Ca^{2+} channels open. The resulting Ca^{2+} influx triggers exocytosis of synaptic vesicles, resulting in the release of transmitter. The synaptic vesicle is rapidly retrieved by endocytosis and reutilized for the formation of synaptic vesicles". After its release at the presynaptic membrane surface, the neurotransmitter is supposed to diffuse rapidly to the postsynaptic membrane.

A potential problem for this theory has been made explicit by Hucho[169], in raising the question "How does the transmitter molecule released from the presynaptic membrane reach the postsynaptic membrane? The superficially correct answer is by diffusion. But an explanation is needed of how it diffuses past the numerous molecules of acetylcholinesterase present in the synaptic cleft which would theoretically be able to hydrolyse many times the quantity of released transmitter and prevent it from reacting with the postsynaptic membrane."

If the release occurred in part at the postsynaptic membrane, the problem would obviously not arise. But, quite apart from this problem, the details of the release mechanism remain to be explained, and a considerable amount of experimental work has been done, especially on the effect of repeated synaptic activation.

It has been found that, with repetitive excitation at a synapse, there is a facilitation effect: successive pulses produce a proportionately larger effect at the postsynaptic membrane, sometimes presumed to be the result of residual internal calcium, which is in fact observed. In their experiments, Katz and Miledi[170] found facilitation factors up to 70. However, there is a sharp cut off of transmitter release following each pulse, and there is no simple relation between the degree of facilitation and the amount of transmitter available. A mathematical model for the release of neurotransmitters at synapses, in reasonable agreement with experiment and to some extent independent of the detailed mechanism, was developed by Dodge and Rahamimoff[171]. The influx of calcium raises the internal concentration in the expected way; and assuming that four calcium ions bind (internally) on a receptor to secure the release of a neurotransmitter molecule, the amount of transmitter released will increase as the fourth power of the calcium concentration at low concentrations; but there is a saturation level depending on the number of receptors. Barton, Cohen and Van der Kloot[172] proposed a modified model with a finite base level of internal calcium; then the number of calcium ions binding to a receptor site could be more than 4, and experiments performed at low concentrations do not enable the precise number to be predicted.

The influence of variations in the potential on the release of neurotransmitter has often been neglected. That electrostatic considerations are important is evident from the experimental investigations of Parnas, Parnas and Dudel[173], who have shown that in addition to presynaptic calcium release, there must be a voltage-dependent factor, and that depolarization has a direct effect on the release machinery.

We conclude that while there is more to be learned about synaptic transmission, the arrival of an electrical potential at the presynaptic membrane of such a synapse is undoubtedly accompanied, as elsewhere in the activating fiber, by an influx of calcium ions. This influx is primarily responsible for the release in the synaptic cleft of an additional number of ACh molecules. As a consequence, the preexisting equilibrium with AChR in the postsynaptic membrane is disturbed and excess ACh molecules become bound to their receptors in the postsynaptic membrane. In this reaction, previously bound calcium ions are released which, driven by strong electrostatic forces, enter the postsynaptic cell through the protein channels described earlier. Finally, the influx of calcium ions tends to initiate the development of a potential in the postsynaptic cell by a mechanism which we have already described and will be considered in detail later.

Neurochemical Transmitters

Today it is known that a number of different neurotransmitters determine the character and behavior of many, perhaps most, of the synaptic junctions in the brain. Because the functioning of the brain critically depends on the biochemical interactions of these and other neurotransmitters, they are discussed in detail below. But it is important to recognize that, in addition to the 'chemical' synapses, there are many tight electrical junctions of the type illustrated in Figure 2.8. They have been observed at axon-axon, axon-soma, axon-dendrite, and even dendrite-dendrite connections [64], and could prove to be even more numerous than the foregoing type.

There is a wide variety of neurochemical substances, and in many instances a particular neurotransmitter is found to be associated with specific neurons and parts of the nervous system with a recognized function. Thus, some are invariably found in association with inhibitory neurons and others with excitatory neurons, and the variety of each type appears to be well adapted to the chemical control of distinct functions of the brain. The presence of a particular neurotransmitter at a synapse is the result of the action of enzymes in the presynaptic neuron. The neurotransmitter is stored in vesicles which from time to time fuse with the presynaptic membrane, so that it is released into the synaptic cleft. There, its action is a consequence of its ability to bond with a corresponding molecular receptor in the postsynaptic membrane. In most instances, the receptor molecule has been identified, and it has been verified that the binding of the neurotransmitter to the receptor affects the release of calcium at the surface of the postsynaptic membrane. We shall discuss briefly some of the more important of these substances:

(1) We have already mentioned acetylcholine (ACh), which was one of the earliest neurotransmitters to be identified. It is widely distributed in the mammalian nervous system[174], and its action is more or less typical of neurotransmitter action at excitatory chemical synapses, though it is active in some types of neuro-muscular junctions as well. The action of ACh depends on its affinity for ACh receptor molecules (AChR) embedded in the surface. There are two types of AChR: the nicotinic variety nAChR, found in many synaptic membranes, and the muscarinic variety mAChR, found at some neuromuscular junctions.

(2) The amino acid L-glutamate is another widely distributed neurotransmitter that depends on its affinity for the N-methyl-D-aspartate (NMDA) and also the α-amino -3-hydroxy -5-methyl -4-isoxazole proprionate (AMPA) receptors. These receptors forms part of the membrane surface and are permeable to calcium, but are typically blocked by magnesium ions, for which they have an affinity. The action of L-glutamate depends on its ability to displace the magnesium, thus permitting the entry of calcium. Neurotransmitter mechanisms of this type are known to be effective in particular at synapses where long-term potentiation occurs[175–176]. L-glutamate is also an important transmitter at the neuro-muscular junctions of animals, including crustaceans and insects[177]. Other amino acids, such as aspartate have a similar excitatory action, as have cyclic adenosine monophosphate (cAMP) and cyclic guanosine monophosphate (cGMP).

(3) The catacholamines, adrenaline (A), noradrenaline (NA) and dopamine (DA) are all derived from the amino acid phenylalanine and are the transmitters of the sympathetic system that is responsible for involuntary actions and certain emotions. It is the production of NA that has the important function of inducing the partial arousal accompanied by the rapid eye movements (REM) that occur every hour or two during sleep, and which may be important for the formation of long-term memory.

From our point of view, dopamine is one of the most interesting of the neurotransmitters, since it is implicated in the mechanisms of motivation, incentive and reward which often have unconscious origins in the limbic system but have an important affect on learning, cognitive behaviour, and other forms of conscious activity. Insufficiency of dopamine, on the other hand, produces symptoms of restlessness, lack of volition and poor memory. The effect of drugs such as cocaine and d-amphetamine is probably due to their action on dopamine receptors. Dopamine is a favoured neurotransmitter of neurons associated with the hypothalamus and activation of the medial prefrontal cortex.

(4) The hormones, epinephrine, norepinephrine and histamine: These are of two types, one of which mobilizes calcium while the other activates adenosine triphosphate (ATP). The latter is involved with the adenylate cyclases Ca-ATPase, Na/K-ATPase and H/K-ATPase[178] in active transport ion pumping as described in Section 2.4.

An equally important role is played by the neurotransmitters associated with local inhibitory neurons called interneurons. In the absence of these, much of the nervous system of an animal would be in a state of uncontrolled activity; a fine balance of excitatory and inhibitory action is obviously vital for the control of motor and brain functions. Inhibitory neurotransmitters differ from those listed above primarily by releasing chloride instead of calcium ions in interaction with their receptors in the postsynaptic membrane. The chloride then enters through channels little more than 5 Å in diameter in these receptors and depresses the potential in the postsynaptic neuron.

We complete our list with some recognized inhibitory neurotransmitters.

(5) Gamma aminobutyric acid (GABA) is an inhibitory transmitter which interacts with GABA receptors of two different kinds – type A that activates chlorine channels, and type B that leads to increases of both chloride and potassium concentrations in the synaptic cleft[179].

(6) Glycine resembles GABA in its action, both being derived from amino acids.

(7) Serotonin (5-HT) is implicated in the induction of sleep, as NA is implicated in partial arousal, and in such aberrant mental states as severe depression[180]. The effect of hallucinatory drugs such as LSD appears to be due to the similarity of their molecular structure and consequent interference with the action of serotonin.

We shall next consider in more detail the potentials that carry information between different parts of the brain.

Chapter 3

Properties of Neural Potentials

3.1 Graded and Action Potentials

In the resting state, the electrical potential within a cell is determined primarily by the active transport of ions across the membrane. As described in Section 2.4, this implies the transfer of sodium and calcium from the internal to the external electrolytic fluid, and transfer of potassium in the opposite direction, in the course of the metabolic activity of the ATPase molecules embedded in the cellular membrane. Although there is no resultant movement of electric charge, the effect of the active transport is to produce quite large gradients of the ionic concentrations across the cellular membrane. The potassium remains in approximate electrochemical equilibrium across the membrane, but there are important gradients of the electrochemical potentials of the other ions. There is also a preponderance of negative charge associated with protein at the internal surface of the membrane and within the cytoplasm; this changes, if at all, very slowly and does not contribute to the ionic currents in the cell. Consequently the internal electrical potential is typically 60 mV lower than in the extracellular fluid, and the cellular membrane is strongly polarized.

In the absence of synaptic activation, the potential within a cell is thus determined by the constitution of the cell and the active transport of ions across the membrane. There are channels through the membrane, many of them associated with protein molecules in the cell wall. But these channels are so narrow that, for reasons to be explained in Section 3.5, they do not normally allow the diffusion of ions back into the cell. However, there is an upper limit to the potential difference that the membrane can sustain, and the active transport of ions across it in the outward direction must ultimately be compensated by the transfer of ions in the opposite direction. In quiescent states of the living animal, a considerable fraction of this activity probably occurs in conjunction with periodic potentials commonly observed in the extracellular fluid, and these certainly play a part in maintaining the potential of cell at its resting level.

At the resting level, nevertheless, the membrane of a cell remains in a metastable state vulnerable to small perturbations. The degree of polarization associated with the resting level can easily be changed locally. At synapses, usually with the participation of neurochemicals, this change is initiated by an influx of calcium ions through channels in the neural membrane, as described in Section 2.5. Synaptic activation from other cells may occur on the soma, or cell body, with a direct effect on the intracellular potential, or at various localities distributed over the dendrites leading into the cell. The mode of conduction of ionic currents along the branches of a dendritic tree towards the soma has been studied by Rall[181] and Tuckwell[182]. The cumulative effect of the various synaptic stimuli may merely *potentiate*, or raise the potential within the cell, but if continued will ultimately be followed by a firing, with the depolarization of the adjacent membrane, and the transmission of an action potential along the axon of the cell.

Within the living animal the firing is very likely to occur synchronously with activation arising from the fluctuations of potential in the extracellular fluid. Though usually less than a few mV in amplitude, the latter serve to alternately polarize and depolarize the membrane, and polarization may well have the effect of destabilizing an already precarious state of equilibrium. The precise conditions under which this occurs will be the subject of quantitative studies from the point of view of classical theory in Section 4.5 and from the point of view of quantum mechanics in Chapter 7. As a result of these studies it will become clear that, at the right frequency, extracellular potentials as small as 1 nV, at the quantal level, may initiate an action potential. In confirmation of this, it has been known for some time from experiment that very small periodic fluctuations of potential in the extracellular field can determine whether or not an action potential results.

The immediate result of destabilization is the creation of positive or negative graded potential pulses of a few mV amplitude, which rapidly attenuate as they spread along the neural fibre unless reinforced by others. But if, as a result of such reinforcement, the potential in the lower soma rises above some threshold value unique to the neuron, the membrane there suddenly becomes much more permeable to calcium and sodium ions.

Explosive depolarization then produces an action potential spike that shoots to 40 mV or more above the threshold and propagates unchanged in amplitude throughout the axon at a speed of around 120 m/sec. In the region of its origin, however, the potential drops precipitately to 20 mV or so below the original resting level and remains in a refractory state for the 5 to 50 msec required for metabolic processes to restore it to this level before another action potential can be generated.

Motor neurons stimulated intracellularly with inward and outward directed currents of increasing magnitude typically exhibit all of these responses, as shown in two different ways in Figure 3.1.After an action potential, a cell passes through a series of refractory states in which the potential gradually returns to its resting level. During the refractory period the cell is insensitive to external stimuli of any kind, but thereafter it is sensitized and a further action potential may follow. Thus, the spacing of action potentials, which characterizes the information being transmitted, is affected by the refractory period, but can also vary depending on the magnitude as well as the frequency of the stimuli received. The potential in the critical region of the soma can be held below threshold by inhibitory hyperpolarizing pulses; but becomes increasingly sensitive to activation on approaching this value, where extremely small changes in ionic composition may lead to the development of a spike or action potential. The magnitude (60 mV) of the overshoot of the action potential in the Figure is a feature of the experimental conditions; though there is a overshoot of the action potential in a living animal, it is normally very much smaller.

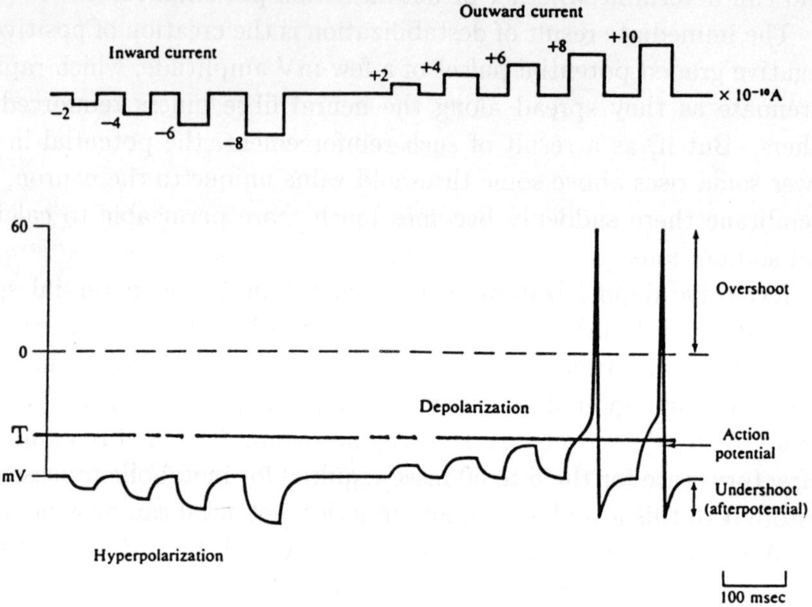

Fig. 3.1 Observed variation of potential in the output of a motor neuron subjected to trans-membrane negative inhibitory and positive excitatory current pulses, illustrating hyperpolarization for the former and depolarization for the latter when a well-defined threshold (T) is exceeded. Depolarization results in an overshoot above the zero level, followed by an undershoot, leaving the neuron in a temporary refractory state.

There are various ways of modelling graded and action potentials. For an account of the early history of this subject, the reader is referred to the work of Cole[183]. The first attempt at a realistic description of the non-linear ionic processes associated with an action potential was due to Hodgkin and Huxley, and will be discussed in Section 5.1. A somewhat simpler and more faithful model for an action potential was developed subsequently by Fitzhugh[184]. In 1975 the authors[45] introduced a quantum-mechanical model of a single neuron, and also of a network of such neurons, exhibiting the non-linear characteristics of action potentials. We shall describe this model briefly in Section 3.4; it provides a simple application of the principles of quantum mechanics and motivates the more detailed physically based classical treatment, developed subsequently by the authors, to be presented in Section 4.6. Models like these, which attempt to describe every detail of the ionic potentials and currents, are still not too difficult for application to realistic neural networks of modest size, and some examples will be found in Chapter 5.

However, with larger networks there are advantages in simplicity, and in the 1980s an extensive development of neural network theory occurred[85,9], based on a very simple model neuron with just two states. A generalization of this model with any number of states and other more realistic features will be described in Chapter 6.

3.2 Rhythmic and Chaotic Potential Waves

Following neuroanatomical and neurophysiological investigations of the structure and function of the nervous system, experimental studies of the electrical activity in the brain of the living animal have provided some of the most fruitful insights into cortical action. By the late 1920's, as related in Section 2.3, it was known that variations of potential near the cortical surface could be detected in attenuated form by electrodes attached to the scalp. Soon afterwards, Berger[148], with the aid of the electroencephalogram (EEG), discovered periodic fluctuations of potential of about 10 Hz in human subjects, known as the α-rhythm We have already noted that somewhat different information, conveyed by the small magnetic fields[185] that are generated by ionic currents near the cortical surface, can be obtained by the use of the magnetoencephalogram (MEG). Still further information, not restricted to superficial phenomena, are obtained from electrically sensitive probes[186] inserted into the brain, where the action potentials of individual neurons may be observed as 'spikes'. These spikes, however, are recorded only from locations very near the membrane surface, and are rapidly attenuated with distance from the membrane. Elsewhere the potentials observed may be roughly classified as rhythmic or chaotic. The rhythmic potentials, whether spontaneous or induced, may in turn be classified according to behavioural correlates or the observed shapes and frequency bands. The frequencies fall within

(1) the alpha band, with frequencies around 10 Hz;
(2) the beta band, with frequencies around 20 Hz;
(3) the gamma band, with frequencies around 40 Hz;
(4) the delta band, with frequencies around 2 Hz; and
(5) the theta band, with frequencies between 4Hz and 8Hz.

Rhythmic potentials may appear either in the form of waves, or as spindles repeated at regular intervals. The band width may be fairly narrow; nevertheless, the frequencies are rarely sharply defined, and the amplitude of a component of the potential with a particular frequency is usually very small indeed. Also, although well correlated wave forms of approximately the same shape may be widely distributed over the cortical surface, and sometimes an apparent velocity of propagation of the order of 1 m/s can be detected, there is considerable dispersion and the mode of transmission is obviously very different from the way sound and light are transmitted in homogeneous media.

Electroencephalography and magnetoencephalography, supplemented by information obtained from probes, have provided a detailed picture of the electrical activity associated with various types of behaviour and response to sensory stimuli. For a time, however the significance of the experimental data obtained in this way was poorly understood, and there may have been an impression that all extracellular potentials were a mere by-product of the internal activity of neurons and other cells. It was, for instance, readily concluded that the thalamus was the source of the α-rhythm, since many of the potentials synchronized with the α-rhythm were relayed through this nucleus. It is now usual to make a distinction between the α-spindles, that appear as regularly spaced spikes on an EEG, and the α-waves that have a more sinusoidal shape. The spindles are often associated with thalamic activity. There is good evidence[187] that spindles are generated by pyramidal cells activated by impulses relayed by, though not originating in the thalamus. On the other hand, the α-waves are observed even when the thalamus is inactive, and in 1977 the first evidence appeared[188] for a source of the α-rhythm in layers IV and V, containing large pyramidal cells, in the cortex of the dog.

It was soon recognized that the rhythmic potentials are associated with particular states of mind. The α-spindles[189] are found especially in the period of awakening after sleep. The α-waves, on the other hand, appear in relatively tranquil states of awareness, and the β- or γ-waves in somewhat more agitated states. These rhythms all disappear rapidly[190] when voluntary motor action is called for, as in response to a sensory stimulus; the disappearance is clearly the result of desynchronization by the global activity that follows. The very slow δ-waves are most commonly found during deep sleep, but are punctuated with spindles that are associated with thalamic activity and become more frequent in light sleep.

An extensive study has been made of *event-related* or *evoked* potentials on EEG records obtained from human subjects who are required to respond in some way, as by the movement of a finger of one hand, in response to a sensory stimulus[191–192]. As related by Kornhuber[193], a voluntary movement "is preceded by patterns of excitation in the association cortex, which are recognized as the readiness potential in diffuse scalp recording", and "the first event preceding a movement of the right finger is not a potential in the left motor cortex, but a bilateral readiness potential, widespread over precentral and parietal regions. A second potential, 90-80 msec before movement, is also bilateral and widespread. A third potential, 50 msec before, is limited to the hand area of the contralateral motor cortex". Subsequently, it was found possible to characterize the components of evoked potentials[194], in terms of function, or sign and latency (*i.e.,* the time after the application of the sensory stimulus in cs or ms). These components are related to (i) sensation (negative, N1), (ii) perception (positive, P3), expectancy (contingent negative variation, CNV) and intention or readiness (*Bereitschaftspotential,* BP). Still more recently, attention has been given to the DC components of these potentials, whose significance was discussed in Section 2.3, and to the mode of generation and propagation of the potentials across the cortical surface[195,82]. It is evident that experimental studies of this kind are gradually affording insight into the workings of consciousness.

Perhaps the most interesting type of periodic potential is the rather slow θ-rhythm, found mainly in the limbic system, particularly in the hippocampus and the septum[195], though of course other frequencies are often found there as well. An early review of relations between the θ-rhythm and various types of cortical function was made by O'Keefe and Nadel [197]. More recently, Lopes da Silva[24] has emphasized the role of the θ-rhythm in the 'gating' and synchronization of potentials in the cortex, and we shall develop these ideas further in Section 3.4.

It was slowly recognized that extracellular potentials may and do affect neuronal activity. Positive experimental and other evidence[77,198] that communication between neurons is possible through the extracellular fluid had in fact been available for some time. But it was not until 1992, while introducing a symposium[199] on electroencephalography, that Mountcastle was able to say (*loc.cit.* p.xviii) "Rather suddenly, however, a paradigm change is upon us, for the proposition that slow wave events are active agents for signal transmission now stands as a testable hypothesis, with some evidence to support it", and quite extensive experimental evidence to support it, derived mainly from the study of EEG activity, was summarized (*loc.cit.* pp. 435-457) by Başar. The evidence comes from observations of synchrony and coherence, oscillation and resonance, and of *chaos*, which, in the technical sense, is distinguished from the random character of 'noise'.

The observations that action potentials of various types of neurons are synchronous with extracellular rhythmic potentials[152] suggest that it may not always be meaningful to distinguish between cause and effect in the relation between rhythmic neuronal and extracellular activity. This conclusion will be reinforced by physically based calculations in Sections 4.4 and 4.5 to follow showing that, on the one hand, oscillatory potentials of up to a few mV in amplitude are a natural feature of the superficial *Debye* layers of an electrolytic fluid, and on the other hand, very small potentials with a sharply defined frequency are transmitted with considerable amplification in both directions by channels in the neural membrane. Although the potentials, including rhythmic potentials, recorded by an EEG are small in amplitude compared with an action potential, they are to some degree manifestations of *non-linear* processes and exhibit the characteristics of all such phenomena. We shall review these briefly before proceeding to a discussion of chaotic potentials.

A system regulated by linear processes is particularly simple, not only in its mathematical description but in its physical behaviour. A change in the initial configuration of any such system is reflected by a proportionate change in the configuration at any subsequent time: output is linearly related to input. A pendulum not far removed from its state of rest is a simple example; the electrolyte in contact with a neural membrane is another, provided that it is likewise sufficiently near to its resting configuration. However, linear processes are the exception rather than the rule in nature, and even the motion of a pendulum is regulated by non-linear *anharmonic* processes that make the position of the pendulum virtually unpredictable after a sufficiently long time. What is a 'sufficiently long time' depends on the initial configuration and other dynamical conditions. The same is true of ionic oscillations in the neighbourhood of a neural membrane, but the non-linear effects are different and the 'sufficiently long time' may be quite short. Under special conditions, non-linearity may manifest itself in a variety of forms. Sometimes there is an *attractor*, and the final configuration, far from being unpredictable, is stable and independent of the initial state of the system. But, where there is more than one attractor, it is possible for the system to be attracted to one relatively stable configuration, then after some time, to another, and never reach a state of equilibrium. The long term behaviour of the system again depends very sensitively on the initial conditions.

Most of these conclusions were reached by Poincaré at the end of the last century, but modern computers were needed for the full appreciation of their implications. So-called *strange attractors* were found by Lorenz[200] in the course of computer modelling the non-linear behaviour of fluids. So long as they were based on classical mechanics the non-linearities did not, in principle, affect the possibility of making accurate predictions for any length of time, on the basis of sufficiently accurate information concerning the initial configuration. It is this predictability in principle that has disappeared with the advent of quantum mechanics. Quantum mechanics places limits not only on the completeness and accuracy of information concerning the initial configuration of a system, but also and more fundamentally on the possibility of making accurate predictions. This is so especially where sub-microscopic events may affect the outcome, as they do ultimately in nearly all non-linear processes.

Another well known consequence of classical mechanics, wherever non-linearities are concerned, is the appearance of periods that are double the fundamental period of a periodic process. In its application to rhythmic potentials, the doubling of a natural period would provide a facile explanation for the relations between the α-rhythm, the β-rhythm and the γ-rhythm. There could be some truth in such an explanation, but, as we shall see in Section 4.5, there is a deeper explanation in terms of the physical processes regulating the transmission of frequencies by the neural membrane.

In the mathematical theory of non-linear rhythmic processes, the appearance of periods that are higher multiples of the fundamental period is the normal precursor of chaos[201–202]. This mathematical theory is based on the study of difference and differential equations that, at best, describe an idealization of physical processes. But, as Başar has emphasised[28] in a volume largely devoted to the analysis of the non-rhythmic fluctuating potentials of the cortex, highly irregular fluctuations cannot be interpreted as random noise, but often conceal 'strange attractors' with well defined frequencies, usually much greater than that of the alpha-rhythm. Noise is devoid of useful information, but chaotic activity in the cortex is highly correlated and its underlying periodic components could be even more effective than the rhythmic potentials in the acquisition, creation and transmission of information.

The identification of phenomena with chaotic, as distinct from random, characteristics in the brain does not imply that they are predictable in detail, even in principle. Again, because quantum mechanics limits the information that can be obtained concerning the state of any system, exact prediction is impossible. There is always new information to be gained. However, the fact that in chaotic potentials much of this information is correlated is undoubtedly significant in the search for understanding of the functioning of the brain.

3.3 Long Term Potentiation and Memory

We shall next discuss a phenomenon that is now generally accepted as the key to understanding the formation of memory in the cortex. Even before the discovery of LTP (long term potentiation), it had been known with some certainty that the hippocampus, one of the subdivisions of the limbic system or allocortex, played an important part in the retention of memory. The allocortex is believed[124] to be a survival of the cortex of primitive animals present on the earth quite early in the evolution of the animal species, perhaps an indication of the importance of memory in the struggle for survival. It is usual to make a distinction between working memory, which lasts for a few seconds, and long term memory, which may last for life. In making this distinction we could well associate working memory with transient changes in the concentrations of ions and neurotransmitter substances, and the formation of long-term memory with structural changes in the brain. However, structural changes cannot be effected in a few seconds or even a few hours. The hippocampus is known to play a part in the process. It has been known for a long time from clinical studies[143] that patients with hippocampal damage lose the capacity to form long term memory, but sustain no loss of memory of events before the damage was inflicted. From such studies it became clear that memory was not stored in the hippocampus, but that the hippocampus played an indispensable role in the formation of long term memory.

A theory of the formation of memory in general terms was suggested by Hebb [101]. Briefly stated, this was to the effect that the transmission of information by synapses in the brain is facilitated by use. No specific mechanism was known, however, until the discovery in 1973 of LTP in the dentate area of the hippocampal formation by Bliss and Lomo[92]. It was found that, following certain types of stimuli, excitatory cells in this area remained in a sensitized or potentiated state, in which they would respond very much more readily to subsequent activation through the transmission of a potential. Potentiation in this context implies an elevated, though still very low, concentration of calcium in which a cell is nearer to its firing threshold.

Following the initial discovery of LTP, similar phenomena were found in other areas of the cortex[95], and over a period of time the details of the mechanism have gradually become fairly clear. Much experimental work was done on hippocampal slices *in vitro*, where it was found possible[203] to induce LTP by a prolonged sequence of stimuli with a particular frequency. Considerable evidence has been obtained[204] that it is the combination or *association* of a weak synaptic stimulus and a lengthy equally spaced (periodic) sequence of stimuli that is most effective in such experiments. It is hard to resist the suggestion[205] that the periodic stimulus is an analogue of the θ-rhythm, the regular fluctuation of 4-7 Hz observed under various conditions in the extracellular environment of the hippocampal formation in the living animal.

The details of the synaptic transmission responsible for LTP have been investigated[175–176], and are not unusual. Again most of the experimental work relates to the hippocampal formation. Activation of an excitatory presynaptic cell results naturally in an influx of calcium from the synapse to this cell, and a local increase of potassium in the synaptic cleft. The neurotransmitter substance is L-glutamate, which becomes bound to AMPA and NMDA receptor molecules in the surface of the post-synaptic cell, and it is therefore natural that NMDA antagonists will inhibit the development of LTP. The binding of L-glutamate by receptor molecules is responsible for the influx of calcium to the postsynaptic cell, and while this is often the precursor of an action potential, in this context it results in potentiation. Activation of inhibitory interneurons (basket cells), on the other hand, leads to the binding of GABA transmitter molecules by GABA receptor molecules in the postsynaptic membrane and an influx of chloride to the postsynaptic cell.

Experimentally, LTP has been found to persist for periods ranging from several minutes to many hours. The fact that it is not permanent is sufficient to confirm that, while cells experiencing LTP play a part in the formation rather than the preservation of long term memory, some independent mechanism must be responsible for maintaining the cells in a hypersensitive state. An apparent mechanism of this type was uncovered by Fifkova and others[97–98], who found that, under the conditions of LTP, there was an actual growth of dendritic spines, amounting to 30-40%, on postsynaptic cells. Such structural changes are evidently favoured by potentiation. However, there has also to be a mechanism for the timely reactivation of these cells, if this sensitization is to be effective.

The reactivation of hippocampal cells is most likely to be related to activity in other parts of the brain[206]. Behavioural studies of living animals, in conjunction with electroencephalography, have shown a close correlation between the appearance of the θ-rhythm in the hippocampus and the initiation of voluntary motor action in the neocortex.

On the other hand, passive or involuntary motor action does not have the same effect, and learned motor activity is sustained even after the hippocampus is disabled.

Some insight into the need for frequent reactivation of the cells that are implicated in the formation of long term memory may be gained from clinical studies[207,208] of those who have experienced TGA (transient global amnesia); these amount to as many as 1 in 4000 of the population and include one of the authors. The sudden onset of an attack of TGA is easily recognized by an observer, because of the inability of the subject to retain the memory of current events for more than a few seconds. The symptoms gradually disappear after a period that is usually less than a day. Up to the time of the attack, memory is normal. Throughout the attack, normal memory is retained of events that occurred more than two or three days before the attack. After the attack, memory is normal except for events occurring *up to two or three days before, as well as during the attack.* The last observation is consistent with the need for a period of progressive consolidation of memory in the cortex, considerably longer than a single period of LTP, in the process of formation of long term memory. It seems clear that such consolidation must be interrupted by the dysfunction of the same part of the cortex that is responsible for the formation of long term memory, in most instances the hippocampal formation. Though the consolidation need not be a fully conscious process, it does not appear to be active during slow wave sleep, and it is possible that one of the functions of the REM (rapid eye movement) sleep and dreaming, that punctuates slow wave sleep, is to allow consolidation to take place.

It is common experience that memory does not normally consist of discrete impressions of isolated events, which divorced from their context would have little significance or value. Instead, memory consists of continuous or almost continuous sequences, often in close correspondence with sequences of external events conveyed to the conscious observer by the senses. These observations are relevant to the development of a model of the formation of sequential memory, such as will be presented later in Section 6.5. It must be supposed that a given sensory impression I_1 is part of a sequence I_0, I_1, I_2, ... , properly ordered in time. Representatives of the different types of cortical units affected by this sensory input are given labels R_0, R_1, R_2, ... , S_0, S_1, S_2,

... , H_0, H_1, H_2, ... , corresponding to sequences of sensory receptor units, sensory association units and hippocampal units, respectively. The first neuron capable of detecting the particular sensory impression I_1 of the sequence belongs to the sensory receptor unit R_1. The firing of the output neuron of R_1 activates the sensory association unit S_1, which, on firing, activates a hippocampal unit H_1 synchronously with the θ-rhythm. The hippocampal unit is therefore left in a potentiated state. The sensory association unit S_2 is activated by I_2, and also by S_1, so that it also fires and activates another hippocampal unit H_2 synchronously with the θ-rhythm. This hippocampal unit is also left in a potentiated state, and so the process continues. The independent activation and firing of S_0, S_1, S_2, ... may be repeated as the result of the conscious or unconscious activity of the cortex, and it is this repetition that constitutes the short term or working memory of the sequence of sensory impressions.

Perhaps 90 minutes later, again as the result of conscious or unconscious activity of the cortex, the unit S_1 may again fire, and, provided that the firing in synchronous with the θ-rhythm, the hippocampal unit will be further potentiated; it will therefore, ultimately fire and contribute to the activation of S_2 synchronously with the θ-rhythm. Thus, with the participation of hippocampal units, the activation and firing of S_0 is necessarily followed by the sequential firing of H_0, S_1, H_1, S_2, H_2, ... At this stage, what may be called medium term memory of the sequence of impressions has been formed. Finally, perhaps after several days, as a result of the progressive sensitization of the synapses of S_0 onto S_1, of S_1 onto S_2, ... , the sequential firing of S_0, S_1, S_2, ... is possible without the participation of hippocampal units. At this stage, long term memory of the original sequence of sensory impressions has been established. A model of this type appears to be entirely consistent with the known facts concerning the formation of memory.

3.4 A Quantum Theory of Potentials

In Section 1.3 we have seen that an important question, associated with certain interpretations of quantum mechanics and quantal paradoxes such as the paradox of Wigner's friend, is whether the animate brain is subject to the same underlying physical laws as ordinary matter. The authors' interest in this question led them to devise a quantum mechanical model of the action of a single neuron[45] and investigate its application to an early example of a neural network[39,209]. The object of such an investigation was to examine whether a quantum-mechanical model of this kind could reproduce the more fundamental characteristics of networks in the biological brain. The model took it for granted that the internal activity of a neuron could be affected not only by synaptic action but also by activation from the extracellular fluid, and assimilated the evidence, discussed in Section 3.2, that rhythmic potentials with a particular frequency were involved.

An exposition of quantum mechanics that is more than adequate for the present purpose is given in the final Chapter of this book; here we shall make a beginning by collecting some of the more immediately useful ideas and results. A quantum mechanical variable should be regarded as an *operator*, and represented by a square array of numbers forming a *matrix*. A dynamical variable describing the behaviour in time of a simple system can be represented by a simple matrix F with elements F_{jk} that are real or complex numbers; the subscripts j and k usually take integral values between 1 and some upper limit L, possibly infinite. The sum of the diagonal elements, $\sum_{j=1}^{L} F_{jj}$ of F is called the *trace* of F and is denoted by $\mathrm{tr}(F)$. The ordinary product FF' of two simple matrices F and F' is a simple matrix with elements $(FF')_{jk} = \sum_{l=1}^{L} F_{jl}F'_{lk}$; obviously, FF' is different from $F'F$ in general. On the other hand, the direct product $F \otimes F'$ of any two matrices F and F' is a matrix with elements $(F \otimes F')_{jj'kk'} = F_{jk}F'_{j'k'}$; the ordinary product of $F_1 \otimes F'_1$ and $F_2 \otimes F'_2$ is $F_1F_2 \otimes F'_1F'_2$. An observable quantity, such as a potential, is represented by an *hermitean* matrix F, for which the element F_{kj} is the complex conjugate $\overline{F}_{jk}$ of F_{jk}. If F and F' are hermitean matrices, so is $i[F, F']$, where $[F, F'] = FF' - F'F$ is the *commutator* of F and F'.

The fundamental observable of any system at rest is its total energy H, and in quantum mechanics this is therefore represented by an hermitean matrix. For reasons given in Section 7.2, the energy is the agent of change in time. For our present purposes we adopt what is known as the Heisenberg representation, where any dynamical variable

F satisfies the *commutation relation* [see (7.4.3)]

$$i\hbar\frac{dF}{dt} = [F, H]. \tag{3.4.1}$$

When H is a known function of the dynamical variables, this serves as a differential equation to determine F as a function of the time t.

The state of the system is also described by a matrix P_0, called the statistical matrix or sometimes the density matrix. Since P_0 determines the probability some selected observable has any particular value, $\mathrm{tr}(P_0) = 1$, and the *expectation value*, or most probable value $< F >$ of any dynamical observable F in the Heisenberg representation at time t is given by

$$< F >= \mathrm{tr}(FP_0). \tag{3.4.2}$$

In the Schrödinger representation, the statistical matrix depends explicitly on the time, and [see (7.2.11)]

$$i\hbar\frac{\partial P}{\partial t} = [H, P], \tag{3.4.3}$$

where $P = P_0$ at time $t = 0$.

We consider the application of this to a composite system consisting of part or the whole of the nervous system N of an animate observer, and an external stimulus S. For a part of the nervous system the stimulus takes the form of excitation from the extracellular fluid; for the entire nervous system it could be a beam of light, impinging or about to impinge on the senses of the observer. The energy of the composite system is

$$H = H_N + H_S + V_{NS}, \tag{3.4.4}$$

where H_N and H_S are the contributions to the energy of the nervous system and the stimulus in isolation, and V_{NS} is the energy of interaction of the stimulus with the nervous system. We shall denote the statistical matrices of N and S by P_N and P_S respectively. Before the interaction, the statistical matrix P is the direct product $P_N \otimes P_S$, but during and after the interaction it must be expressed as a sum (usually infinite) of direct products: $P = \sum_j P_{N,j} \otimes P_{S,j}$, where $\sum_j P_{N,j} = P_N$ and $\sum_j P_{S,j} = P_S$. Thus, P_N is always a *partial trace* $\mathrm{tr}_S(P)$ of P and P_S is the other partial trace $\mathrm{tr}_N(P)$.

The objective information that can be gained, in principle, from the nervous system of the observer at time t is given by an adaptation of the quantal formula (7.3.2),

$$I = -\mathrm{tr}_N(P_N \log P_N). \tag{3.4.5}$$

This information changes at a rate determined by the interaction energy; the rate of change is most easily computed in the *interaction representation*, the detailed theory of which is given in Section 7.3; it will not be needed here. We note simply that the rate of change of this information is given by

$$i\hbar \frac{dI}{dt} = -\mathrm{tr}_N\{\log P_N \mathrm{tr}_S([V_{NS}, P_N]\}. \tag{3.4.6}$$

In the following we shall develop an explicit formula for the energy observable H_N, first for a model neuron, and then for an entire nervous system! For for the sake of simplicity, we shall take into account only the changes in the electrical and electrochemical energy of the sodium and potassium ions, whose numbers are most significant in determining the electrical potential and other important variables of the model.

A Quantized Model Neuron

In modelling the action of a single neuron, it is sufficient for most purposes to consider the *exchange* of sodium and potassium ions between the interior of the cell and the extracellular fluid, across the cellular membrane. As this exchange does not affect the total number of sodium and potassium ions on either side of the membrane, only the internal and external numbers N^{i} and N^{e} of sodium ions need be considered. In quantum mechanics, these are matrices that can be expressed in the form

$$N^{\mathrm{i}} = c^{\mathrm{i}*}c^{\mathrm{i}}, \qquad N^{\mathrm{e}} = c^{\mathrm{e}*}c^{\mathrm{e}}, \tag{3.4.7}$$

where, as in (7.3.17), $c^{\mathrm{i}*}$ and c^{i}, also $c^{\mathrm{e}*}$ and c^{e}, may be interpreted as creation and annihilation matrices, satisfying

$$\begin{aligned} c^{\mathrm{i}}N^{\mathrm{i}} &= (N^{\mathrm{i}}+1)c^{\mathrm{i}}, \qquad N^{\mathrm{i}}c^{\mathrm{i}*} = c^{\mathrm{i}*}(N^{\mathrm{i}}+1), \\ c^{\mathrm{e}}N^{\mathrm{e}} &= (N^{\mathrm{e}}+1)c^{\mathrm{e}}, \qquad N^{\mathrm{e}}c^{\mathrm{e}*} = c^{\mathrm{e}*}(N^{\mathrm{e}}+1). \end{aligned} \tag{3.4.8}$$

These, and (3.4.7), are the essential relations, but they are not sufficient to determine the matrices uniquely. If it is assumed that there is no upper limit to the values of $N^{\rm i}$ and $N^{\rm e}$,

$$c^{\rm i}c^{\rm i*} = N^{\rm i} + 1, \qquad c^{\rm e}c^{\rm e*} = N^{\rm e} + 1. \tag{3.4.9}$$

The eigenvalues (possible results of a measurement) of $N^{\rm i}$ and $N^{\rm e}$ are then automatically non-negative integers.

There are four main contributions to the energy of the model neuron in interaction with the extracellular fluid:

(1) If χ is the difference in electrochemical potential of a sodium and a potassium ion, the variable part of the energy associated with these ions is $\chi(N^{\rm i} + N^{\rm e})$, with $N^{\rm i}$ and $N^{\rm e}$ given by (3.4.7).

(2) The interaction energy, responsible for the exchange of ions across the membrane, is of the form $\lambda(c^{\rm i*}c^{\rm e} + c^{\rm e*}c^{\rm i})$.

(3) A time-dependent, and therefore non-conservative contribution, of the form $c^{\rm i*}v(t) + v^*(t)c^{\rm i}$ from other neurons that form synapses on the cell.

(4) To these we must add the variable electrostatic energy of interaction of the ions within the cell, and the interaction energy responsible for the exchange of ions across the cellular membrane. On the basis of the Debye-Hückel theory of electrolytes (see Section 4.3), the electrostatic energy is of the form $\mu N^{\rm i} \exp[\alpha(M - N^{\rm i})]$, since the electrostatic potential is a linear function of $N^{\rm i}$. This contribution to the energy is non-linear, and has the consequence that, under suitable conditions, a large change in the state of the neuron can be brought about by a small change in $N^{\rm i}$.

By combining these four contributions, and using the expressions for $N^{\rm i}$ and $N^{\rm e}$ given in (3.4.7), we obtain the variable part of the energy of a single neuron and its extracellular environment in the form

$$\begin{aligned} H_N = {} & \chi(c^{\rm i*}c^{\rm i} + c^{\rm e*}c^{\rm e}) + \lambda(c^{\rm i*}c^{\rm e} + c^{\rm e*}c^{\rm i}) + \\ & + (c^{\rm i*}v + v^*c^{\rm i}) + \mu c^{\rm i*}c^{\rm i} \exp[\alpha(M - c^{\rm i*}c^{\rm i})]. \end{aligned} \tag{3.4.10}$$

This expression can be used to study the effect on the neuron of a stimulus coming from a synapse or the extracellular fluid. One approach would be to determine the behaviour in time of the statistical matrix

P_N of the neuron and its immediate environment. But here our primary interest is in the macrosopic behaviour of the system, and this requires only a knowledge of the time dependence of the membrane potential V, which is the difference between the external and internal potentials φ^{e} and φ^{i}, and is therefore given by

$$\varphi = \varphi^{\mathrm{e}} - \varphi^{\mathrm{i}} = (\chi/e)(c^{\mathrm{e}*}c^{\mathrm{e}} - c^{\mathrm{i}*}c^{\mathrm{i}}), \tag{3.4.11}$$

where e is the ionic charge. To determine the time dependence of V, we first use (3.4.1) and (3.4.8) to obtain

$$i\hbar\frac{dc^{\mathrm{i}}}{dt} = [c^{\mathrm{i}}, H_N] = \chi c^{\mathrm{i}} + \lambda c^{\mathrm{e}} + \mu c^{\mathrm{i}}[e^{\alpha} - (e^{\alpha}-1)c^{\mathrm{i}*}c^{\mathrm{i}}]\exp[\alpha(M - c^{\mathrm{i}*}c^{\mathrm{i}})] + v(t),$$

$$i\hbar\frac{dc^{\mathrm{e}}}{dt} = [c^{\mathrm{e}}, H_N] = \chi c^{\mathrm{e}} + \lambda c^{\mathrm{i}}. \tag{3.4.12}$$

A semi-classical approximation is possible for large values of N^{i} and N^{e}. The above pair of matrix equations can be replaced by ordinary differential equations and solved by the usual numerical methods for the complex variables c^{i} and c^{e}, together with their complex conjugates, $c^{\mathrm{i}*}$ and $c^{\mathrm{e}*}$ respectively. It is then an easy matter to compute the potential corresponding to various initial conditions and various values of the parameters of the model with the help of (3.4.10).

Figure 3.2 below shows several examples of output from a computer program constructed for this purpose [see Appendix A3.4]. The variation in time of the potentials corresponding to various initial conditions is shown. The lower oscillatory curve models the effect on a neuron of rhythmic excitations from the extracellular fluid, and others model the action potential that can result from such interchanges when a threshold is reached. As shown in the original papers[45], a great variety of outputs can be obtained from different choices of the time dependent term $v(t)$ in the first equation of (3.4.12), so as to model the excitatory and inhibitory synaptic stimuli which affect a neuron in the biological context.

A Quantized Neural Network

It is not difficult to formulate a generalization of this model to simulate the action of a neural network of any size. If the individual neurons of the network are distinguished by a subscript j that takes values 1, 2, 3, ... , the energy of the entire network takes the form

$$H_N = \sum_j (H_j + \sum_k V_{jk}), \tag{3.4.13}$$

where

$$H_j = \chi_j(c_j^{i*}c_j^{i} + c_j^{e*}c_j^{e}) + \lambda_j(c_j^{i*}c_j^{e} + c_j^{e*}c_j^{i}) + \\ + \mu_j c_j^{i*}c_j^{i}\exp[\alpha(M_j - c_j^{i*}c_j^{i})] \tag{3.4.14}$$

is the energy of the j-th neuron in isolation, and V_{jk} is the energy acquired by this neuron by virtue of synaptic input from the k-th neuron. The simplest choice that provides for the transfer of energy involved is

$$V_{jk} = \nu_{jk}c_j^{i*}c_k^{e}, \tag{3.4.15}$$

where $\nu_{jk} = 0$ if there is no synapse from the k-th to the j-th neuron, but otherwise ν_{jk} determines the *synaptic weight* corresponding to this interaction. It is obviously possible to provide also for external input to the network, by the introduction of time-dependent terms analogous to those involving v and v^* in (3.4.10). There are now equations like (3.4.12) for each neuron; for the j-th neuron, we have

$$i\hbar\frac{dc_j^{i}}{dt} = \chi_j c_j^{i} + \lambda_j c_j^{e} + \mu_j c_j^{i}[e^{\alpha} - (e^{\alpha}-1)c_j^{i*}c_j^{i}]\exp[\alpha(M_j - c_j^{i*}c_j^{i})] + \sum_k \nu_{jk}c_k^{i}),$$

$$i\hbar\frac{dc_j^{e}}{dt} = \chi_j c_j^{e} + \lambda_j c_j^{i}. \tag{3.4.16}$$

This set of differential equations, given by the authors in (1975)[45], could be regarded as early precursors of the neural network equations in common use today. In a semi-classical approximation, they can again be treated as ordinary differential equations, and following numerical integration the potentials

$$\varphi_j = \varphi_j^{e} - \varphi_j^{i} = (\chi_j/e)(c_j^{e*}c_j^{e} - c_j^{i*}c_j^{i}), \tag{3.4.17}$$

are easily determined. Typical output from the computer program is shown in Figure 3.2.

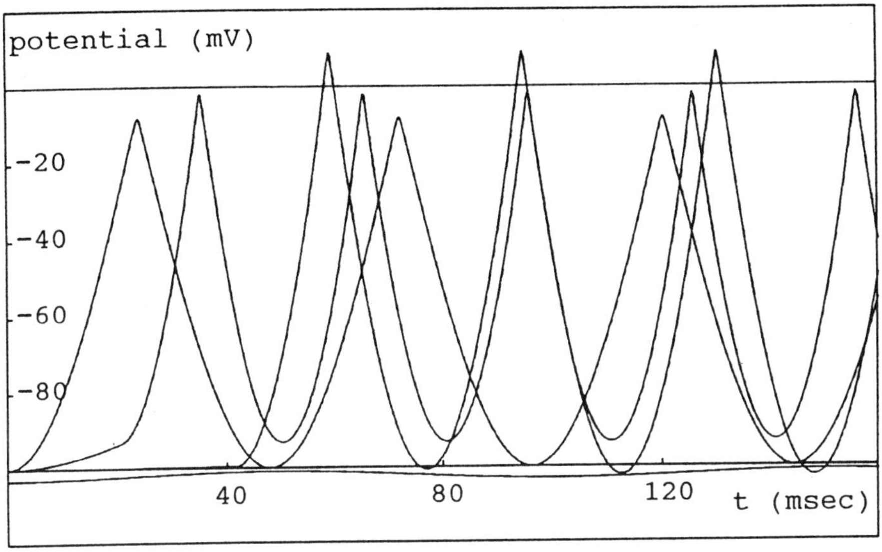

Fig. 3.2 Computer plot displaying the action potentials for three neurons with sequential synaptic connections, the second and third initially in a resting state. Sub-threshold variations in potential for a fourth neuron are also shown.

The Figure shows the variations of potential in four neurons. The firing thresholds are determined by the values of the M_j in the non-linear terms of (3.4.14) and (3.4.16). In the lower curve, the non-linear term is small and ineffective so that the oscillations are small, and the firing threshold is not reached. Initially the potentials in the other three neurons are also below threshold, but it is supposed that a stimulus is applied to the first soon after time $t = 0$, and the program models the sequential firing of the three neurons as a result of the synaptic activation of the second by the first, and of the third by the second. Very much larger networks have been modelled in a similar way, but when the principles are known it is possible to obtain equivalent results without the solution of differential equations, as we show in Chapter 6.

3.5 Neural Aspects of Consciousness

Although by now the structure and functions of the various parts of the nervous system are relatively well understood, there is still much to be explained about the many aspects of consciousness and thought. Consciousness is clearly related to the information processing capacity of the central nervous system of animals, but is not simply the information processor. It is also closely related to, though not synonymous with thought: since Descartes, thought has been widely recognized as a fundamental condition for conscious existence. But thought seems to mean different things to different people; for some, like Descartes and Jaynes[210], it must be expressed in spoken or unspoken language, and is therefore restricted to humans beyond a rather early age; other animals (including, presumably, parrots and dolphins) are supposed not to think and, by extension, are not conscious. Eccles[15] is disposed to extend consciousness to mammals other than humans, but no further. Here we are unwilling to accept such restrictions, and therefore make explicit the criteria that tend to support our more generalized concept.

In Section 1.2 we defined consciousness in terms of awareness and volition. Ultimately we shall be led to a precise definition of, and a consequent distinction between, these two but they are closely related, and for the present we shall take it for granted that awareness implies the existence of a form of consciousness.

Athough awareness is certainly an important part of human experience, it is not continuously active in human beings; they are not aware when asleep, under anaesthesia, or suffering from severe concussion. There are two main types of sleep. As we have seen in Section 3.2, slow wave sleep is characterized by slow rhythmic variations of the extracellular potential in the cortex, usually punctuated with spikes known as 'sleep spindles'. These occupy most of an EEG (electroencephalogram) record made during sleep. They are identified by the absence of eye movement and most other motor activity, though of course not of the activity essential for life. It has been conjectured that this sleep is needed to restore neural function, but in excess it is known to have an adverse effect on the formation of memory, and in Section 3.3 we have suggested a reason for this. Slow wave sleep is interspersed with regular periods of REM (rapid eye movement) sleep, characterized by various forms of cortical activity. The motor activity may include a range of other movements and is accompanied by activity, not only in various associated nuclei, such as the pontine, geniculate and occipital nuclei, but also in the entorhinal cortex and the hippocampus with its theta-rhythm.

Since the hippocampus plays an important part in the formation of long-term memory, the last suggests a role for REM sleep, or more probably the interruption of slow wave sleep, in the reinforcement of the memory of waking experience. The periods of REM recur at intervals of an hour or two during sleep, and have been found to be invariably accompanied by dreams; these clearly represent the reenactment of diverse impressions drawn from the memory of waking experience. Since some dreams are remembered, REM sleep may be classified as a state of virtual awareness. On the other hand, we regard arousal from sleep as the restoration of full awareness.

The phenomena associated with falling asleep and arousal are found not only in humans and other mammals, but in birds and marsupials, and even in reptiles, amphibia, fish and insects; they appear to be almost universal characteristics of the central nervous system. REM sleep has been observed in representatives of nearly all classes of animals[211]. This suggests that in animals other than humans the process of arousal from sleep should also be interpreted as the restoration of awareness, in no way dependent on language. However, there may well be different grades of consciousness depending on the architecture of the central nervous system, and other distinctions worth making.

We have referred to REM sleep as a state of virtual awareness. Dreams are generally not retained in memory unless reinforced soon, usually following arousal. This implies that there is a form of awareness that leaves no impression in long-term memory, which we call *transient* awareness. Apart from dreams, a good deal of the normal waking experience of animals falls into this category; often the transience may be attributed to inattention or forgetfulness, or in its more severe manifestations to some form of amnesia. One of the advantages of human language is that it can assist the conversion of conscious experience that might well have been transient to a more enduring form.

It follows that some degree of awareness is experienced by many even if not by all living creatures. However, a material machine whose behaviour is completely predictable is not regarded as aware, even if its mode of operation is highly ingenious and has all the attributes of intelligence. In Section 1.5 we have already noted that a computer differs from most other machines and resembles the central nervous system in its capacity to process information. But in most computers the output is uniquely related to the input and the latter is therefore, in principle, completely predictable, whereas the motor output of the central nervous system is, to the external observer, very much less predictable. The computer is at present a machine that in operation merely reflects the intelligence of the designer and programmer.

We conclude that awareness and thus a form of consciousness are displayed by most animals; that they are properties, though not necessarily exclusive properties, of the nervous system in its role as a processor of information; that transient awareness is not necessarily associated with the formation of long-term memory; and that neither awareness or consciousness can be properly be attributed to any material system whose behaviour is completely predictable. So much follows from a reasonable interpretation of common usage, but carries no explicit implication of what awareness is or how it works. Volition, the other primary aspect of consciousness, is normally understood to be the manifestation of spontaneous decision making in the brain, and is also to some extent unpredictable.

These characteristics, as we have argued (Section 1.2), are not only necessary but exclusive attributes of all quantum mechanical processes. Moreover, quantum mechanics can be regarded as the theory of information processing at the most fundamental level, forcing us to consider the possibility that consciousness is associated with quantum mechanical processes in the central nervous system.

The same possibility has been suggested in general terms by many other investigators, but there is no agreement on the nature of the essential quantum mechanical processes. Eccles[146] has taken up an interesting idea of Margenau[31] that the probability field of quantum mechanics may provide the means for a non-material mind or self to interact with the brain. However, in the search for microsites at which this interaction could occur, Eccles (*loc. cit.)* and Beck and Eccles[212] have promoted the role of exocytosis (release of neurotransmitter substances into vesicles) at synapses for the quantum mechanical control of the brain, while Penrose[12] has suggested that quantum gravity could affect the microtubules which are found within many cells. The recent literature[213–217] abounds with other more or less plausible suggestions, most of which assign an important role to quantum mechanics.

These suggestions were made, however, in the absence of a clear idea of the nature of consciousness. Margenau's concept of a 'probability field', though inspired by quantum mechanics, was too general to suggest a mechanism for the interaction of the mind, regarded as the seat of consciousness, and the animal cortex, or brain. We do not believe that any new idea is necessary, provided that the probability field is identified, in the most obvious way, with the extracellular field of the nervous system. This field is partly generated by and partly determines the ambient ionic charge throughout the brain, and as we have already seen (in Section 3.2), there is good evidence that the extracellular field does in many instances exercise decisive control over the information processing activity of the brain. In the context of quantum mechanics, the extracellular field is indeed a probability field, in the sense that it has components that cannot be predicted exactly, even in principle. The smallest components, known as quanta, may be regarded as probability waves, and each wave has a characteristic wave length and frequency.

In most contexts of macroscopic physics quantal effects associated with an electromagnetic field are not only random but so small that, averaged over a short period of time, they are completely unobservable. For this reason, classical (unquantized) electromagnetic theory is sufficient in such contexts, and in principle allows exact predictions to be made. It therefore remains to be established that the control of ionic activity in the animal cortex by the extracellular field implicates processes in which quantum mechanical effects are significant. To this end, we shall review those elements of the biological structure that allow the extracellular field to influence systematically the activity of the animal cortex.

At the cellular level, the pumping of sodium and calcium from the a cell, described in Section 3.1, eventually produces a metastable state, with a potential difference up to 100 mV between the intracellular and extracellular fluids. In this metastable state, a small influx of calcium at a synapse can trigger the comparatively large response seen in a graded potential, and ultimately the even larger response seen in an action potential. The electrostatic metastability of the cell is comparable with the metastability of inorganic devices, such as Geiger counters and cloud chambers, used to detect events at the microscopic level where quantum mechanics is undoubtedly important. Similarly, activation of the cell by very small fluctuations in the extracellular field may contribute to the initiation of graded and, ultimately, of action potentials in a cell; and these potentials may generate and transmit a relatively large amount of information derived partly from the field and partly by way of the synapses from other cells. A cell may also affect and contribute significantly to the information carried by the extracellular field.

The essential features of the cell in information processing are, firstly, its capacity for extremely large amplification of potentials transmitted in either direction through channels in the membrane; and, secondly, the large measure of correlation between the ionic currents in different channels. The mathematical analysis of these functions of the cellular membrane will be given in the following Chapter. Here we shall point out the close parallel between the development of an evoked potential in the cell due to the influx of ions though the membrane and the formation of a trail of water droplets revealing the passage of a charged particle through a cloud chamber. These processes are both initiated at the quantal level. The cloud chamber contains vapour in a metastable (supersaturated) state, so that water droplets are formed on molecules ionized by interaction with the moving charge. Each water droplet contributes to evidence of the passage of a charged particle through the supersaturated vapour; in a similar way the amplification of a single quantized component of the extracellular potential, in transmission through a particular channel in the neural membrane, contributes to evidence that a cell has experienced activation by quanta of the extracellular field. But the appearance of a single water droplet in a cloud chamber would have little significance, and similarly the activation of a cell by a single channel of its membrane would usually have little effect. The quantum parallelism implied by the activation of more than one channel is therefore also important. A well documented example was noted by Bohr[25], in discussing the biological implications of quantum mechanics: there is good evidence that cells of the visual cortex can be activated by very few of the electromagnetic quanta present in a light beam of very low intensity. However, an isolated activation could easily be dismissed as insignificant.

At the level of one of the columnar cortical units that are organized around a single output (pyramidal or Purkinje) cell, there is a multiplicity of excitatory (spiny stellate or granular) cells capable of receiving input relayed from distant cells, but also a sufficient number of local inhibitory cells providing feedback to ensure that output from the unit is significantly influenced by the extracellular field. The output cell has the function of summing potentials and information received in various ways: directly through the extracellular fluid, by way of synapses from cells in other parts of the cortex, and above all from many of the cells of the unit to which it belongs. The summation of information may be compared with the summation of the information about the passage of a charged particle provided by individual water droplets in a cloud chamber; and this observation may be relevant to the question of why it is necessary have the participation of so many cells in a cortical unit to secure the output of a single cell. The function of the excitatory stellate and granular cells and the inhibitory cells of the cortex is easily understood in these terms. Columnar units of the sensory and motor association cortices have a even more complex organization, with internal excitatory (Martinotti and neurogliaform) cells. These cells could have several different roles, which certainly include interactions with the extracellular field in the layers in which they are to be found.

At the highest level, we have seen that the animal cortex may be subdivided into the allocortex (which includes the hippocampus), the cerebellum and the cerebrum. From the present point of view, this way of subdividing the cortex is relevant because of the specific type of rhythmic (sinusoidal) potential associated with each subdivision. As we have seen in Section 3.3, the hippocampal formation is the seat of the theta-rhythm and is known to have an important function in the formation of long-term memory. In the cerebral cortex the alpha-rhythm is associated with relaxed states of mind, and the beta-rhythm with somewhat more excited states of mind. It is known (see Bullock and Başar[195]) that such components of the potential with characteristic frequencies are propagated across large areas of the cortical surface.

Finally, we have referred to the rather recent discovery[218] that rapidly fluctuating or chaotic EEG potentials, at one time regarded as devoid of significance, on closer analysis prove to have a potentially important content of information. Potential fields of all these types evidently cannot be regarded as mere by-products of cellular activity, but are closely correlated with it and form an essential part of the overall electrical activity of the cortex.

We have also seen that the sinusoidal potentials are rapidly obscured or interrupted at certain times, notably when attention is given to sensory excitation or the initiation of motor output. Though less obvious, the strange attractors concealed in the subsequent chaotic fluctuations are potentially rich in information that can be communicated to individual neurons. Since the acquisition of sensory information and the decision to perform any motor function both require conscious participation, the accompanying phenomena are of great importance for any theory of consciousness. As we have already noted, field components with a particular frequency are made up of quanta, and the various rhythms and attractors may therefore be regarded as the manifestation of quantum mechanical effects at the highest level. From the mathematical point of view, non-linearity is an important condition for the emergence of chaotic phenomena and strange attractors, and the interaction between the extracellular field and the neural network is indeed highly non-linear.

The conscious attention given to sensory excitation may be characterized as the acquisition of information, and the conscious decision to initiate motor action as the creation of information. However, it is also possible for information to be consciously retrieved from or committed to memory, without the assistance of the senses or voluntary motor action. Our conclusion, then, is that consciousness in animals may be identified with the activity already described at various levels, but more specifically that which accompanies the acquisition or retrieval, and the creation or memorization of information. As we have already remarked in the previous Chapter, this activity is initiated in the frontal and parietal association cortices, though it is intimately related to other activity throughout the nervous system, where the acquisition of sensory information and the creation of information by motor action is learned. At the cellular level, the conscious activity of the cerebral cortex is not completely predictable but may be influenced by individual quanta of the extracellular field.

The distinction between conscious and unconscious activity is not sharp. There is much unconscious activity that is concerned with the processing and not with the intake and output of information. This includes the activity required for the formation of memory, with the participation of the hippocampus; for the retrieval of information from memory; for the influence of emotions, with the participation of the limbic system; for the learning and smooth execution of motor functions, with the participation of the cerebellum; and for the performance of autonomous functions such as breathing and heartbeat. It is very probably an advantage from the point of view of natural selection that much of this activity should not intrude into the conscious mind.

We defer the development of a general theory of consciousness to the final Chapter of this volume. For the present, we merely note that a better understanding of the meaning and requirements of consciousness enables us to assess the possibility of finding and recognizing consciousness outside the animal cortex, or of creating artificial consciousness. If consciousness is defined in the way we have suggested, the possibility does indeed arise wherever information is processed on a macroscopic scale, provided that quantal effects are allowed to influence input and output, and probably the processing as well. Most non-linear phenomena, such as turbulence, are ultimately unpredictable, and liable to be influenced by events at the microscopic level where quantal effects are important. However, memory has an important role in information processing and is deficient in most natural phenomena. If consciousness should appear there, it would be of the transient type experienced by animals deprived of long-term memory. In view of the apparent difficulty of recognizing consciousness even in animals with memory but without the power of speech, it is very likely that any isolated manifestations of the phenomenon in nature would go unnoticed.

However, the possibility of simulating or creating consciousness in the laboratory is by no means excluded. It is already possible to simulate conscious behaviour by the suitable programming of a computer with sequential processing. Examples of this will be given later, in

Section 6.5. The quantal effects are simulated with the help of pseudo-random input determined only by the precise time at which the program is started; and though it would not be difficult to substitute real quantal input for the pseudo-random input, it is hard to see how this would affect the performance of the computer. The verisimilitude of the simulation depends only on the amount of memory available and the ingenuity of the programmer.

But information processing in the animal cortex is not sequential; it is extensively parallel, and complex on a scale not yet approached in artificial sequential or parallel processors. If the creation of artificial consciousness is to be achieved, it would appear that an approach most likely to succeed should be based on the selective imitation of the biological model. Some progress in this direction has already been made, and will be described in Chapter 6 below.

Chapter 4

The Ionic Transfer of Information

4.1 Communication in the Nervous System

The general impression that we have obtained from the study of the nervous system in the preceding Chapters is that it is simple in essence, though complex in detail. The simplicity is in its constitution as a set of symbiotic cells of similar material and structure. The complexity arises partly from the differentiation of the cells in terms of form and function, and partly from the elaborate system of communication that has been developed between different cells in the course of evolution.

An understanding of the activity of the nervous system is beset by a number of puzzles; but perhaps the most intriguing of these concerns the nature of consciousness, which we have linked to quantum mechanics and will be considered later. Quantum mechanics is, of course, a theory of information derived from the sub-microscopic domain; but for the present we shall restrict attention to the macroscopic, especially the electric, phenomena that also present a number of unfamiliar features. Since these are associated with the cellular membrane, it might be supposed that they are within the province of biochemistry and neurophysiology. However, it is known[219] that similar phenomena are found at the surfaces of many inorganic materials, and that artificial membranes exist that work in much the same way as their biological counterparts. It is therefore a reasonable inference that the complexities of organic chemistry and physiology are irrelevant to the understanding of the electric properties of the cellular membrane.

On the other hand, it seems that the biological applications of the physically based theory of electrolytes, and particularly the theory of surface phenomena in electrolytes, are poorly understood. This theory was developed before the advent of quantum mechanics, but although it is in part a microscopic theory, its essential features are the same for classical and quantum mechanics.

Our approach to the understanding of the biological phenomena is based on the conviction that the fundamental laws obeyed are the same as the laws obeyed by ordinary matter. We shall therefore begin with a discussion of these laws, from a contemporary point of view. The fundamental concepts are *information* and *action*.

The quantitative theory of *information*, to be described in the next Section, is due mainly to Shannon[46] in the classical context, and to Brillouin[220] in the quantal context. As we shall make clear in Chapters 7 and 8, information in the quantal context is defined in a subtle way that does not contradict the classical definition where it is applicable, but has important additional implications for a theory of consciousness. However, it is the classical concept that is most firmly rooted in our conscious experience, which tends to accept that there are no limits to the information that can be acquired concerning the external world. Shannon's classical definition of information is objective, in the sense that it concerns information to be gained. The quantity can be measured in bits, but even then is not necessarily an integer, since most information is not certain but is determined by a set of probabilities. It is precisely on account of the ability of the classical definition to assess the information concerning uncertain events that it has an important application to thermodynamics and statistical mechanics. On a suitably chosen scale, the information to be gained concerning a system is the same as the *entropy* of the system as defined in thermodynamics. For most people, information is a more intuitively meaningful concept than entropy; and an understanding of their equivalence a valuable insight!

Action is the fundamental concept of mechanics, which can be based entirely on what is known as the *principle of least action.* This is as true of quantum mechanics as it is of classical (Newtonian) mechanics, so that conceptually it affords a point of view from which the difference between the classical and quantal theories is minimal.

The principle of least action affords a natural expression to the idea that the laws of nature are independent of the sentient observer. Moreover, it assures the existence of a fundamental set of observables for any system. These are its energy, momentum, angular momentum and central vector. The first three are *conserved*: the total amount of energy, momentum and angular momentum of an isolated system, or of the universe as a whole, does not change with time. The central vector of an isolated system, defined as the product of its mass and the position vector of the centre of mass of a system, varies linearly with the time. It is therefore possible to define *energy* as the agent of change in the time, *momentum* as the agent of change with the position, *angular momentum* as the agent of change with the orientation, and the *central vector* as the agent of change with the velocity of the observer.

The interactions between two or more systems are also subject to the principle of least action, though they remain more of a problem. The Maxwellian laws governing the electromagnetic interactions between systems carrying an electric charge are very well understood, and can be formulated as what is known as a gauge theory in terms of the action principle. Electromagnetism is now recognized as a special application of a more general gauge theory applicable to the weak interactions responsible for the decay of radioactive nuclei, and very likely to the strong interactions responsible for nuclear forces. The only other known type of interaction is that due to gravity, where it was found that Newton's theory could not be formulated in a way independent of the observer; at the fundamental level, this has therefore given way to Einstein's theory of gravitation. Although some might disagree, we believe that the laws of radioactive decay, nuclear forces, and gravitational forces have no great relevance for the understanding of the nervous system, even when the phenomenon of consciousness is included. We shall, in fact, find it necessary to consider only the electromagnetic interaction of charged systems. The theory of electrolytes, reviewed in Section 4.3, is based partly on electrostatics, and partly on thermodynamics and statistical mechanics.

Unlike the microscopic laws, the macroscopic laws are not all time-reversible, as anyone may appreciate very easily by running a videotape backwards. The laws of electromagnetism, including the laws of electrostatics, are time-reversible but the generalized form of Ohm's law that relates ionic currents to the gradients of the electrochemical potentials is time-irreversible. The dynamical theory of electrolytes makes use of the generalized Ohm's law, and so is time-irreversible.

Further, irreversible processes in many contexts are predominantly dissipative and do not permit the kind of oscillatory behaviour in which a system, such as a pendulum or a planet, returns to its initial configuration without the expenditure of a great deal of energy. The oscillatory potentials of the brain that were discussed in Section 3.2 have therefore presented something of a puzzle, insofar as they were not regarded as serving any important purpose in the nervous system. However, the ionic theory of electrolytes is very similar to the ionic theory of plasmas[221] in physical theory, where oscillatory phenomena abound. Although their temperatures may be very different, an electrolyte closely resembles a plasma in the presence of ions relatively free to move in response to electromagnetic forces. In plasmas the oscillatory phenomena are associated with *resonances*, and it is reasonable to expect that resonances should appear also in electrolytes under suitable conditions. This expectation will be confirmed in the physically based theory of Section 4.4 to follow

Because of the high electrical conductivity of ionized media, the potential within an electrolyte is normally very uniform, and electrostatic oscillations are not normally observed in ordinary electrolytes. However, in the neighbourhood of the neural membrane, in what we shall call the Debye layer, very large gradients of potential are normal, and resonant oscillatory phenomena are not only possible but commonly observed. The potentials, currents, energy and information associated with these resonances will be determined in Section 4.4. In the electrolytic channels through the membrane, large gradients of potential are also common, and resonant oscillations, matching the oscillations at the membrane surfaces in frequency and amplitude are also to be expected. This is again confirmed by the theory of Section 4.5, but there it will be found that there are certain important additional features affecting the amplitudes and frequencies transmitted. To be more specific, the amplitude changes very rapidly with distance from the membrane surface and the transmission of oscillatory potentials by the membrane depends critically on the frequencies involved.

The theoretical analysis of ionized systems also requires unstable variations of potential under some conditions. Such instabilities are predicted and found experimentally, in conjunction with oscillatory behaviour, in plasmas. These instabilities are invariably associated with metastable states of low entropy, produced at a considerable cost in energy. This is true also in the biological context, where the metastability is achieved naturally by the expenditure of metabolic energy and the pumping of calcium and sodium from the cell. The nervous system uses a variable but considerable fraction, of the order one half, of the total energy intake of the body

As we have already noticed in the previous Chapter, the reduced internal calcium and sodium levels within a cell are to some extent offset by a much higher concentration of potassium than in the extracellular environment, but also by the negative charge associated with protein within the cell. The differences in the composition of the extracellular and intracellular fluids imply a difference in electrostatic potential across the cell membrane, and the internal potential is usually of the order of 100 mV lower than outside the cell. However, the pumping of positive calcium and sodium ions under the influence of metabolic processes cannot continue indefinitely without compensation. The compensation may occur by diffusion of ions through channels in the membrane, but this is difficult since the width of the channels (of the order of 5 Å) is less than the diameter of the hydrated ions, which need to be stripped of their water molecules before they can pass. However, when the difference reaches a certain level the electrostatic forces become irresistible, and diffusion occurs. If there is a sufficiently rapid rise in the external level of calcium, an instability develops, and there is a sudden influx first of calcium, then of sodium ions tending to restore the balance. This influx is offset in part by an efflux of potassium, and these transient ionic currents are accompanied by a fluctuation in the electric potential. This is the somewhat catastrophic event that we have referred to as an 'action potential', or a 'firing' of the cell. The mechanism of such a potential will be discussed in detail in Section 4.6.

Although the fluctuation in potential is usually greater within the firing cell, there is a significant fluctuation amounting to a few millivolts in the extracellular fluid near the cell membrane that is easily detected by a suitable probe. The firing of a cell is therefore, at least potentially, an extracellular signal transmitted by the cell to others in its neighbourhood. However, the changes of potential and ionic concentrations in the extracellular fluid near a firing cell are such as to increase the electrostatic and ionic stability not only of the firing cell but of a near neighbour, so that the latter is actually less likely to fire, at least synchronously, or very soon after. This is perhaps fortunate, since if every cell in a symbiotic cluster were actively transmitting information to its neighbours, the resulting confusion would resemble that in a group of people who were all speaking simultaneously!

Nevertheless, where there is some advantage in nourishment, survival or reproductive capacity to be derived from communication between cells, natural selection will, over a period of time, enhance any feature which tends to facilitate the means of communication. It is not hard to imagine how this has affected the development of features favouring communication by potentials between certain cells, identified as neurons, in the nervous system of animals. These cells do not normally have large areas of membrane surface in close relation to one another, and even there, as we have seen in Section 2.5, the special facilities afforded by neurotransmitter molecules are required to ensure effective transmission.

The remaining Sections of this Chapter present the detailed mathematical reasoning that lends precision to the foregoing considerations. But for the benefit of the reader who wishes to by-pass the quantitative analysis, a summary of essential results is provided at the end of Section 4.6.

4.2 The Classical Theory of Information

It is hardly possible to discuss in any detail the action of the brain, or of any type of computer or network of computers, without introducing the idea of information. In ordinary language, the word is used in a sense that is generally understood, but lacking in precision. It is mainly due to the initiative of Shannon[46] (see also Szilard[222] and Brillouin[220] that the idea of information has been refined and given a quantitative meaning. Though its application to computing was obvious, for a long time there was little appreciation of the fundamental importance of this quite simple idea in many different areas of the physical, biological and social sciences; this is true particularly of the neurosciences, where it is still only slowly gaining currency. In statistical thermodynamics the *entropy* of a macroscopic system is a measure of the lack of information concerning the system at the microscopic level. For this reason, information is sometimes called *negentropy*, but here we adopt the view that in a wider context information is a more meaningful concept. Later, we shall find that it may be used to illuminate some otherwise puzzling aspects of quantum mechanics, especially in the area of the theory of observation. But its classical application to thermodynamics is relevant to the purpose of the present Chapter, and we shall therefore introduce it here as an easily assimilated but powerful mathematical tool that will also find various uses subsequently. The essential results in the application to statistical thermodynamics are, however, summarized at the beginning of the next Section.

The theory of information is most useful in the great majority of applications where information is incomplete, and is an extension of the theory of probability. Let us suppose that the result or outcome O of an experiment E on some material system is not known for certain, but that there are R different possible outcomes o_1, o_2, ... o_R. The experiment in this context may be very simple, consisting of nothing more than an the observation of an event: this could well be so if the event were, for instance, a horse race! Also, it is not necessary that the experiment should ever be performed; information usually changes with time and is of most interest as long as the actual result is not known. However, we may suppose that at any time, based on what is known concerning similar systems, we can assign a probability to each of the possible results: the probability of the r-th outcome o_r will be denoted by p_r. This means simply that if the same experiment were performed on a sufficiently large set of N indistinguishable systems, the outcome o_r should be expected in about p_rN experiments. An imaginary set of indistinguishable systems of this kind is called an *ensemble*. The probabilities, the entire set of which we shall denote by P, must obviously satisfy

$$\sum_{r=1}^{R} p_r = p_1 + p_2 + ... + p_R = 1. \tag{4.2.1}$$

Typically, an individual outcome o_r is a number or a set of numbers, and the mean or expectation value $< O >$ of the outcome of the experiment then defined by

$$< O >= \sum_{r=1}^{R} p_r o_r = p_1 o_1 + p_2 o_2 + ... + p_R o_R. \tag{4.2.2}$$

The information I_A actually available concerning an experiment of the type described is now defined as a multiple k of the expectation value of $\log(Rp_r)$:

$$I_A =< k \log(RP) >= k \sum_{r=1}^{R} p_r \log(Rp_r), \tag{4.2.3}$$

where log denotes the natural logarithm, and k determines the unit in terms of which information is measured. When only the s-th result o_s is deemed possible, then $p_s = 1$ and $p_r = 0$ when r is different from s ($p_r = \delta_{rs}$), so that $I = \log(R)$ is then the maximum information to be derived by performing a suitable experiment. More generally, the missing information, or information that could, in principle, be gained by performing the experiment, is

$$I = -k < \log(P) >= -k \sum_{r=1}^{R} p_r \log(p_r). \tag{4.2.4}$$

In certain applications, including those most relevant to our present interests, the information to be gained is a better defined concept, when N and R are allowed to tend to infinity, than the information available, which depends on the values of N and R in the above discussion. In statistical thermodynamics it is assumed that there is standard information to be gained concerning a system, depending only on a set of thermodyamical variables and the region occupied by the system; then I becomes the entropy of the system, in suitable units, and is usually denoted by S.

Though the above definition of information may at first seem artificial, it has the following intuitively sensible consequences:

(1) The information defined in (4.2.3) is non-negative. It is zero in the unlikely event that nothing is known relevant to the result of the experiment. For then all results of the experiment E are equally likely, all the p_r have the value $1/R$, and $I_A = 0$, *i.e.*, there is no *a priori* information, and the information to be gained from E is $I = k\log(R)$. Otherwise, it is not hard to show that the information is positive but does not exceed $\log(R)$. In particular, if the experiment has only two possible results ($R = 2$), the maximum information is $k\log(2)$, and this unit of information in called a bit. Thus, quite generally, we may choose $k = 1/\log(2)$ if the information is measured in bits.

(2) Information concerning independent experiments is additive. This is a consequence of the fact that the probabilities of independent events are multiplicative. For if $\widehat{\mathrm{E}}$ is an experiment, completely independent of E, with the possible outcomes $\widehat{o}_1$, $\widehat{o}_2$, ..., and $\widehat{p}_s$ is the probability of the outcome $\widehat{o}_s$, then the probability that the results of the separate experiments E and $\widehat{\mathrm{E}}$ are o_r and $\widehat{o}_s$, respectively, is $p_r\widehat{p}_s$. It is then a consequence of the definition in (4.2.1) that if the information to be gained from $\widehat{\mathrm{E}}$ is $\widehat{I}$, then the information to be gained from both experiments is $I + \widehat{I}$. In particular, if each of the two experiments has only two possible results, the maximum information is 2 bits. There is an obvious application of these ideas to experiments consisting of the retrieval of elements from the binary memory of a computer.

In the present Chapter, some results drawn from the statistical thermodynamics of electrolytes will be needed; but here these results will be obtained from information theory to illustrate what are clearly much more general principles. The need for a statistical theory in this area arises because of the complexity of an electrolyte at the microscopic level. Even in the absence of ions in solution, the structure of water is complicated by the fact that its molecules are electric dipoles, with centres of positive charge near the oxygen atoms and negative charge near the hydrogen atoms. Moreover, the dipole moment of a water molecule is changed by an electric field, which may include the dipolar fields of other molecules with various orientations in the vicinity. The charge associated with an ion in solution not only polarizes but attracts water molecules in its immediate neighbourhood. Ions in solution are therefore hydrated, and have an effective diameter considerably increased by the shell of water molecules that are normally associated with it as it diffuses through the electrolyte. It is obviously impossible, even in terms of classical physics, to obtain the information necessary for the detailed description of such a system at the ionic level. Nevertheless, a very useful description of the microscopic structure of an electrolyte, based on statistical thermodynamics, was introduced by Debye and Hückel[223] and will be developed in the next Section. Here we shall summarize the general principles of statistical thermodynamics, which were developed much earlier by Gibbs[224]. A more detailed discussion of the application of these principles to plasmas and other ionized systems has been given elsewhere[221].

At first we shall consider only systems in or very near thermodynamical equilibrium. The information available concerning a particular system is in this context precisely that of macroscopic thermodynamics. This information includes in general the geometrical and kinematical parameters of the region containing the system, including its volume (V), its angular velocity of rotation ($\mathbf{u}$), possibly zero, and its translational velocity ($\mathbf{v}$). But it also includes the values of a set of *intensive* variables, such as the absolute temperature T and the electrochemical potentials $(\chi_1, \chi_2, ...)$ of the different constituents of the system. The *statistical ensemble* in this context is a set of indistinguishable systems for all of which these variables have the same value.

There is also a set of *extensive* quantities, that always includes the macroscopic energy (H), the macroscopic momentum ($\mathbf{P}$), the macroscopic angular momentum ($\mathbf{J}$), the work function (W) and the macroscopic masses $(M_1, M_2, ...)$ of the different constituents of the system. The thermal energy (Θ) is given by

$$\Theta = H - \mathbf{u} \cdot \mathbf{J} - \mathbf{v} \cdot \mathbf{P} + W - \sum_a \chi_a M_a. \tag{4.2.5}$$

The thermal energy is also an extensive quantity and is in fact the part of the entire energy of the system associated with the random motions and interactions at the ionic and molecular level that are inaccessible to observation. It is therefore related to the *deficit* of information (I) as defined in (4.2.4). The precise relation is given in (4.2.7) and (4.2.8) below.

The extensive quantities can be expressed as three-dimensional integrals of corresponding densities over the region occupied by the system:

$$H = \int \rho_H d^3x, \qquad W = \int p d^3x, \qquad M_a = \int \rho_a d^3x \qquad (a = 1, 2, ...), \tag{4.2.6}$$

where ρ_H is the energy density, p is the hydrostatic pressure, and ρ_a is the mass density of the a-th constituent of the system. It is a fundamental problem of statistical mechanics to express these densities in terms of T, χ_1, χ_2, ... We shall not consider this problem here, but shall regard the densities of the extensive thermodynamical quantities as known functions of the intensive quantities. The functional dependence can of course also be found by experimental measurement.

All extensive quantities have the important property that they are additive: thus, if Θ and $\widehat{\Theta}$ are the thermal energies of two disjoint systems, their combined thermal energy is $\Theta+\widehat{\Theta}$; but, in addition, if the two systems are in thermal contact, it is possible with the help of thermodynamics to determine the separate thermal energies (Θ and $\widehat{\Theta}$) of the two systems from the value of $\Theta + \widehat{\Theta}$. Now, as we have already noted, the definition of entropy S in terms of the deficit of information I in (4.2.4) implies that S is additive, and the relation adduced above between S and Θ must therefore be

$$S = k\beta\Theta = k\beta(H - \mathbf{u} \cdot \mathbf{J} - \mathbf{v} \cdot \mathbf{P} + W - \sum_a \chi_a M_a), \tag{4.2.7}$$

where the coefficient of proportionality β is an intensive variable. The nature of this coefficient can be established in the following way. We consider, as before, two disjoint systems, for which the total deficit of information is in general $S + \widehat{S} = k(\beta\Theta + \widehat{\beta}\widehat{\Theta})$. But if the systems are in thermal contact, this can depend only on $\Theta + \widehat{\Theta}$; thus, $\beta = \widehat{\beta}$ is a condition for their joint thermal equilibrium, and it follows that β is some function of the empirical temperature. It is essentially this result that is used to define the absolute temperature (T):

$$\beta = 1/(kT), \tag{4.2.8}$$

where k is a constant depending on the choice of units. If thermodynamical units are adopted for information, k is Boltzmann's constant.

In such units, the deficit of information is identical with the thermodynamical entropy. The value $k = 1.380662\times10^{-16}$erg /°C of Boltzmann's constant may be inferred from the 'ideal gas law'

$$p_a = (k/m_a)M_aT/V, \tag{4.2.9}$$

where p_a is the partial pressure exerted by the a-th constituent of any system when its density is sufficiently small, and m_a is the molecular mass of that constituent.

In the following we shall consider only systems at rest, so that **u** and **v** are both zero in (4.2.7), and the terms involving the macroscopic momentum and angular momentum will disappear. A differential form of the relation (4.2.7) is obtained by considering a small local extension of the boundary of the region containing the system; this does not affect the intensive variables, but S, H, W and M_a are changed by amounts dS, dH, pdV and dM_a respectively. With the help of (4.2.8) we then infer

$$TS = H + W - \sum_a \chi_a M_a,$$

$$TdS = dH + pdV - \sum_a \chi_a dM_a. \tag{4.2.10}$$

Gibbs' formulation of these relations,

$$TS = U + W - \sum_a \mu_a M_a,$$

$$TdS = dU + pdV - \sum_a \mu_a dM_a \tag{4.2.11}$$

where U is the internal energy and μ_a the chemical potential of the a-th constituent of the system, follows when terms involving the electrostatic potential φ are eliminated by writing

$$dH = dU + \varphi \sum_a (e_a/m_a)dM_a, \qquad \chi_a = \mu_{a+}(e_a/m_a)\varphi, \tag{4.2.12}$$

where (e_a/m_a) is the charge/mass ratio for the a-th constituent. The form (4.2.10) has the advantage that χ_a, like the temperature, is independent of position in thermodynamic equilibrium, whereas φ and μ_a may vary from point to point in an extended system.

For a region small enough to allow the pressure to be treated as independent of position, $W = pV$, so that by considering variations of T and the μ_a we obtain also the Gibbs-Duhem relation

$$SdT = Vdp - \sum_a M_a d\mu_a. \tag{4.2.13}$$

It follows that, if S_a is the deficit of information concerning the a-th constituent, and p_a is the partial pressure associated with this constituent, then

$$S_a dT = Vdp_a - M_a d\mu_a \tag{4.2.14}$$

If the density of the a-th constituent is sufficiently small, the partial pressure is given by (4.2.9), so that

$$\mu_a = (kT/m_a)\log(M_a/\rho_a^0 V), \qquad S_a = (kTM_a/m_a)[-\log(M_a/\rho_a^0 V)], \tag{4.2.15}$$

where ρ_a^0 is a constant that may be identified as the value of the mass density ρ_a at any suitable place and time. At any point and at any time time, it can be seen from (4.2.15) that

$$\rho_a = M_a/V = \rho_a^0 \exp(-\beta m_a \mu_a). \tag{4.2.16}$$

As will appear in the next Section, this relation between the ionic densities and the chemical potentials (μ_a) plays an important role in the theory of electrolytes. In the biological applications, the ionic concentrations are sufficiently small to validate the use of (4.2.9); however, corrections for the higher concentrations are available for use where needed[225].

The above are all well known results of macroscopic thermodynamics. The additional insight provided by information theory is that the extensive quantities defined there are to be regarded as expectation values of corresponding microscopic quantities, and are collectively equivalent to quantified information concerning a macroscopic system. To be more precise, suppose H, W and M_a are expectation values of corresponding microscopic quantities H_r, W_r and M_{ar}, so that, for instance, H is the mean or expectation value of the energy H_r measured in a conceptual experiment on a particular system of an ensemble, assuming it were possible to make measurements at the microscopic level of the total energy. But, according to (4.2.4), S is to be regarded as the expectation value of $-k\log(p_r)$, where p_r is the probability that the particular values H_r etc. should be realized The macroscopic relation (4.2.7) may therefore be regarded as a consequence of taking the expectation value of the corresponding microscopic relation

$$-\log(p_r) = (H_r + W_r - \sum_a \chi_a M_{ar})/(kT). \tag{4.2.17}$$

This is a generalized form of Boltzmann's law, according to which the probability that a system will be found in a microscopic state of energy H_r is proportional to $\exp(-\beta H_r)$, where $\beta = 1/(kT)$.

We have supposed above that the system considered is in thermodynamic equilibrium, but we now discuss the rather easy generalization for systems that are not in equilibrium. The absolute temperature (T) and the electrochemical potentials (χ_a) are no longer independent of time and do not have the same value throughout an extended system, so that the information must now be sufficient to determine these quantities as functions $T(t, \mathbf{x})$ and $\chi_a(t, \mathbf{x})$ of the time t and the position $\mathbf{x}$. It is clear that, in quantitative terms, this information is much greater than implied by thermodynamical equilibrium. However, if we restrict attention to a region that is so small that the variation of the intensive quantities within the region can be neglected, all of the above results continue to apply. It is convenient in these circumstances to redefine the extensive quantities H, W and M_a as the energy per unit mass, the work function per unit mass, and the mass of the a-th constituent per unit mass; it is then possible to express W in terms of the pressure and total mass density ρ, and the M_a in terms of the mass density ρ_a of the a-th constituent:

$$W = p/\rho, \qquad M_a = \rho_a/\rho, \tag{4.2.18}$$

where it is now obviously true that $\sum_a M_a = 1$. The volume per unit mass is $V = 1/\rho$.

Also, the appearance of differentials can be avoided in identities like (4.2.10) if they are replaced by derivatives with respect to the time:

$$T\frac{dS}{dt} = \frac{dH}{dt} + p\frac{dV}{dt} - \sum_a \chi_a \frac{dM_a}{dt}. \tag{4.2.19}$$

At this stage we are concerned only with systems at rest, but if the system is supposed to be in motion the time derivatives should be regarded as derivatives following the motion.

The densities of the entropy, the internal energy and the mass of the a-th constituent are clearly ρS, ρU and $\rho_a = \rho M_a$. With each of these densities of extensive quantities we can associate a flux density. Flux densities are vectors, and the statement, for instance, that σ is the flux density of entropy implies that the rate of transfer of entropy across a small area δA, perpendicular to the unit vector $\mathbf{n}$, is $\sigma \cdot \mathbf{n}\delta A$, where the dot denotes a scalar product. It follows from Gauss' theorem in vector analysis that the rate of efflux of entropy per unit volume is $\nabla \cdot \sigma$ (sometimes written div σ), and hence that

$$\Gamma = \rho \frac{dS}{dt} + \nabla \cdot \sigma \tag{4.2.20}$$

is the rate of increase of entropy per unit volume.

Except in thermodynamical equilibrium, the information concerning any system left to itself can only decrease, as a result of thermal conduction and diffusion, which are responsible for the gradual attenuation of the dependence of $T(t, \mathbf{x})$ and $\chi_a(t, \mathbf{x})$ on time and position. Differences of temperature and electrochemical potentials can only be maintained by external intervention that amounts to providing an influx of information, or to inducing an efflux of entropy, through the boundary of the region occupied by the system. According to (4.2.10), the gradient of entropy (∇S) is given by

$$T\nabla S = \nabla H + p\nabla V - \sum_a \chi_a \nabla M_a, \tag{4.2.21}$$

and is zero across the boundary only under *adiabatic* conditions, which imply that the normal components of $\nabla H + p\nabla V$ and the ∇M_a are zero at the boundary.

If $\mathbf{q}$ is the flux density of internal energy, the relation corresponding to (4.2.20) may be written

$$-p\rho \frac{dV}{dt} = \rho \frac{dH}{dt} + \nabla \cdot \mathbf{q}, \tag{4.2.22}$$

where the left side clearly represents the work done per unit volume by the hydrostatic pressure. Finally, if $\mathbf{u}_a$ is the diffusion velocity of the

a-th constituent of the system, $\rho_a \mathbf{u}_a$ is the flux density of the mass of this constituent, and the rate of its creation is

$$\Gamma_a = \rho \frac{dM_a}{dt} + \nabla \cdot (\rho_a \mathbf{u}_a). \tag{4.2.23}$$

In the absence of chemical or nuclear reactions, both sides of this equation must be zero. Like the time derivatives in (4.2.19), there is a relation

$$T\sigma = \mathbf{q} - \sum_a \mu_a \rho_a \mathbf{u}_a \tag{4.2.24}$$

between the flux densities of entropy, internal energy and mass. Then it follows with the help of (4.2.19), (4.2.20), (4.2.22) and (4.2.23) that the rate of loss of information per unit volume is

$$\Gamma = -\sigma \cdot \nabla T/T - \sum_a \rho_a \mathbf{u}_a . \nabla \chi_a . \tag{4.2.25}$$

We have identified thermal conduction and diffusion as processes responsible for an irreversible loss of information at the macrosopic level, and now complete this Section with a statement of the empirical laws of thermal conduction and diffusion. The flux densities of entropy (σ) and of mass ($\rho_a \mathbf{u}_a$) of the a-th constituent of the system are both zero in thermodynamical equilibrium, and otherwise depend on the gradients (∇T and $\nabla \chi_a$) of the intensive variables that are also zero in equilibrium. If the latter are not too large, the dependence must be linear, so that

$$\sigma = -\lambda \nabla T/T - \sum_a \lambda_a \nabla \chi_a, \qquad \rho_a \mathbf{u}_a = -\lambda_a \nabla T/T - \sum_b \lambda_{ab} \nabla \chi_b, \tag{4.2.26}$$

where the coefficients λ, λ_a, and λ_{ab} (of thermal conduction, thermal diffusion, and diffusion, respectively) are functions of the intensive variables; they can be determined either by the methods of irreversible statistical thermodynamics or by direct measurement. When these relations are substituted into (4.2.25), the resulting expression for the rate of loss of information is

$$\Gamma = \lambda (\nabla T/T)^2 + 2 \sum_a \lambda_a \nabla \chi_a \cdot \nabla T/T + \sum_{a,b} \lambda_{ab} \nabla \chi_a \nabla \chi_b . \tag{4.2.27}$$

This is necessarily positive, because the coefficients of thermal conduction and diffusion cannot be negative, and the other coefficients satisfy various determinantal inequalities to ensure that no recovery of information lost to the microscopic domain can be expected. The irreversible conversion of the energy associated with the gradients of temperature and electrochemical potential into heat is a consequence of the second law of thermodynamics, and though this has only a statistical validity, the chances of observing a violation of the second law in a macroscopic system are minuscule.

4.3 The Theory of Electrolytes

Since both intercellular and intracellular transmission of information by the nervous system occurs in an electrolytic medium, it is hardly possible to gain an understanding of the fundamental processes involved except in terms of the theory of electrolytes. This is based on electrostatics but also to a considerable extent on statistical mechanics, and we therefore begin with a summary of some essential results derived from the considerations of the last Section. We consider in particular an electrolyte consisting of any number of different kinds of ions in aqueous solution. Again we distinguish different types of ions and molecules by an affix a, for which the substitutions K, Na, Ca, Cl, H_2O, ... may be made (or K^+, Na^+, Ca^{++}, Cl^-, H_2O, ... to indicate the charge carried by the potassium, sodium, calcium and chloride ions and water, respectively). A water molecule in an electrolyte has centers of positive charge associated with its hydrogen atoms, and a center of negative charge associated with its oxygen atom, so that overall it has an electric dipole moment and is attracted to neighboring ions. At the sub-microscopic level, therefore, a water molecule is sometimes best regarded as a pair of ions, H^+ and OH^-. The number of water molecules that are attracted to a particular ion is known as its hydration number. In the following table we list estimates of the size and hydration numbers of some of the more important ionic components of electrolytes[226].

Ion or molecule	Mean radius (10^{-8} c.)	Hydration number
K^+	1.33	4
Na^+	0.95	5
Ca^{++}	0.99	12
Mg^{++}	1.00	14
Cl^-	1.81	1
H_2O	1.38	

Table 4.1 Radii and hydration numbers of principal ions and water molecules in biological electrolytes.

An important concept is the number density (n_a) of particles of the a-th type; this is in general a function $n_a(t, \mathbf{x})$ of the time t and the position $\mathbf{x}$, and defined so that $n_a d^3x$ is the probability of finding the mass centre of a particle of the specified type in a sufficiently small volume d^3x centred at the point $\mathbf{x}$. If m_a is the effective mass, and e_a the electric charge, of particles of the a-th type $\rho_a = m_a n_a$ is their contribution to the mass density and $\epsilon_a = e_a n_a$ is their contribution to the charge density. The resultant mass density ρ and charge density ϵ are obtained by summation over the different constituents of the electrolyte:

$$\rho = \sum_a m_a n_a, \qquad \epsilon = \sum_a e_a n_a. \tag{4.3.1}$$

It is a consequence of statistical thermodynamics [see (4.2.16)] that, if the density of the a-th constituent is sufficiently small,

$$n_a = n_a^0 \exp(-\beta m_a \mu_a), \tag{4.3.2}$$

where n_a^0 is a constant, μ_a is the chemical potential per unit mass for the a-th constituent, and $\beta = 1/(kT)$, where k is Boltzmann's constant and T is the absolute temperature. In biological systems the concentrations of the ions in solution is sufficiently low for this to provide a valid approximation for the charge densities in (4.3.1), so the charge density is

$$\epsilon = \sum_a \epsilon_a, \qquad \epsilon_a = e_a n_a^0 \exp(\beta m_a \mu_a). \tag{4.3.3}$$

In thermodynamical equilibrium, another expression can be obtained for the ionic charge densities ϵ_a by using the relation $\chi_a = \mu_a + (e_a/m_a)\varphi$

in (4.2.12):

$$\epsilon_a = e_a n'_a \exp(-\beta e_a \varphi), \tag{4.3.4}$$

where $n'_a = n^0_a \exp(\beta e_a \chi_a)$ is also a constant in thermodynamical equilibrium. Under the same conditions, by a suitable choice of the constants n^0_a in (4.3.2) we can interpret the n'_a as number densities at some point where the charge density and potential are both zero, so that

$$\sum_a e_a n'_a = 0. \tag{4.3.5}$$

A second, more general relation between the electrostatic potential and the charge density is provided by Coulomb's law of electrostatics. In its simplest form, this states that the potential at the point $\mathbf{x}$ due to an electric charge e at the point $\mathbf{x}-\mathbf{r}$ is $e/(\kappa r)$ in a medium of dielectric constant κ; this is valid even if the charge is in motion, provided that its velocity is negligible compared with the velocity of light. The potential due to a system of charges is the sum of the potentials due to the individual charges, and it follows that the expectation value $(\varphi)$of the potential at the point $\mathbf{x}$ is given by

$$\varphi = \int [\epsilon(\mathbf{x}-\mathbf{r})/\kappa r] d^3x \qquad \text{or} \qquad \nabla^2\varphi = -4\pi\epsilon/\kappa, \tag{4.3.6}$$

where $\nabla^2 = \partial^2/\partial x_1^2 + \partial^2/\partial x_2^2 + \partial^2/\partial x_3^2$ is Laplace's differential operator.

By combining this result with (4.3.4), we obtain the Debye-Hückel equation

$$\nabla^2\varphi = -4\pi \sum_a (e_a n^0_a/\kappa) \exp(-\beta e_a \varphi). \tag{4.3.7}$$

for thermodynamical equilibrium.

If we assume an absolute temperature of $\sim$ 300°K, a charge $e_a = e_{\mathrm{K}} = 4.80324 \times 10^{-10}$ esu, and a potential of 25 mV, $\beta e_a \varphi \approx 1$. So, if the potential is less than $\sim$ 20 mV, the exponential function in (4.3.7) may be approximated by $1 - \beta e_a \varphi$ and the equation reduces to

$$\nabla^2\varphi = a_D^{-2}\varphi, \qquad a_D^{-2} = (4\pi/\kappa) \sum_a e_a^2 n_a^0, \tag{4.3.8}$$

where a_D is called the Debye shielding length, and has a value that is typically somewhat less than 10 Å in the nervous system of animals.

The solution depends on the information available. Given only that there is an ion of the a-th type at distance r from the point $\mathbf{x}$, (4.3.8) reduces to

$$\frac{1}{r}\frac{d^2}{dr^2}(r\varphi) = a_D^{-2}\varphi,$$

and has the solution

$$\varphi = (e_a/r)\exp(-r/a_D) \qquad (r \geq d) \tag{4.3.9}$$

that reduces to e_a/r for small r. However, this Debye-Hückel potential is good only for sufficiently large values of r, partly because the approximation leading from (4.3.7) to (4.3.8) is valid only when φ is sufficiently small, and more significantly because it ignores the finite size of the ion. We shall therefore regard (4.3.9) as valid when r is not less than the ionic diameter d, and where necessary assume that φ has the constant value $(e_a/d)\exp(-d/a_D)$ for $r \leq d$. It will be noticed that, according to (4.3.9), the expected potential due to an ion in an electrolyte falls quite rapidly to zero at large distances; this result can be attributed to the tendency of an ion to attract other ions, including H^+ or OH^- ions, of opposite charge, so that the expected total charge within a sufficiently large sphere surrounding an ion is zero.

In the biological context, it may be necessary to take account of the more specific information concerning the electrolytic environment, especially that concerning the cellular membranes. The relevant electrostatics and statistical mechanics have been discussed by Vaccaro and Green, and Ellis [227,150]. The extracellular fluid occurs in layers, 100-200 Å (1 Å $=10^{-8}$ cm) in thickness, between the external surfaces of neighbouring cells. Partly as a result of the extrusion of sodium and calcium ions by the cells, and partly because of the negative charge associated with protein within the cell, the intracellular potential is normally about 100 mV below that of the extracellular environment. There, a small excess of positive charge ensures that the nervous system as a whole is electrically neutral, or very nearly so. Because of the potential difference, the membranes are polarized, with an external negative surface charge that is only partly neutralized by the positive ions attracted to the cell. The extracellular potential near the external surface of the cellular membrane (-φ_e, say) is a little below that within the adjacent electrolyte. If the distance between the external surfaces of two neighbouring cells is $2d_e$, the relevant solution of (4.3.8) is

$$\varphi = -\varphi_e \cosh[(z_e - d_e)/a_D]/\cosh(d_e/a_D), \tag{4.3.10}$$

where z_e is the distance from the external surface of one of the cells. As the denominator $\cosh(d_e/a_D)$ is very large, this potential is nearly zero except within a few Ångstrom of the cell membranes, but for small values of z_e it is closely approximated by $-\varphi_e \exp(-z_e/a_D)$. A similar result can be given for the potential near the internal surface of the cell membrane, but since the electrochemical potentials of sodium and calcium vary rapidly across the membrane, a new zero $-\varphi_0$ has to be adopted for the potential within the cell, and φ must be replaced with $\varphi + \varphi_0$ in (4.3.8). The solution is then

$$\varphi = -\varphi_0 + \varphi_i \cosh[(z_i - d_i)/a_D]/\cosh(d_i/a_D), \tag{4.3.11}$$

where z_i is now the distance from the internal surface. As will be seen later, the constants φ_e, φ_0, and φ_i can be determined from a knowledge of the internal and external ionic concentrations and one further condition, usually the requirement that the electrochemical potential of potassium should be continuous across the membrane.

We shall now generalize these results for electrolytes that are not necessarily in thermodynamical equilibrium. To obtain the time dependent solutions of (4.3.6) we shall need to consider the variation with time of the charge density. This can always be expressed with the help of (4.3.3) in terms of the chemical potentials, and in thermodynamical equilibrium the latter depend only on the position $\mathbf{x}$, but more generally they vary with time. We suppose that the electrolyte as a whole is always at rest at the macroscopic level. Nevertheless, there is in general a velocity of diffusion ($\mathbf{u}_a$) associated with particles of the a-th type, so that these have individual contributions $\rho_a \mathbf{u}_a$ to the momentum density and $\epsilon_a \mathbf{u_a}$ to the electric current density $\mathbf{j}_a$. These vectors should be regarded as functions of time (t) and position ($\mathbf{x}$), as required by the conservation equation

$$\frac{\partial \epsilon_a}{\partial t} + \nabla \cdot \mathbf{j}_a = 0, \tag{4.3.12}$$

which follows from (4.2.22), if no ions of the a-th type are being created. From (4.2.26) we can obtain a form of Ohm's law that will be used consistently throughout this Chapter. If we disregard thermoelectric effects, represented by the term involving the temperature gradient ∇T in (4.2.26) , the current density $\mathbf{j}_a$ is proportional to the gradient $\nabla \chi_a$ of the electrochemical potential $\chi_a = \mu_a + e_a \varphi / m_a$, and is therefore given by

$$\mathbf{j}_a = \sigma_a \nabla (\varphi_a - \varphi), \qquad \varphi_a = -m_a \mu_a / e_a \tag{4.3.13}$$

where σ_a is the conductivity for ions of the a-th type, and φ_a is the chemical potential per unit (negative) charge. We are assuming here that the diffusion velocity is not affected by gradients of electrochemical potentials other than $\nabla \chi_a$; this simplification is valid, because of the relatively small ionic concentrations in the nervous system. We shall make use of the chemical potential φ_a in preference to μ_a in the following, because it obviously differs from the electric potential only by a constant in thermodynamical equilibrium (for which $\mathbf{j}_a = 0$).

By the summation of (4.3.12) with respect to a, we obtain

$$\frac{\partial \epsilon}{\partial t} + \nabla \cdot \mathbf{j} = 0, \tag{4.3.14}$$

where, as in (4.3.3), ϵ is the total charge density, and $\mathbf{j}$ is the total current density; this is the formulation of the overall conservation of charge. Similarly, by the summation of (4.3.13) with respect to a, we have the generalized Ohm's law

$$\mathbf{j} = \sum_a (\sigma_a \nabla \varphi_a) - \sigma \nabla \varphi, \qquad \sigma = \sum_a \sigma_a, \tag{4.3.15}$$

where σ is overall conductivity of the electrolyte.

The ionic conductivities σ_a are proportional to the corresponding charge densities ϵ_a, assuming again that the latter are not too large; we therefore introduce the constants γ_a by writing

$$\sigma_a = \epsilon_a / (\gamma_a k T); \tag{4.3.16}$$

then, by substituting (4.3.13) into (4.3.12), we obtain

$$\frac{\gamma_a k T}{e_a} \frac{\partial (\log \epsilon_a)}{\partial t} = \nabla^2 (\varphi_a - \varphi),$$

or, with the help of (4.3.3) and (4.3.13),

$$\gamma_a \frac{\partial \varphi_a}{\partial t} = \nabla^2(\varphi_a - \varphi) \qquad (4.3.17)$$

By combining (4.3.1), (4.3.2) and (4.3.6) we have also

$$\nabla^2 \varphi = (4\pi/\kappa) \sum_a e_a n_a^0 \exp(-\beta e_a \varphi_a), \qquad (4.3.18)$$

and these last two differential equations are sufficient, with the appropriate boundary conditions, to determine all the potentials.

4.4 Potentials, Energy and Information

As an introduction to the various specialized applications that will be made of the results so far obtained in this Chapter, we shall find it useful to discuss the solutions of the equations (4.3.17) and (4.3.18) for the electric potential (φ) and ionic potentials (φ_a). These equations we first rewrite in the form

$$-\nabla^2 \varphi = \gamma_a \frac{\partial \varphi_a}{\partial t} - \nabla^2 \varphi_a = (4\pi/\kappa) \sum_b e_b n_b^0 \exp(-\beta e_b \varphi_b), \qquad (4.4.1)$$

recalling that κ is the dielectric constant (~ 80 for aqueous electrolytes) and $\beta = 1/(kT)$ is inversely proportional to the absolute temperature (T). The coefficients γ_a may be interpreted as ionic resistances, and as the n_b^0 are fixed values of the ionic number densities, the $e_b n_b^0$ are the corresponding charges densities. The analysis that follows is applicable in electrolytic fluid near either the external or the internal surface of a cellular membrane, and for the sake of simplicity we shall suppose that the membrane surface is flat. The effect of geometrical parameters such as the curvature of the membrane surface is usually small but not hard to take into account.

The general method of solution expresses the potentials φ and φ_a in terms of a number of components:

$$\varphi = \sum_r \varphi^{(r)}, \qquad \varphi_a = \sum_r \varphi_a^{(r)}, \qquad (4.4.2)$$

where $\varphi^{(r)}$ and $\varphi_a^{(r)}$ are simply periodic with period ω when they are sufficiently small, but as in many non-linear problems, for larger values acquire a series of harmonics. In the non-linear context, to be discussed in Section 4.6, they can always be determined to any desired degree of accuracy using numerical methods. But to initiate the numerical procedure it is convenient to make use of the analytical solutions that can be obtained after approximating the exponentials in (4.4.1) by $1 - \beta e_b \varphi_b$. As we have already pointed out in the last Section, this linearization is permissible, provided that the ionic potentials φ_a do not exceed ~ 10 mV. With this approximation, the equations for the ionic potentials reduce to

$$\gamma_a \frac{\partial \varphi_a}{\partial t} = \nabla^2 \varphi_a - \sum_b C_b \varphi_b, \qquad C_b = (4\pi\beta/\kappa) n_b^0 e_b^2, \tag{4.4.3}$$

The constants C_a are evidently proportional to the ionic concentrations, but weighted with the squares of the ionic charges (e_b). From the solution of the above, the electric potential can be obtained with the help of the equation

$$\nabla^2 \varphi - \sum_b C_b \varphi_b = 0 \tag{4.4.4}$$

that is obtained with the same approximation from (4.4.1); in thermodynamic equilibrium, this reduces to the Debye-Hückel equation.

In the following we shall find particular solutions $\varphi_a^{(r)}$ and $\varphi^{(r)}$ ($r = 1, 2, ...$) of the linearized equations (4.4.3) and (4.4.4) that correspond to components of the non-linear solution shown in (4.4.2), and have an angular frequency $\omega = \omega^{(r)}$ corresponding to each value of r. For a particular value of r, the solution is obtained by expressing $\varphi_a = \varphi_a^{(r)}$ as the real part of a complex function ψ_a that is an eigenfunction of the differential operators in (4.4.3), thus:

$$\varphi_a = \Re \psi_a, \qquad \frac{\partial \psi_a}{\partial t} = i\omega\psi_a, \qquad \nabla^2 \psi_a = (q + i\omega p)\psi_a, \tag{4.4.5}$$

where i is the imaginary unit. Though $\omega = \omega^{(r)}$, $q = q^{(r)}$ and $p = p^{(r)}$ and therefore also $\psi_a = \psi_a^{(r)}$ may be substituted for different values of r; we shall show the dependence on r only where necessary. We shall find that q can be regarded as the inverse square Debye shielding distance in a dynamical context, and the parameter p may also be given a physical meaning, as a measure of the mean resistance of the electrolyte corresponding to the solution defined in (4.4.5).

It will appear below that ω, p and q may not be chosen independently, as there are two relations connecting them. It will be shown, moreover, in the next Section, that the choice of ω is restricted to one of a number of characteristic frequencies determined by the geometry of the membrane.

When ψ_a is substituted for φ_a in (4.4.3), we obtain the algebraic equations

$$[q + i\omega(p - \gamma_a)]\psi_a = \chi, \qquad \chi = \sum_b C_b \psi_b. \tag{4.4.6}$$

to determine the ionic potentials. We shall assume that ω is real, since otherwise the solution would become unacceptably large for either large positive values or large negative values of the time t. We may assume that p and q are also real; let us write

$$\chi = c\exp(i\omega t - \mathbf{k}\cdot\mathbf{x}), \qquad \mathbf{k}^2 = q + i\omega p; \tag{4.4.7}$$

where c is a complex constant and the vector $\mathbf{k}$ is also complex. We choose the origin of the coordinate vector $\mathbf{x}$ on the surface of the cellular membrane, and the sign of $\mathbf{k}$ must be chosen to make the real part of $\mathbf{k}\cdot\mathbf{x}$ positive within the adjacent electrolytic fluid, so that the potentials decrease exponentially with distance from the membrane. The solution of (4.4.6) for ψ_a is then

$$\psi_a = \frac{\chi}{q + i\omega(p - \gamma_a)}, \tag{4.4.8}$$

which obviously satisfies (4.4.5). But when this is substituted into (4.4.6), the condition

$$\sum_b \frac{C_b}{q + i\omega(p - \gamma_b)} = 1 \tag{4.4.9}$$

is obtained, and this should be regarded as a necessary relation between $q + i\omega p$ and ω. The corresponding solution of (4.4.4) for φ is

$$\varphi = \Re\psi, \qquad \psi = \frac{c\exp(i\omega t - \mathbf{k}\cdot\mathbf{x})}{q + i\omega p}. \tag{4.4.10}$$

The condition (4.4.9) is known as a dispersion equation since, as can be seen from (4.4.7), it is essentially a relation between the angular frequency ω and the (complex) wave-vector $\mathbf{k}$. It may be separated into the two real equations

$$\sum_b \frac{qC_b}{q^2 + \omega^2(p - \gamma_b)^2} = 1, \qquad \sum_b \frac{(p - \gamma_b)C_b}{q^2 + \omega^2(p - \gamma_b)^2} = 0. \qquad (4.4.11)$$

For given values of the C_b and γ_b, there is a solution for each value of ω. The most convenient method of solution is to choose some value of p, and use the second equation of (4.4.11) to determine q/ω; the first equation can then be used to determine q, and hence the corresponding value of ω. The resulting values are most easily obtained from a computer subroutine constructed for this purpose [see Appendix A4.4]. As a rule we are interested only in solutions with real values of ω, since others either grow exponentially with time, and are thus not only unstable but unphysical, or decrease exponentially with time and are therefore soon insignificant.

When p and q are known, magnitude of the vector $\mathbf{k}$ can determined with the help of (4.4.7):

$$\mathbf{k} = \mathbf{w} + i\omega\mathbf{v}/\mathbf{v}^2, \qquad q = \mathbf{w}^2 - \omega^2/\mathbf{v}^2, \qquad p = 2\mathbf{w}\cdot\mathbf{v}/\mathbf{v}^2; \qquad (4.4.12)$$

while the directions of both $\mathbf{w}$ and $\mathbf{v}$ are determined by the geometry of the membrane surface. For $\mathbf{v}$ may be interpreted as the velocity of propagation of the component of the potentials with frequency ω, and is therefore usually in a particular direction parallel to the surface, while $\mathbf{w}$ is along the outward normal to the surface. The velocity of propagation of the potential is then given by

$$\mathbf{v}^2 = \omega^2/[(q^2 + \omega^2 p^2)^{\frac{1}{2}} - q]. \qquad (4.4.13)$$

We note that when the frequency ω is given the value 0 in (4.4.12), q and p are given by

$$q = \sum_b C_b = a_D^{-2}, \qquad p = a_D^2 \sum_b \gamma_b C_b, \qquad (\omega = 0) \qquad (4.4.14)$$

where a_D is the Debye shielding length, as defined in (4.3.8). Thus, at zero frequency, q is the inverse square Debye length, and p is the mean ionic resistance. When the frequency is different from zero, we shall continue to interpret q as an effective inverse shielding length, and p as an effective resistance. With this interpretation, it can be seen from (4.4.11) that the shielding length increases with frequency, and can easily exceed the thickness of the neural membrane, typically ~ 80 Å. Although the frequency in the above analysis can have any value, we shall see in the next Section that the transmission of potentials across the membrane is limited to certain characteristic frequencies. The present considerations show that we should be particularly interested in those frequencies for which q is small, so that the ionic forces are exerted over relatively large distances in the electrolyte.

Even if the frequency is such that the effective resistance p has a value sufficiently near to one of the ionic resistances γ_a, it is possible that q is small (and the effective shielding length is correspondingly large), though it is clear from the first equation in (4.4.12) that this can only happen if the corresponding value of C_a (and therefore the concentration of ions of the a-th type) is sufficiently small. Under these conditions, the entire denominator in (4.4.9) is small, and, in the terminology of dispersion theory, the condition for a *resonance* is satisfied. We note here that resonances are necessarily associated with ions present in small concentrations, and shall see later in this Chapter that the activation of these resonances plays an essential part in the development of graded and action potentials.

When the ionic potentials reach values of 10 mV, the accuracy obtained by linearization of the exponential factors in (4.4.1) is no longer very good, and for higher values the use of the non-linear equations becomes increasingly important. Since values of more than 50 mV are attained in action potentials, we shall need a non-linear generalization. In the non-linear domain, it is no longer possible to express the potentials as the real parts of complex functions ψ_a and ψ. We therefore require that the r-th components $\varphi^{(r)}$ and $\varphi_a^{(r)}$ of the potentials, expressed as in (4.4.2) should satisfy the conditions

$$\nabla^2\varphi^{(r)} = p^{(r)}\frac{\partial\varphi^{(r)}}{\partial t} + q^{(r)}\varphi^{(r)}, \qquad \nabla^2\varphi_a^{(r)} = p^{(r)}\frac{\partial\varphi_a^{(r)}}{\partial t} + q^{(r)}\varphi_a^{(r)}, \tag{4.4.15}$$

which are obviously consistent with (4.4.10) and (4.4.5) without involving complex quantities. Then the non-linear equation (4.4.1) will be satisfied by (4.4.2), provided

$$p^{(r)}\frac{\partial\varphi^{(r)}}{\partial t}+q^{(r)}\varphi^{(r)}=$$

$$(p^{(r)}-\gamma_a)\frac{\partial\varphi_a^{(r)}}{\partial t}+q^{(r)}\varphi_a^{(r)}=-(4\pi/\kappa)\sum_b e_b n_b^0\exp(-\beta e_b\sum_s\varphi_b^{(s)}). \tag{4.4.16}$$

These coupled differential equations are easily solved by numerical methods to express local values of the components $\varphi^{(r)}$ and $\varphi_a^{(r)}$ of the potentials as functions of the time. A computer subroutine for this purpose is included in the program used for modelling action potentials [see Appendix 4.6] in the nervous system as described in the later Sections of this Chapter. For the present, we notice that, so long as $\varphi^{(r)}$ and $\varphi_a^{(r)}$ are sufficiently small, it is unnecessary to perform the numerical integrations, since the results must coincide with the analytical results obtained from (4.4.5), (4.4.8) and (4.4.10) above. In any event, the values of $p^{(r)}$ and $q^{(r)}$ in (4.4.16) are obtained by the algebraic solution of the equations (4.4.11) in the manner described.

Currents

A variety of other quantities of both theoretical and experimental interest can be derived from the potentials; these include the ionic currents, energy and information. The expressions to be obtained for the currents have a validity independent of the linearization introduced in (4.4.3), and are therefore well adapted for application to the ionic currents that accompany an action potential as well as currents of smaller magnitude.

According to (4.3.13), the contribution to the electrical current of ions of the a-th type is given by

$$\mathbf{j}_a=\sigma_a\nabla(\varphi_a-\varphi). \tag{4.4.17}$$

In particular, this expression can be used to compute the current within the axon of a neuron, where it is necessarily directed along the internal surface, away from the soma towards the synapses with other neurons. We introduce a longitudinal coordinate z in this direction, so that, if v is the velocity of propagation of a potential along the axon, φ is locally a function of $z - vt$ and

$$\mathbf{v}\cdot\nabla\varphi = v\frac{\partial\varphi}{\partial z} = \frac{\partial\varphi}{\partial t}. \tag{4.4.18}$$

To a good approximation, φ_a satisfies the same equation, and the longitudinal currents can therefore be expressed in terms of the time derivatives of the potentials:

$$j_a = \frac{\sigma_a}{v}\frac{\partial(\varphi_a - \varphi)}{\partial t}. \tag{4.4.19}$$

The velocity of propagation v can be found from the differential equation

$$\frac{\partial^2\varphi}{\partial t^2} = v^2\frac{\partial^2\varphi}{\partial z^2} = v^2\nabla^2\varphi = -(4\pi v^2/\kappa)\sum_b e_b n_b^0 \exp(-\beta e_b \varphi_b) \tag{4.4.20}$$

which is obtained from (4.4.18) with the help of (4.4.1). It should be remembered that, like (4.4.18), this equation is valid only during the passage of the action potential. Most of the solutions of this equation are unstable for large values of the time, and v must be chosen so that, with a given initial value, φ returns to approximately the same value after the passage of the action potential.

Energy

The energy of the nervous system, as for any other system, is a conserved quantity, so that any resultant gain or loss in a particular region is across a conceptual boundary that separates it from its environment. The total energy can be obtained by the addition of the energies associated with individual cells and the energy of the extracellular fluid. In turn, the energy of any of these components of the nervous system can be broken down into energy associated with individual ions and molecules, and still further into kinetic energy and potential energy associated with these microscopic constituents. The potential energy includes the energy of the electrostatic field generated by the ions. Another way of representing the energy is as a sum of the electrochemical energy, the thermal energy which has both kinetic and potential components, the gravitational energy and the energy of mass motion. The last two may vary as the result of motor activity of the body, but can usually be ignored in the study of the nervous system, and we shall also ignore the thermal energy that is maintained at a relatively steady level by metabolic and other processes regulating the temperature of the bodily environment. In the present context, we are therefore concerned primarily with electrochemical energy.

The equations (4.4.3) satisfied by the electrochemical potentials are not unchanged when the sign of the time t is reversed, as might be expected since ionic diffusion is not a reversible process and part of the electrochemical energy associated with it is dissipated in the form of heat. However, we have seen that the equations have oscillatory solutions, and it is the *available* energy associated with the oscillations in which we are primarily interested. The density of available energy can be obtained by a modification of the Lagrangian technique used where energy is rigorously conserved. A Lagrangian density $\mathcal{L}$ is given by

$$\mathcal{L} = (\kappa/4\pi)\sum_a [\tfrac{1}{2}\gamma_a(\overline{\chi}_{a,t}\varphi_a - \overline{\chi}_a\varphi_{a,t}) - \nabla\overline{\chi}_a\cdot\nabla\varphi_a - \overline{\chi}_a\sum_b C_b\varphi_b], \quad (4.4.21)$$

where $\varphi_{a,t}$ and $\overline{\chi}_{a,t}$ denote the derivatives of the chemical potentials per unit charge φ_a and the Lagrangian parameters $\overline{\chi}_a$, respectively, with respect to time. The equations satisfied by φ_a and $\overline{\chi}_a$ are

$$\frac{\partial}{\partial t}\frac{\partial\mathcal{L}}{\partial\varphi_{a,t}} + \nabla\cdot\frac{\partial\mathcal{L}}{\partial\nabla\varphi_a} = \frac{\partial\mathcal{L}}{\partial\varphi_a}, \qquad \frac{\partial}{\partial t}\frac{\partial\mathcal{L}}{\partial\overline{\chi}_{a,t}} + \nabla\cdot\frac{\partial\mathcal{L}}{\partial\nabla\overline{\chi}_a} = \frac{\partial\mathcal{L}}{\partial\overline{\chi}_a},$$

and reduce to

$$\gamma_a\varphi_{a,t} = \nabla^2\varphi_a - \sum_b C_b\varphi_b, \qquad -\gamma_a\overline{\chi}_{a,t} = \nabla^2\overline{\chi}_a - C_a\sum_b\overline{\chi}_b. \quad (4.4.22)$$

The first of these is clearly the same as (4.4.3), as required, and the second shows that $\overline{\chi}_a$ is related to a *time-reversed* electrochemical potential $\overline{\varphi}_a$ by

$$\nabla^2\overline{\chi}_a = C_a\overline{\varphi}_a = -4\pi(\overline{\epsilon}_a - \overline{\epsilon}_a^0)/\kappa, \quad (4.4.23)$$

in linearized approximation, where $\overline{\epsilon}_a$ is a time-reversed charge density associated with ions of the a-th type. This makes it clear that $\overline{\chi}_a$

is essentially the time-reversed form of the electrostatic potential χ_a associated with ions of the a-th type. The potential φ is therefore given by

$$\varphi = \sum_a \chi_a \tag{4.4.24}$$

But in time-reversible theories the energy density $\mathcal{H}$ can be derived from the Lagrangian density, using the formula

$$\mathcal{H} = -\mathcal{L} + \varphi_{a,t}\frac{\partial \mathcal{L}}{\partial \varphi_{a,t}} + \overline{\chi}_{a,t}\frac{\partial \mathcal{L}}{\partial \overline{\chi}_{a,t}},$$

and this can be expressed in two different forms:

$$\mathcal{H} = \mathcal{H}_1(\varphi, \overline{\chi}) = (\kappa/8\pi)\sum_a [(\nabla\cdot(\nabla\overline{\chi}_a\varphi_a + \overline{\chi}_a\nabla\varphi_a) + \gamma_a(\overline{\chi}_{a,t}\varphi_a - \overline{\chi}_a\varphi_{a,t})],$$

$$\mathcal{H} = \mathcal{H}_2(\varphi, \overline{\chi}) = (\kappa/4\pi)\sum_a (\nabla\overline{\chi}_a \cdot \nabla\varphi_a + \overline{\chi}_a \sum_b C_b\varphi_b), \tag{4.4.25}$$

which are equivalent because of (4.4.22). But the physical energy density cannot depend on time-reversed quantities, and we therefore define the energy within the region R occupied by the electrolyte in the present theory as

$$H = \int \mathcal{H}_1(\varphi, \chi) d^3x = (\kappa/8\pi)\int \sum_a \gamma_a(\chi_{a,t}\varphi_a - \chi_a\varphi_{a,t})d^3x + H_S, \tag{4.4.26}$$

where the three-dimensional integration is over the interior of R, and

$$H_S = (\kappa/8\pi)\sum_a \int (\nabla\overline{\chi}_a\varphi_a + \overline{\chi}_a\nabla\varphi_a)\cdot \mathbf{dS}$$

is the surface energy, obtained when the first term in the expression for $\mathcal{H}_1(\varphi, \chi)$, as given by (4.4.25), is converted by Gauss' theorem to a surface integral.

The result of (4.4.26) allows the energy associated with a particular resonance to be calculated. We use (4.4.5) and (4.4.23) to express φ_a in terms of χ_a, thus:

$$\varphi_a = \nabla^2\chi_a/C_a = (p\chi_{a,t} + q\chi_a)/C_a,$$

and since $\chi_{a,t,t} = -\omega^2 \chi_a$, (4.4.26) reduces to

$$H = (\kappa/8\pi) \int \sum_a (p\gamma_a/C_a)({\chi_{a,t}}^2 + \omega^2 {\chi_a}^2) d^3x + H_S. \qquad (4.4.27)$$

Disregarding the surface energy, this is the energy of the field in an oscillatory mode with frequency ω. In general there will be more than one resonance and the energy is expressed as a sum of such terms.

Information

The available information I, which is essentially electrochemical and excludes contributions from the internal energy, is obtained in a similar way from the expression $\mathcal{H}_2(\varphi, \chi)$ derived from (4.2.25):

$$kTI = -\int \mathcal{H}_2(\varphi, \chi) d^3x = (-\kappa/4\pi) \int \sum_a (\nabla \overline{\chi}_a \cdot \nabla \varphi_a + \overline{\chi}_a \sum_b C_b \varphi_b) d^3x, \qquad (4.4.28)$$

where k is Boltzmann's constant, T is the absolute temperature and I is in thermodynamical units. We note that, although $\mathcal{H}_1(\varphi, \overline{\chi})$ and $\mathcal{H}_2(\varphi, \overline{\chi})$ are the same, $\mathcal{H}_1(\varphi, \chi)$ is in general different from $\mathcal{H}_2(\varphi, \chi)$, because $\overline{\chi}$ and χ are different functions of the time. As we have seen in the last Section, information to be gained is the same as the entropy, in thermodynamical units, and we shall show that I, as defined above, is in fact the electrochemical contribution to the entropy.

With the help of (4.4.4) and (4.4.24), we can rewrite (4.4.28) as

$$kTI = (\kappa/4\pi) \int \sum_a C_a \varphi_a (\varphi_a - \varphi) d^3x + kTI_S, \qquad (4.4.29)$$

where

$$kTI_S = (-\kappa/4\pi) \int \sum_a (\nabla \overline{\chi}_a \varphi_a) \cdot \mathbf{dS}$$

is a surface contribution. Finally, as shown in (4.4.23), $C_a \varphi_a$ can be expressed in terms of the charge densities, and we have

$$kT(I - I_S) = -\int \sum_a \epsilon_a (\varphi_a - \varphi) d^3x = -\int \sum_a \rho_a \chi_a d^3x. \qquad (4.4.30)$$

in terms of the ionic mass densities ρ_a and the electrochemical potentials $\chi_a = \mu_a + e_a\varphi/m_a$. This is what should be expected from the definition of the entropy in (4.2.10); equation (4.4.29) is well adapted to the calculation of the information in a particular neuron, and has been used for this purpose[51] in modelling simple nervous systems.

4.5 Interactions with the Extracellular Fluid

The results of the previous Section enable us to examine in more quantitative detail the interactions of the extracellular and intracellular fluids in the nervous system of animals. We have already discussed the active transport, or pumping, of sodium and calcium from the interior to the exterior of cells as part of their metabolic activity, and will be more concerned here with the occasional or periodic transfer that necessarily occurs in the opposite direction. We have emphasised that an influx of calcium and sodium, and a compensating efflux of potassium ions, is part of the mechanism of the graded and action potentials that accounts for a great deal of the internal electrical activity of the nervous system. But we have also suggested that the periodic fluctuations of potentials observed in the extracellular fluid are not simply the byproduct of the internal activity, but is another manifestation of the transfer of ions across cell membranes that is largely independent of the internal activity and should be regarded as much a cause as the effect of this activity.

In this Section we shall model the exchange of ions through the electrolytic channels that is a common feature of the unmyelinated cell membrane. These channels are not more than a few angstroms in diameter, and they cannot be detected by ordinary microscopy. However, their existence was confirmed by observing the passage of radioactive tracer ions across the membrane, and more recently by the detection of currents by microelectrodes near specific locations in the membrane. As we shall see in Section 5.1, the flux of ions across the membrane was postulated by Hodgkin and Huxley as an essential part of the interpretation of their 'voltage clamp' experiments.

There has, however, been some difficulty in understanding why the channels through the membrane, though normally impenetrable to ions, can in certain circumstances allow the free transfer of ions between the extracellular and intracellular fluids. The original idea was that the entrance to the channels was normally blocked by 'gates' that, by some unspecified mechanism, could open for short periods to allow ions to pass. But this idea is difficult to reconcile with the possibility of the continuous exchange of ions that is required to account for periodic external potentials, and the small but persistent influx of potassium across the membrane that is known to occur whenever the potential gradient is sufficient. The electronic structure of molecules suggests that the 'gating' mechanism must be electrostatic rather than mechanical. The hydrated ions are too large to pass through the channels, which therefore offer considerable resistance to transfer. A quite strong steady electrostatic field is necessary to separate an ion from its entourage of water molecules, but an alternating field is more effective, and a strong impulsive field is even more effective in this respect.

Graded and action potentials will be discussed in the following Section. The fluctuations of potential to be considered here do not exceed a few mV in amplitude, and we may therefore make use of the linearized equations (4.4.3) and (4.4.4) of the previous Section. Again we shall look for periodic solutions of these equations of frequency ω, but within the channels can no longer assume that the resting concentrations of the steady state are independent of position. Experimental studies indicate that the membrane has a surface that is depressed near the entrance to the channels, so that the length of the channels is appreciably less than that of the thickness of the membrane. The actual channels are approximately cylindrical. Therefore, to investigate the potentials within a particular channel we introduce cylindrical coordinates z and r within the channel, where z measures the distance from the point in the channel midway between the two membrane surfaces, and r the radial distance from the middle of the channel. With these coordinates, Laplace's operator is

$$\nabla^2 = \frac{\partial^2}{\partial z^2} + \frac{1}{r}\frac{\partial}{\partial r} r \frac{\partial}{\partial r}. \tag{4.5.1}$$

The dependence on r can be removed from the equations by writing

$$\frac{1}{r}\frac{\partial}{\partial r} r \frac{\partial \varphi}{\partial r} = -\alpha^2 \varphi, \qquad \frac{1}{r}\frac{\partial}{\partial r} r \frac{\partial \varphi_a}{\partial r} = -\alpha^2 \varphi_a. \tag{4.5.2}$$

The solution of these equations is proportional to the Bessel function $J_0(\alpha r)$, where the choice $\alpha = 2.406/r_c$ ensures that φ and φ_a vanish for $r = r_c$, on the surface of the channel. For a non-cylindrical geometry it would, of course, be possible to adopt other coordinates systems, but the results would be similar except that they would involve functions other than the Bessel functions that are appropriate here. On substitution from (4.5.1) and (4.5.2), (4.4.3) and (4.4.4) reduce to

$$\frac{\partial^2 \varphi}{\partial z^2} - \alpha^2 \varphi = \frac{\partial^2 \varphi_a}{\partial z^2} - \alpha^2 \varphi_a - \gamma_a \frac{\partial \varphi_a}{\partial t} = \sum_b C_b \varphi_b. \tag{4.5.3}$$

We note that the coordinate z increases across the membrane from a value $-\frac{1}{2}d$ in the extracellular fluid to $\frac{1}{2}d$ in the cytoplasm (intracellular fluid), if d (~ 50 Å) is the length of channel.

To determine the dependence of φ and φ_a on z, we must take explicit account of the fact that the charge-weighted concentrations C_b of the resting state in (4.5.3) are functions $C_b(z)$ of position within the channels. However, for $z = -\frac{1}{2}d$ and $z = \frac{1}{2}d$, they must make a smooth approach to the values C_b^{e} and C_b^{i}, respectively, in the external and internal electrolytic fluids. To a good approximation, therefore they may be expressed in the form

$$C_b(z) = C_b^{\text{m}} + C_b^{\text{d}} \sin(\pi z/d), \tag{4.5.4}$$

where $C_b^{\text{m}} = \frac{1}{2}(C_b^{\text{e}} + C_b^{\text{i}})$ is the mean value at $z = 0$, and $C_b^{\text{d}} = \frac{1}{2}(C_b^{\text{i}} - C_b^{\text{e}})$ is the difference between this value and the value in the cytoplasm.

As in the previous Section, to solve the linear equation (4.5.2) for the ionic potentials, we first express the φ_a as the real parts of corresponding complex functions with a simply periodic dependence on the time and the coordinate x:

$$\varphi_a = \Re \psi_a, \qquad \frac{\partial \psi_a}{\partial t} = i\omega \psi_a. \tag{4.5.5}$$

It then follows from (4.5.2) that

$$\frac{\partial^2 \psi_a}{\partial z^2} - (\alpha^2 + i\omega\gamma_a)\psi_a = \chi, \qquad \chi = \sum_b C_b \psi_b. \tag{4.5.6}$$

With C_b given by (4.5.4), this is a generalization of Mathieu's equation [228], and can be solved in by similar methods. It is known that differential equations of this type have a solution only when the parameters involved satisfy special conditions. In this instance the frequency must satisfy a condition depending on the concentration differences C_a^{d} and the geometry of the channels, determined here by d and α, and the discrete values of ω allowed by this condition are called *eigenvalues.* Other frequencies will not be transmitted by the channel that we are considering. Since the solutions $\chi(z)$ are complex, there are in fact two independent conditions to be satisfied if potentials are to be transmitted across the membrane. The other condition may obtained from the form of the general solution of (4.5.6),

$$\chi = \sum_{j=-\infty}^{\infty} \chi_j \exp(\lambda_j z), \qquad \lambda_j = (ij + \epsilon)\pi/d;$$

$$\psi_a = \sum_{j=-\infty}^{\infty} \psi_{aj} \exp(\lambda_j z). \tag{4.5.9}$$

The real component $\epsilon\pi/d$ of λ_j is a parameter that corresponds to the inverse Debye shielding length within the channel, and the following analysis shows that it depends on the frequency, so that ϵ, like ω, must satisfy an eigenvalue condition. In the intracellular and extracellular fluids, ϵ is related to the mean resistance p of a resonance, as defined in (4.4.5) of the previous Section, so that the latter is also determined for a component of the potential transmitted by a particular channel of the membrane. However, since there are many channels with different geometrical parameters, a whole range of values of p is possible.

By substitution in (4.5.6), we find that

$$\psi_{aj} = \frac{\chi_j}{\lambda_j^2 - \alpha^2 - i\omega\gamma_a}, \tag{4.5.10}$$

and

$$(1 - f_j)\chi_j = g_{j-1}\chi_{j-1} - g_{j+1}\chi_{j+1},$$

$$f_j = \sum_b \frac{C_b^{\mathrm{m}}}{\lambda_j^2 - \alpha^2 - i\omega\gamma_b}, \qquad g_j = \frac{1}{2}\sum_b \frac{C_b^{\mathrm{d}}}{\lambda_j^2 - \alpha^2 - i\omega\gamma_b}. \tag{4.5.11}$$

When $C_b^{\rm d} = 0$, the above difference equation for χ_j is satisfied by $f_j = 1$, which will be recognized as the dispersion equation (4.4.9), if the real and imaginary parts of $\lambda_j^2 - \alpha^2$ are denoted by q and $i\omega p$. But whereas the dispersion equation, valid within the extracellular and intracellular fluids, could be satisfied for almost any real value of ω, this is not true of the difference equation. Most solutions of both types are unacceptable, because for general values of ω and ϵ, the χ_j increase like j^2 for large values of j, so that the infinite series in (4.5.9) are badly divergent, irrespective of the values of the other constants in the equations. However, for special values of ω and ϵ, there are convergent solutions for which the χ_j decrease like j^{-2} for large values of j; these are easily obtained numerically, to a very good approximation, by neglecting χ_j for $\mid j \mid > J \sim 8$, then choosing any small but non-zero value of χ_j and obtaining solutions of the remaining set of linear equations. A computer program is easily constructed to obtain the pair of eigenvalues of ω and ϵ, using values of the the external and internal ionic concentrations $C_a^{\rm e}$ and $C_a^{\rm i}$ and the resistances γ_a given in the Table 4.2. A computer program also allows graphs of the other resonances shown in Table 4.2 to be seen on the computer screen [see Appendix 4.5].

Type of ion	$C_a^{\rm e}$ (dM)	$C_a^{\rm i}$ (dM)	γ_a (10^{12}s/c^2)
K^+	0.030	1.500	1.0
Na^+	1.500	0.125	8.2
Ca^{++}	0.0025	0.00015	11.0
Cl^-	1.250	0.60	13.4

Table 4.2 Values adopted for the external and internal ion concentrations and effective resistances for each of the types of ion transmitted by channels in the neural membrane.

The results, to be described in more detail below, depend as expected on the geometry (radius and length) of the channel. But the calculations also show that for each frequency there is a particular type of ion, depending on the direction of transmission, whose concentration fluctuates most, and with exponential growth from one end of a channel to the other. The channels are therefore identified as calcium, potassium, sodium and chloride channels, as they have been for some time in the literature for experimental reasons. The lowest eigenvalues ω and the corresponding values of the Debye parameter ϵ are listed in Table 4.3.

Type of channel	Angular frequency ω (s^{-1})	Debye parameter ϵ
K^+	0	3.25680
Ca^{++}	31.255	2.86865
Na^+	44.819	3.00013
Cl^-	66.272	3.47015
Na^+	101.727	3.43049
Na^+	184.130	4.09798
K^+	360.643	2.95124

Table 4.3 Ionic character of channel, eigenvalues of the angular frequency, and corresponding Debye parameters for solutions of the generalized Mathieu equation.

The radius of the channels in the membrane is of the order of 5 Å, small compared with the thickness ($\sim$ 50 Å) of the membrane. For such values, there is always an eigenvalue $\omega = 0$ of the angular frequency, and it is obvious from (4.5.10) that, for this particular eigenvalue of ω, the potentials all have the same value. The existence of a static solution of this type helps to explain how it is possible for quite a wide range of differences of the ionic concentrations to be sustained between the ends of the channels in the membrane.

The lowest non-zero eigenvalue of the angular frequency ω obtained from the computer program is $\sim$31 s^{-1}, or 5 Hz, near the lower end of the part of the spectrum corresponding to the θ-rhythm in the cortex; the calculations show that it is characteristic of a calcium channel. As shown in Table 4.3, other modes, with successively higher frequencies, are characteristic of a sodium channel in the θ-band, chloride and sodium channels in the α-band, sodium and potassium channels in the β-band, and there are others with still higher frequencies. The frequencies are the same for inward and outward transmission, so that it is possible to have coherent inward and outward transmission by the same channel. The lowest mode of oscillation is illustrated in Figure 4.1.

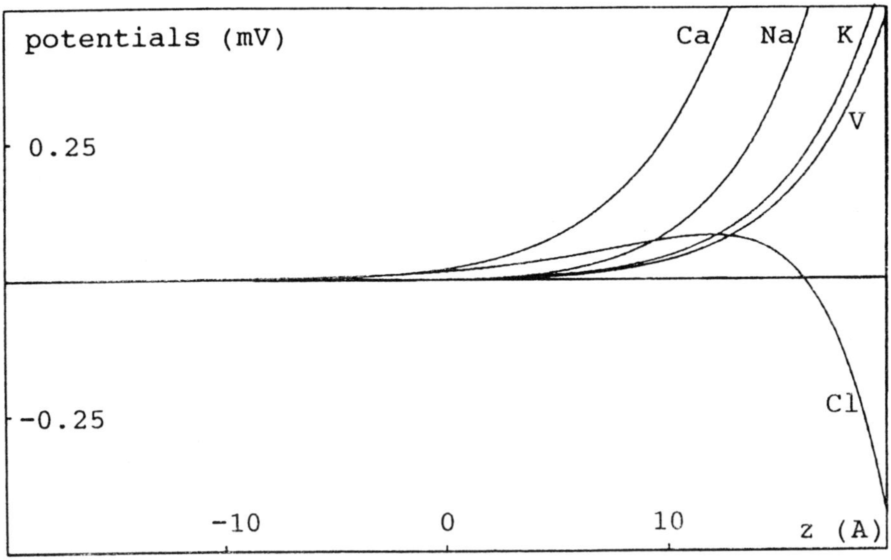

Fig. 4.1 Amplitudes of a small potential (V) and chemical potentials (K, Na, Ca and Cl) as functions of the distance through a calcium channel of the neural membrane, corresponding to a frequency of ~5 Hz.

The figure displays the fluctuations in the potentials φ_a derived from (4.5.5), (4.5.10) and (4.5.11) as functions of the distance z from the midpoint of the channel, increasing with distance from the outer membrane surface. As might be expected from the differential equations (4.5.6), and can be seen from (4.5.9), they all increase exponentially, like $\exp(\pi\epsilon z/d)$ with z, so that it is possible for a tiny fluctuation of the order of 1 nV at the outer membrane surface to be translated into a very much larger and easily detected fluctuation within the cell. The curves all change shape with the phase, but the amplitude of the fluctuations in the calcium concentration is dominant and it is obvious that the frequency of $\sim 31\ \text{s}^{-1}$ which we have chosen as an illustration corresponds to a calcium resonance.

When fluctuations of the potentials of the type discussed in this Section exceed a threshold of about 10 mV, the linearized theory is no longer reliable, and it is necessary to use the non-linear equations as described in the next Section, where it will be shown that the fluctuations at the surface of the membrane develop into graded and action potentials. The results of this Section therefore have important implications for the activation of neurons by potentials in the extracellular fluid, and help to explain why many action potentials are synchronous with extracellular activity.

However, the amplification of small potentials in outward transmission across the membrane is also a consequence of the theory, and the eigenvalues of the frequency are the same as for inward transmission. Depending on the boundary conditions at the internal and external surfaces of the membrane, there are in fact solutions corresponding to simultaneous inward and outward transmission. We thus conclude that fluctuations of potential within individual cells may contribute to potentials with particular frequencies in the extracellular fluid. The frequency of transmission, of course, depends on the differences in the concentration of potassium and other ions between the membrane surfaces, as well as on the geometry of the channels and their immediate surroundings; these may all vary from cell to cell. Together, these effects provide a potentially important method of communication between cells that is complementary to the well recognized transmission of information by action potentials at synapses.

The very rapid growth of small components of the extracellular potential with the right frequency in transmission across the membrane is of fundamental importance for a theory of consciousness based on quantum mechanics. The number of ions within a channel is initially very small, so that the amplification of a potential of ~ 1 nV to an easily detected potential at the opposite surface of the membrane can be correctly described as an escalation of events initiated at the quantal level. A purely quantum mechanical account of this process will appear in Chapter 7. For the present we note that the process is a necessary consequence of large differences in the concentrations across the membrane, or in other words, of the *electrostatic metastability* of the cell.

4.6 Graded and Action Potentials

In the resting state, the electrical potential within a cell is determined primarily by the active transport of ions across the membrane. As we have pointed out in Section 2.4, this implies the transfer of sodium and calcium from the internal to the external electrolytic fluid, and transfer of potassium in the opposite direction, in the course of the metabolic activity of the ATPase molecules embedded in the cellular membrane. Although there is no resultant movement of electric charge, the potassium remains in approximate electrochemical equilibrium across the membrane, and the higher internal concentration of potassium implies a lower electric potential than in the extracellular fluid. The lower potential is to some extent stabilized by the negative charge associated with protein within the cell, which of course moves, if at all, very slowly, and does not contribute to the ionic currents in the cell. There is, however, a limit to the potential difference that can be sustained by the membrane, and the active transport of ions across it must be compensated by the transfer of ions in the opposite direction though channels in the membrane, as described in the previous Section. It seems likely that, in quiescent states, a considerable fraction of this activity is associated with the periodic potentials that are observed in the extracellular fluid, and that this activity is actually necessary to limit the potential difference across the membrane to a value not exceeding $\sim$100 mV. Nevertheless, at this level, the membrane remains in a highly excitable or *metastable* state.

A metastable state is one that is easily disturbed by quite small perturbations. The unmyelinated cell membrane is subject to a variety of perturbations propagated though the extracellular fluid, and these are often from neighbouring cells. We have previously described the mechanism by which the concentration of calcium at synapses on the external surface of the neural membrane can be raised locally by the interaction of neurotransmitter and neurotransmitter receptor molecules. The resulting influx of calcium through the channels in the membrane leads to a rapid increase in the internal level of calcium, which is normally very low. A local and quite small increase in the concentration of calcium at the internal surface of the membrane may result in a relatively large increase (of several millivolts) in the electrical potential, sufficient to cause a departure from the metastable state, and this is the normal precursor of a graded or an action potential. These potentials are not adequately described by the linear analysis of the previous Sections, and we shall therefore develop methods to solve the equations of the electrolytic fluid that take account of their nonlinearity.

We recall that, according to (4.4.1), the electrochemical potentials φ_a satisfy the partial differential equations

$$\gamma_a \frac{\partial \varphi_a}{\partial t} - \nabla^2 \varphi_a = (4\pi/\kappa) \sum_b e_b n_b^0 [\exp(-\beta e_b \varphi_b) - 1], \tag{4.6.1}$$

in which t is the time, κ is the dielectric constant, $\beta = 1/(kT)$ is inversely proportional to the absolute temperature T (k is Boltzmann's constant), the e_a are the ionic charges and the γ_a are ionic resistances. In fact the above equation differs from (4.4.1) in that 1 has been subtracted from the exponentials, but this subtraction has no effect, provided that the densities n_b^0 are chosen to satisfy the condition $\sum_b e_b n_b^0 = 0$ for electrical neutrality. It is obvious from (4.4.1) that the above equations can also be used to determine the electrical potential φ, if we allow the subscript a to take the value 0, setting $\varphi_0 = \varphi$, and $\gamma_0 = e_0 = 0$. By elimination of the right side of (4.6.1), we see that

$$\nabla^2(\varphi - \varphi_a) = -\gamma_a \frac{\partial \varphi_a}{\partial t}, \tag{4.6.2}$$

a result that can be used to obtain $\varphi - \varphi_a$, and hence φ, in terms of any of the φ_a.

The non-linear equations (4.6.1) must be solved by a combination of analytical and numerical methods. It is important to notice in advance that the solutions, based as they are on the classical electromagnetic theory of a system of charges, are not necessarily stable: even a system consisting of just two charges of opposite sign is inherently unstable. In classical electrostatics there is nothing to prevent the attraction between a positive and a negative charge from inducing a catastrophic collapse of the entire system, with the emission of an unlimited amount of energy in the form of radiation. In reality such a collapse does not occur, because of quantum-mechanical effects that become increasingly important as the distance between the charges diminishes. There is consequently a closest distance of approach of two ions in an electrolyte, which is roughly the sum of the 'radii' of the ions and is determined by quantum mechanical considerations. The mean radii of the more important ions in the present context were given in the table of Section 4.3. These considerations show that there is a lower limit to the electrochemical potential experienced by a positive ion, and an upper limit to the electrochemical potential experienced by a negative ion. When these limits are imposed in the numerical integration of the equations (4.6.1), any instability of the equations is removed in a physically meaningful way.

However, it is a matter of experience that the stable solutions are essentially determined by two of the electrochemical potentials, which can be chosen to be those of ions (such as potassium and chloride within a cell, or sodium and chloride in the extracellular fluid) present in larger concentrations. When these have been found, the electrical potential is obtained by integration of (4.6.2). However, at small amplitudes, where the linearization of the equations (4.6.1) is valid, the linearly independent solutions satisfy the condition (4.4.9). If a linear superposition of these solutions is used to begin the integration of the non-linear equations, with physically reasonable initial conditions, instabilities are very rarely encountered. A computer program for the purpose is provided [see Appendix 4.6].

The solutions for the potentials generated by the computer program are functions of the time, but can also be used to find corresponding solutions depending on position. In solving the equations, we express each potential φ_a as the sum of a number of terms $\varphi_a^{(r)}$ ($r = 1, 2, ...$), which satisfy an equation similar to (4.6.1), except that for $r > 1$ the densities $n_a^{(0)}$ are replaced by

$$n_b^{(r-1)} = n_b^{(0)} \exp\{-\beta e_b(\varphi_b^{(1)} + .. + \varphi_b^{(r-1)})\}, \tag{4.6.3}$$

thus:

$$\gamma_a \frac{\partial \varphi_a^{(r)}}{\partial t} - \nabla^2 \varphi_a^{(r)} = (4\pi/\kappa) \sum_b e_b n_b^{(r-1)} [\exp(-\beta e_b \varphi_b^{(r)}) - 1]. \tag{4.6.4}$$

If we substitute (4.6.3) into (4.6.4) and sum the latter with respect to r, we obtain the desired equation (4.6.1), provided that

$$\varphi = \sum_r \varphi^{(r)}, \qquad \varphi_a = \sum_r \varphi_a^{(r)}, \tag{4.6.5}$$

To specify further the components $\varphi_a^{(r)}$ of the potentials, we introduce the *ansätze*

$$\nabla^2 \varphi_a^{(r)} = p^{(r)} \frac{\partial \varphi_a^{(r)}}{\partial t} + q^{(r)} \varphi_a^{(r)}, \tag{4.6.6}$$

which are clearly analogous to (4.4.5), wherein p could be interpreted as a mean ionic resistance and $q = a_D^{-2}$ as the generalization of the inverse square Debye shielding length of (4.3.8) for this dynamical context. This analogy ensures that the present non-linear theory will reduce to the linearized theory of Section 4.4 when the potentials are sufficiently small. Although $p^{(r)}$ and $q^{(r)}$ could depend on the time and the position in the electrolyte, their variation is slow and for our present purpose they will be treated as constants. As a first approximation, the relationship between $q^{(r)}$ and $p^{(r)}$ in the non-linear theory may be assumed to be the same as between q and p in the linear theory, though small deviations are not only permissible but useful in controlling the stability of the numerical integration.

On substitution from (4.6.6), (4.6.4) becomes

$$(\gamma_a - p^{(r)})\frac{\partial \varphi_a^{(r)}}{\partial t} - q^{(r)}\varphi_a^{(r)} = (4\pi/\kappa)\sum_b e_b n_b^{(r-1)}[\exp(-\beta e_b \varphi_b^{(r)}) - 1], \tag{4.6.7}$$

If $\varphi_a^{(r)}(t)$ is a solution that does not depend on the position $\mathbf{x}$, then a general solution is of the form

$$\varphi_a^{(r)}(t,\mathbf{x}) = \int\int_0^t G^{(r)}(t-t',\mathbf{x}-\mathbf{x}')\varphi_a^{(r)}(t')dt'\chi_a^{(r)}(\mathbf{x}')d^3x', \tag{4.6.8}$$

where the Green's function

$$G^{(r)}(t,\mathbf{x}) = (4\pi t/p^{(r)})^{-3/2}\exp\{-p^{(r)}\mathbf{x}^2/(2t) - q^{(r)}t/p^{(r)}\} \tag{4.6.9}$$

is the particular solution of (4.6.6) that corresponds to a unit source at time $t = 0$. By a suitable choice of the function $\chi_a(\mathbf{x})$, it can be ensured that $\varphi_a^{(r)}(t,\mathbf{x})$ satisfies any required boundary condition, such as $\varphi_a^{(r)}(t,\mathbf{x}_m) = 0$ when $a > 0$ and $\mathbf{x}_m$ is a point on the surface of the membrane, in the intracellular or extracellular environment, or even within one of the channels through the membrane. When $\chi_a^{(r)}(\mathbf{x}') = 1$, $\varphi_a^{(r)}(t,\mathbf{x})$ reduces to $\varphi_a(t)$. If $\varphi(t,\mathbf{x})$ and $\varphi_a(t,\mathbf{x})$ are stationary solutions of (4.6.1) obtained with the help of the *ansätze* (4.6.6), $\varphi(t - \mathbf{x}\cdot\mathbf{v}/\mathbf{v}^2, \mathbf{x})$ and $\varphi_a(t - \mathbf{x}\cdot\mathbf{v}/\mathbf{v}^2)$ are similar solutions moving with velocity $\mathbf{v}$, usually in a direction parallel to the membrane surface.

We have thus reduced the general problem to one of finding time-dependent solutions of (4.6.7), first for $r = 1$ when the $n_a^{(0)}$ are given constants, and then for $r = 2$, 3, etc. This problem is solved in essence by the computer program noted earlier, and we conclude this Section with a discussion of a typical solution near the internal surface of the membrane, illustrated in Figure 4.2 below.

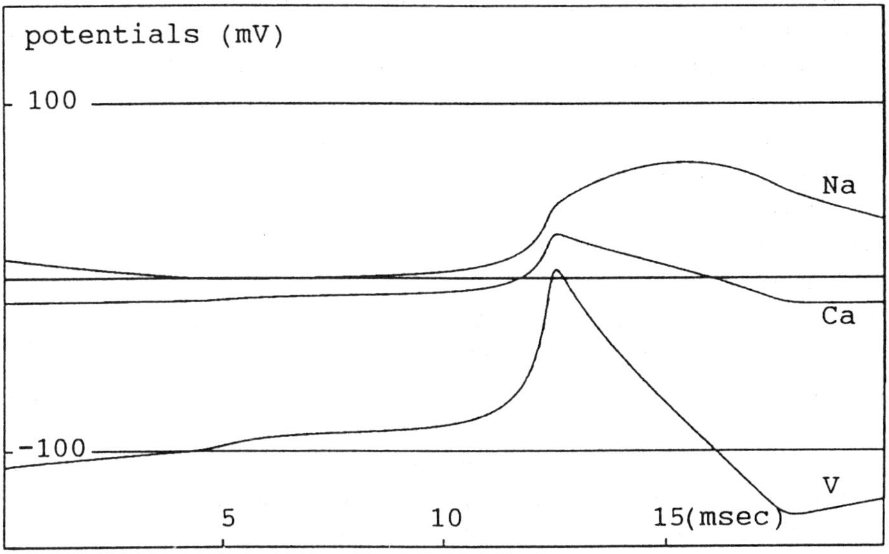

Fig. 4.2 A computed action potential (V) with calcium (Ca) and sodium (Na) potentials on comparable scales superposed.

The above figure is generated by a computer program constructed for the purpose [see Appendix 4.6]. For the sake of clarity we show only the internal electrical potential (as V), and the calcium and sodium chemical potentials (as Ca and Na) on a reduced scale. It should be noticed that an increase in the chemical potentials implies a decrease in the concentrations, and conversely. The potassium electrical potential is somewhat similar in shape to the electrical potential, while the chloride potential also has a similar shape but is opposite in sign. At time $t = 0$, at the left border of the graphs, it may be imagined that a stimulus has been applied, resulting in temporarily depressed levels of calcium and sodium within the cell. This leads first to an influx of calcium, activating the calcium resonance, and producing the characteristic 'shoulder' that precedes a graded or an action potential. The calcium resonance in turn leads to an influx of sodium, which in this instance is relatively small, because the cell is not in a potentiated state. A graded potential of about 20 mV therefore follows. The conditions assumed to obtain this result are very similar to those for the first, except that the cell is slightly potentiated.

Here the potentials pass a threshold, after which a full action potential necessarily follows. During the action potential, a large influx of sodium occurs through the cellular membrane, and there is a corresponding but somewhat more prolonged efflux of potassium. At the end of this process the calcium and sodium levels are again depressed, as they were at time $t = 0$, and depending on the level of potentiation, the whole process leading to an action potential may be repeated once, twice, or many times. Eventually the action potentials are attenuated and disappear.

These studies confirm the importance of the ions present in small but not entirely negligible concentrations: the calcium and sodium ions at the internal surface of the neural membrane, or the calcium and potassium ions at the external surface. The resonances are invariably associated with these ions. It is well known that the presence of other ions, such as magnesium or aluminum, in small concentrations, can seriously affect the efficiency of neural action, and this is easily understood from the study of the resonances associated with the five ions included. By running the computer program that was used used to produce the above figure with a non-zero concentration of a fifth type of ion, it can be seen that, even at very small concentrations, the extra ion creates an additional resonance with important implications for the stability of the action potential.

Summary

Following Shannon, a quantitative definition of information concerning any system, in terms of a set of probabilities, was given in (4.2.3) and (4.2.4). A distinction was made between the information available concerning the system and the information to be gained; in the context of thermodynamics, the latter is the same as the entropy of the system, on a suitable scale. Some important results of thermodynamics and statistical mechanics, including the fundamental identities (4.2.11), and the relations (4.2.16) between the ionic densities and the chemical potentials, were obtained by applying information theory. It was shown in (4.2.27) that there is an irreversible increase of entropy, or loss of information, as a consequence of thermal conduction and diffusion. By similar methods it can be shown that there is also an irreversible increase of entropy associated with viscosity and chemical reactions.

The theory of electrolytes was developed in Section 4.3. The most important results were the mathematical formulation of Coulomb's law of electrostatics in (4.3.6), the equations of conservation of charge for different ions types in (4.3.12), and the generalized form of Ohm's law in (4.3.13). These equations provided the basis for the theory of potentials, currents, energy and information of the intracellular and extracellular electrolytic fluids in subsequent Sections. The physically meaningful solutions can be constructed from particular oscillatory solutions.

In Section 4.4 a complete analysis was made of the equations in a *linearized* approximation, valid for potentials up to about 20 mV, and it was shown that the oscillatory components of potentials can be interpreted as resonances. A resonance implies relatively large fluctuations in the electrochemical potential of a particular ion present *in small concentrations*: calcium and sodium in the intracellular fluid, and potassium in the extracellular fluid of a cell. The resonances correspond to solutions of the dispersion equation (4.4.9). The ionic currents associated with any resonance were obtained in (4.4.17), and the velocity of propagation of the potential in (4.4.20). A Lagrangian technique was developed to determine the *available* energy and information, given by (4.4.26) and (4.4.28) respectively.

In Section 4.5 this analysis was extended to obtain oscillatory solutions for the large potential gradients that exist in an electrolytic channel through the cellular membrane. Admissible solutions were found to correspond to convergent solutions of the difference equation (4.5.10). It was shown that, because of the small diameter of the channel, there is a static solution, so that the membrane can support a large potential difference between its inner and outer surfaces without diffusion. However, there are also fluctuating solutions corresponding to discrete values, or *eigenvalues*, of the frequency in the θ-band, the α-band, and higher frequencies. Because of the electrostatic metastability of the membrane, there is a very large amplification of potentials in transmission, and it is possible for potentials as small as 1 nV with the right frequency to produce observable effects. *These results imply that quantal effects are significant in the transmission of potentials through channels in the membrane.*

In the present Section, the linearized analysis of Section 4 was generalized to obtain nonlinear solutions corresponding to graded and action potentials. The results are in very close correspondence with experiment.

Chapter 5

Insights from Invertebrate Studies

5.1 The Hodgkin-Huxley Equations

Fundamental to the modelling of potentials in the nervous system of a living animal are the equations for the current across the neural membrane. These were first inferred by Hodgkin and Huxley[229] from the analysis of experiments on the giant axon of *Loligo* (the squid). An electrode was inserted into the axon and an attempt made to determine the conductivity of the membrane by suddenly imposing a voltage clamp to the axon in its resting state, or a fixed potential difference between the intracellular and extracellular fluids. A rapid fluctuation in the resulting current across the membrane was observed before a steady state was reached.

From these experiments they formed the important and undoubtedly correct hypothesis that the potential that follows a voltage clamp is accompanied by an influx of sodium ions, and a corresponding efflux of potassium ions, through channels in the neural membrane. The ionic currents through the membrane required by this hypothesis were, however, transient and implied very large variations in time of the conductance of the membrane, assuming the validity of a generalized form of Ohm's law in this context. To establish the notation used by Hodgkin and Huxley, we first formulate the appropriate form of Ohm's law, relating the current to differences of the electrochemical potentials of the various types of ions crossing the membrane.

The current I per unit area can, in fact, be expressed in terms of the potential difference V across the membrane as a sum of four terms:

$$I = I_K + I_{Na} + I_l + C_M \frac{dV}{dt},$$

$$I_K = g_K(V - V_K), \quad I_{Na} = g_{Na}(V - V_{Na}), \quad I_l = g_l(V - V_l). \quad (5.1.1)$$

Here C_M is the capacity per unit area of the membrane surfaces, which is multiplied by the time derivative dV/dt of the potential to obtain the capacitance current; I_{Na} is the component of the current associated with sodium ions crossing the membrane, I_K is the component associated with potassium ions, and I_l is the 'leakage' current associated with other unspecified ions. The coefficients g_K, g_{Na} and g_l are the conductances for the three types of ions, whereas V_K, V_{Na} and V_l are the differences across the membrane of their chemical potentials per unit charge. All potentials are supposed to be measured relative to their 'resting' values, where all components of the current are zero. *It should be noticed that, in the the notation used here, the signs of all currents and potentials are opposite to those used in the early papers of Hodgkin and Huxley.*. This does not affect (5.1.1), but it does affect subsequent equations. The change of notation was found necessary to allow V to *increase* during an action potential from the value 0 assumed for the resting state.

The effect of the voltage clamp on the giant axon of the squid in a resting state was to impose an abrupt change in the potential difference V across the membrane, which was then held at a fixed value until a new resting state was reached. The value of C_M is such that a capacitance current should persist for only a minute fraction of the period of about 10 msec required to pass from one resting state to another, so the first term in (5.1.1) above could be safely disregarded in determining the ionic conductances of the membrane. When this was done, it was found that the potassium and sodium conductances were not even approximately constant in time, but could be expressed in the form

$$g_K = \overline{g}_K n^4, \qquad g_{Na} = m^3 h \overline{g}_{Na}, \tag{5.1.2}$$

where $\overline{g}_K = 36$ m.mho/c^2 and $\overline{g}_{Na} = 120$ m.mho/c^2 were constants, but n, m and h varied with time over characteristic periods immediately following the voltage clamp, and had peak values very much greater than their resting values. The power n^4 of n appearing in the above formula had no special significance, and an even better fit could have been obtained[230] with considerably larger powers of n. However, for a particular value of V, the variation with time of the potassium conductance could be fitted reasonably well by assuming that n in (5.1.2) varied like

$$n = [\alpha_n + \beta_n \exp[-(\alpha_n + \beta_n)t]/(\alpha_n + \beta_n),$$

$$\alpha_n = 0.1(0.1V - 1)/[1 - \exp(1 - V/10)], \qquad \beta_n = .125\exp(-V/80). \tag{5.1.3}$$

The formulas for the factors m^3 and h of the sodium conductance in (5.1.2) were somewhat similar, and could be approximated by assuming

$$m = [\alpha_m + \beta_m \exp[-(\alpha_m + \beta_m)t]/(\alpha_m + \beta_m),$$

$$\alpha_m = (0.1V - 2.5)/[1 - \exp(2.5 - 0.1V)], \qquad \beta_m = 4\exp(-V/18), \tag{5.1.4}$$

and

$$h = [\alpha_h + \beta_h \exp[-(\alpha_h + \beta_h)t]/(\alpha_h + \beta_h),$$

$$\alpha_h = .07\exp(-V/20), \qquad \beta_h = 1/[1 + \exp(3 - V/10)], \tag{5.1.5}$$

In these formulas, the potential V is supposed to be measured in mV and is almost always positive within the axon. A computer program [see Appendix A5.1] enables the graphical display of the current I in (5.1.1) as a function of the time for any value of V, assuming ionic conductances of the above type. By running this program, the reader may personally recreate the results of Hodgkin and Huxley's experiments. It is also possible to vary the numerical parameters so as to fit other experimental data. The reproduction of experimental results in this way raises a number of questions that we shall now attempt to answer in the light of our own and other more recent work; and since they are only partly related, we shall deal with them separately.

(1) A question raised by Cole[231] and others is how closely the conditions of the voltage clamp are related to those of the action potential in the living animal. Quite apart from differences in the initial stimulus that precedes the large exchange of ions between the extracellular and intracellular fluids, there are obvious differences in the behaviour of the actual potential. In the experiments the potential undergoes a large change over a very short period of time, but is subsequently held constant, whereas in the action potential there is a continuous variation of the potential over a period that corresponds to the duration of the ionic currents. It is not obvious, and in fact is not exactly true, that the ionic conductances inferred from the dynamical conditions of the voltage clamp are the same as those obtaining under other dynamical conditions. Nevertheless, we shall verify that after a short initial period the action potential is quite similar to what would be expected if the conductances varied in the same way as in the experiments. Following Hodgkin and Huxley, we may derive an equation for the time dependence of the action potential as described below.

From Ohm's law in the simplified form $\mathbf{j} = -\sigma\nabla\varphi$, obtained from (4.3.15) by neglecting gradients of the chemical potentials, it follows that $\sigma\nabla^2\varphi = -\nabla\cdot\mathbf{j}$, and by integration of this result over the cross section of an axon we obtain

$$\frac{a}{2R_2}\frac{\partial^2\varphi}{\partial z^2} = I, \tag{5.1.6}$$

where a is the radius of the axon, $R_2 = 1/\sigma$ is the specific resistance of the axoplasm, and z measures distance along the axon. Though φ is the potential of the axoplasm, its difference from V is assumed to be approximately constant. On the other hand, if we assume that the action potential propagates with the velocity θ, the wave equation for the propagation of the potential is

$$\frac{\partial^2 V}{\partial z^2} = \frac{1}{\theta^2}\frac{\partial^2 V}{\partial t^2}. \tag{5.1.7}$$

From (5.1.1), (5.1.6) and (5.1.7) we obtain the differential equation

$$\frac{a}{2R_2\theta^2}\frac{d^2V}{dt^2} = C_M\frac{dV}{dt} + \overline{g}_K n^4(V - V_K) + \overline{g}_{Na}m^3h(V - V_{Na}) + g_l(V - V_l) \tag{5.1.8}$$

that can be integrated numerically when n, m and h are known as functions of V. It is assumed that when V varies with time, formulas (5.1.4) and (5.1.5) no longer apply, but n, m and h are solutions of the differential equations

$$\frac{dn}{dt} = \alpha_n(1-n) - \beta_n n, \qquad \frac{dm}{dt} = \alpha_m(1-m) - \beta_m m,$$

$$\frac{dh}{dt} = \alpha_h(1-h) - \beta_h h. \tag{5.1.9}$$

It is easily verified that these are consistent with (5.1.4) and (5.1.5) when V has a constant value, as in the voltage clamp. The solutions of (5.1.8) and (5.1.9) are unstable in general, but they do have solution curves that have a close resemblance to action potentials when V_l and θ are both suitably chosen, as the reader may verify by running the computer program. An example is shown in Figure 5.1.

Curves have been computed by Cronin[232] from the same equations to represent the propagation of an action potential, but these do not provide a very convincing demonstration that a similar mechanism is involved in the voltage clamp and the action potential. However, the above curves are consistent with the relatively large variations of currents of sodium and potassium through the membrane which are a common feature of voltage clamp experiments and the biological action potential.

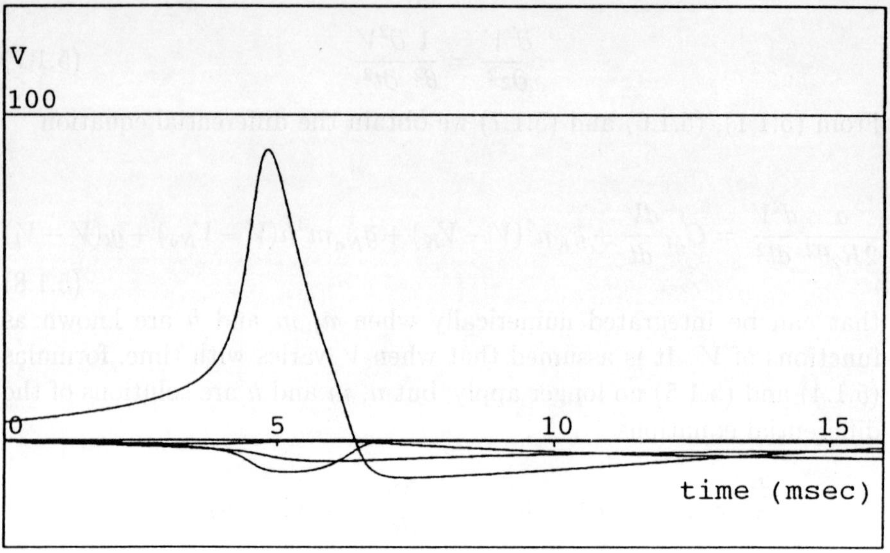

Fig. 5.1 Variation of the membrane potential (V), and of the ionic conductances, with time, as predicted by the Hodgkin-Huxley equations. To avoid the appearance of instabilities, the conductances are given zero values initially.

(2) A very important difference between the voltage clamp and the action potential is in the nature, and the magnitude, of the external intervention that is necessary to secure a comparable effect; actually, no intervention is needed for the propagation of an action potential along any fibre in a living animal. The membrane of the giant axon of the squid separates electrolytic fluids that are far from electrochemical equilibrium with one another, and is maintained in a metastable state by biological action, so that an almost imperceptible influx of calcium ions can precipitate an exchange of ions similar to that predicted by the theory of Hodgkin and Huxley.

In fact later experiments have shown that an important defect of their theory is its failure to take into account the role of the calcium ions. The 'leakage' current in (5.1.1) will certainly not serve this purpose. It was found by Frankenhaeuser and Hodgkin[233] that, in the absence of calcium in the extracellular fluid, no action potential in the ordinary sense is possible, and that the amplitude of the action potential depends very sensitively on the external calcium concentration, even though this is very small. The results of these experiments were explained in part by the subsequent discovery by Katz and Miledi[153] that an action potential within a cell is initiated by an influx of calcium from outside the cell. In the biological context, it is well known[152] that many action potentials are synchronous with periodic fluctuations in the extracellular potential. The physically based theory developed in the previous Chapter (Sections 4.5 to 4.7) accounts for all these facts.

(3) As well as calcium, sodium and potassium, it was found by Mullins[234] that there is a flux of chloride ions across the membrane during an action potential of *Nitella*. Since the chloride ions are normally the only negatively charged ions with a great deal of mobility, it is to be expected that they play an important part in maintaining approximate electrical neutrality within the electrolyte wherever there are significant currents of positively charged ions. As in the last Chapter, therefore, we take the view that at least four types of ionic currents must be considered to formulate an adequate theory of the action potential.

(4) A further problem encountered by the theory of Hodgkin and Huxley arose from the discovery by Sjodin and Mullins[235] of an oscillatory behaviour of the membrane potential of a suitably treated squid axon. Oscillatory potentials, usually repetitive action potentials, are a common feature of nervous activity in many animals, but are not solutions of (5.1.8) and cannot be explained on the basis of that equation, though it is of course possible to assume an oscillatory potential and obtain an oscillatory current[236]. On the other hand, they are a natural feature of the physically based ionic theory. The difficulty with (5.1.8) is that its stable solutions represent predominantly irreversible processes, whereas the action potential has a significant thermodynamically reversible component, as shown by the observation of reversible heat evolution in that context[237].

(5) Finally, it may be asked why the ionic conductance of the axonal membrane to potassium and sodium should vary with time in the manner required by the equations (5.1.2), (5.1.3) and (5.1.4) above. Hodgkin and Huxley pointed out that the functions n, m and h specified in (5.1.3) and (5.1.4) are solutions of the differential equations (5.1.9), but this throws little light on the question. Fitzhugh[184] and Rabinovitch, Thieberger and Friedman[238] have found that the action

potential could be fitted as well or better by the solution of much simpler differential equations than (5.1.8) and (5.1.9).

More recently, considerable progress has been made in the analysis of both the voltage clamp and the action potential in terms of the electrodynamical and electrochemical theory of electrolytes. Vaccaro[239] has shown how the essential results of Hodgkin and Huxley can be reproduced on the basis of this theory. The factors n^4 and m^3h in (5.1.2) are proportional to the membrane conductances, and may be interpreted as relative probabilities that potassium and sodium ions will be transmitted by channels in the membrane. In the previous Chapter, essentially the same theory was used to show that the action potential can be explained in terms of fluctuations in the ionic densities, especially those of ions with low concentrations in the neighbourhood of the neural membrane.

The functions n, m and h were actually chosen to fit the experimental data with reasonable accuracy. The simple explanation that appears to have been generally accepted is that, as a result of a voltage clamp or an action potential, channels in the membrane are temporarily opened to permit the influx of sodium and the efflux of potassium. Today there is little doubt about the existence of such channels. Though their diameter, estimated at a few Ångstroms, does not permit direct observation, the flux of ions leaving or entering the channels has been detected[240] with the help of microelectrodes in the electrolytic fluid near the surface of the membrane.

It appears, therefore, that at least part of the explanation of the surge in the values of the ionic conductances must be sought in the dynamics of the ions within and near the entrances or 'gates' to the channels. Nevertheless, the action potential is a phenomenon that pervades the internal electrolytic fluid and must be consistent with the theory of electrolytes. It is noteworthy that action potentials are found not only in unmyelinated fibres such as the giant axon of the squid, but also in myelinated fibres where the only communication with the extracellular fluid is at the nodes of Ranvier, that occur at infrequent intervals along the fibre. In an electrolyte large variations in ionic conductances are associated with fluctuations in the ionic concentrations, which may be very large under dynamical conditions in the surface layers of an electrolyte. Also, even within the channels the forces acting on the ions are predominantly electrical in nature. We therefore conclude that the fundamental laws governing both the voltage clamp and the action potential must be those of electrodynamics.

5.2 Functions of the Leech Ganglion

Animate systems may be characterized by their ability to create, process and utilize information. Energy is required to sustain the dynamics, as it is for all physical systems, but in any nervous system its role necessarily becomes subordinate to the production, flow and interaction of information. In quantitative terms, the relation between energy and information is highly non-linear, the former dominating events at the interface of the organism and the latter within it, where quite small increments of energy can cause large changes in information.

In Section 4.2 we have provided an introduction to the classical theory of information, based on Shannon's definition of information to be gained in (4.2.4). There is a quantal generalization of this definition, in terms of the statistical matrix, which was used in Section 3.4 to obtain the information I to be gained from observation in a nervous system. The rate of change of information, given in (3.4.6), makes it clear that this information can only change as the result of interactions with some external system; and this point will be developed further in Chapter 7. We have shown that, in a semi-classical approximation, the quantum theory can be developed to provide a description of any serially-connected set of neurons, and that the results are comparable with well- known experimental results, such as those observed in a voltage clamp or an action potential. But, for a complete treatment of the information processing by the nervous system using these methods, it would be necessary to determine the elements of the statistical matrix.

For present purposes, a classical definition of information will suffice; and if we are interested in *available* information, which is essentially electrochemical information, the definition given in (4.4.30) is appropriate. From this definition it follows that the available information changes in any region at a rate given by

$$kT\frac{dI}{dt} = -\int \sum_a \epsilon_a \frac{d(\varphi_a - \varphi)}{dt} d^3x, \tag{5.2.1}$$

where $k = 1/\log(2)$ if the information is in bits, T is the absolute temperature, ϵ_a is the ionic charge density for ions of the a-th type, φ_a is the corresponding chemical potential per unit charge, and φ is the electric potential, so that $\varphi_a - \varphi$ is the electrochemical potential per unit charge. This expression is easily calculated, along with the potentials and their time derivatives, by the methods developed in the last Chapter, including the solution of the linearized equations (4.4.3) and (4.4.4), or their non-linear counterparts (4.6.1). The available information, and its rate of change, can obviously be broken down into chemical contributions from the various ionic species and an additional electrostatic contribution.

Solutions of the non-linear equations governing the potentials are of great interest, not only because they are able to provide a description of a wide range of ionic phenomena but because, although they are based on well established physical principles, they do not require the kind of approximation implicit in more detailed ionic theories, such those based on Boltzmann's equation. They have, in fact been developed for an interconnected set of twelve neurons[45–209] and verified against well-known experimental results, such as the Hodgkin-Huxley voltage clamp results of the preceding Section[239,241–242]. However, in order to obtain solutions within the constraints of present day mathematical and neurophysiological knowledge, a very simple nervous system must be selected.

For several reasons the leech is nearly ideal for such a study. Foremost is the fact that, while supporting an interesting set of behaviors, its nervous system is simple enough to have been extensively documented by Nicholls, Kuffler and others[243–260]. Specifically, the system consists of 21 almost identical ganglia, each of which monitors and controls the muscles and skin of 5 body annuli symmetrically disposed around it. Only the fused ganglia of the head and tail segments are more complex, as indicated in Figure 5.2(a). Moreover, each ganglion except these two, contains an easily identifiable subset of 18 neurons which have been studied extensively by electrophysiological and other techniques and identified with specific sensory modalities and behavioral responses in the above references. They are arranged in two groups of 9 on opposite sides of a longitudinal center plane defining the lateral body halves they innervate, as in Figure 5.2(b).

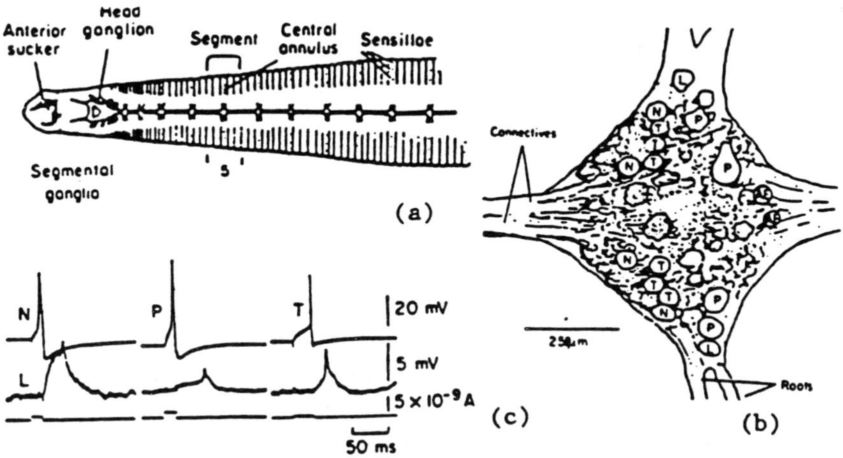

Fig. 5.2 (a) Cross-sectional sketch of the body of the leech, showing the complex head ganglion and 11 of the 21 identical segmental ganglia of its central nervous system; (b) a ventral view of a typical ganglion with T, P, N, L and AE neurons labeled; and (c) typical action potentials of these neurons.

Both groups consist of 7 sensory neurons that respond in 3 different sensitivity ranges (three T-type, two P-type and two N- type) to touch, pressure and noxious pressure respectively, as well as 2 motoneurons that control separate musculatures (one L-type and one AE-type). The AE neurons are known to cause only localized skin ridging. The L neurons, however, produce contractions of the large longitudinal muscle in proportion to the intensity of the stimulus received from the sensory neurons. Consequently, if activated simultaneously they can produce varying degrees of local body shortening, while if one is activated while the other is inhibited, they can act as local generators of wavelike swimming or writhing movements – all basic behavioral modes of the animal. The response of an L motoneuron to the firing of N, P and T sensory neurons is illustrated in Figure 5.2 (c).

The microanatomy of these ganglia is characterized by the simplicity of an early evolutionary stage. All of the approximately 360 cell bodies of each one lie within one of 6 tissue capsules sustained by a single glial cell; and, as in most invertebrate systems, the neurons possess no specialized dendrites or axons. Unlike the axons of the neurons in vertebrates, each of their processes can transmit data in both directions; and it has also been established that all of their interactions are excitatory, T neurons making tight electrical junctions with motoneurons, N neurons forming purely chemical synapses with them, and P neurons acting through synapses of a mixed character.

Since coordinated movements like swimming and crawling with the suckers at head and tail are possible, it is evident that each ganglion must communicate with those on either side of it as well as with the rudimentary brains at the ends, and that some inhibitory synapses mediated by interneurons must be present in these normally excitatory pathways. Considerable progress has been made in modelling these behaviors [254,260–262]; but the foregoing properties are sufficient for the present purpose: analysis of the correlated flow of energy and information through a typical ganglion, as summarized below. Details of the analysis appear in an earlier publication of the authors[50].

If one applies a blunt stylus to an interior segment of the leech and gradually increases the pressure, a well-defined sequence of behavioral responses results. The segment and those immediately adjacent to it suddenly shorten, the skin over this region becomes annularly ridged, the body flattens and, finally, successive zones of contraction confined to either the ventral or dorsal half of the creature sweep along its length from head to tail generating waves that enable motion. One after another the defense mechanisms superimposed by the evolutionary process – passive withdrawal, peripheral toughening, active escape – are activated; and each reflects one upward step in the development of the nervous system.

Figure 5.3 presents the results of quantifying these stimuli and responses. They were obtained by inserting microelectrodes into the cells indicated and monitoring their changes in potential in an intact preparation of the animal, using a piezoelectric stylus to record the contact pressure. It will be apparent that the T, P, N, L and AE cells are activated at increasing levels of threat. Extended firing of the T cells causes the L cells to fire and initiate longitudinal muscle tension immediately; but the T cells are rapidly adapting and will cease firing under constant pressure in less than a second, firing only once or twice again when the pressure is removed. If, however, the pressure is increased, the P cells will begin to fire, increasing the muscle tension, initiating skin ridging and, if continued long enough, causing both to be further increased by the firing of the N cells.

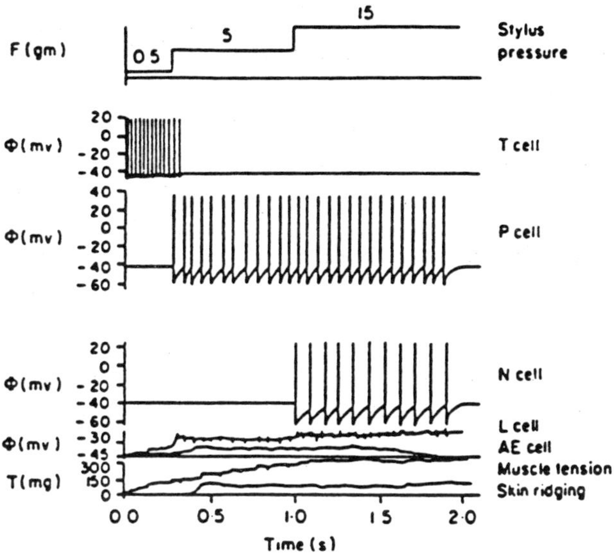

Fig. 5.3 Measured frequencies and magnitudes of action potentials produced by T, P, N, L and AE neurons of an isolated leech segment with the annulus subjected to various exterior stylus pressures.

This amounts to an integrated set of behavioral responses, complex enough to allow this primitive creature to cope with many of the hazards of its environment, yet simple enough to permit analysis. By utilizing the mechanical energy of the stimulating stylus and contracting muscles as boundary conditions, and applying the following equations developed in the reference noted above[50], to describe the coupled flow of energy and information through a neuronal network representative of the T,P,N,L,AE leech system, essentially the same sequence of responses can be predicted. The network on which the model summarized below is based is illustrated in Figure 5.4; and in Figure 5.5 below it may be seen that the results calculated from the model are closely comparable to the experimental results of Figure 5.3.

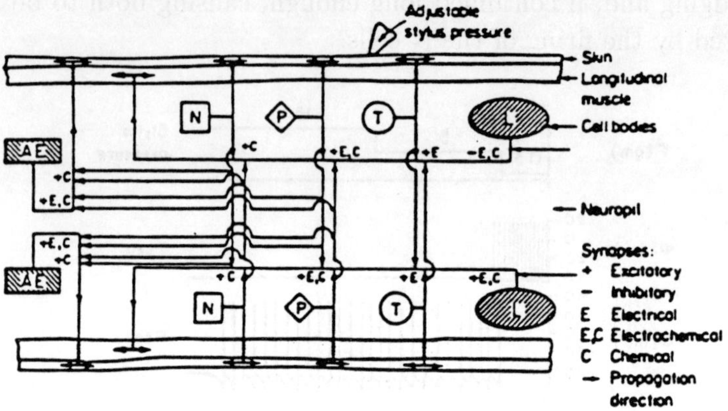

Fig. 5.4 Circuit diagram of the sensory-motor system of the leech with the character of the synapses and the point of application of external pressure indicated.

It should be noted that despite its simplified circuitry and the monopolar character of the 'neurons', this ganglion network has a number of features resembling those of more advanced nervous systems. Perhaps most notable is the fact that the spectrum of synaptic types is much the same, and as for many of the synapses of mammalian systems, ACh has been shown to be the primary neurotransmitter. Even the approximate ion concentrations listed in Table 5.1 are closer to those of mammals than to the values normally quoted for squids and crustaceans[263].

Ions	Concentrations in axoplasm (mM)	Concentrations in blood (mM)
K^+	138	4
Na^+	15	130
Cl^-	10	115
Ca^{++}	<1	<2
$Protein^-$	170	~0

Table 5.1 Concentrations of principal ions in neurons and blood of the leech.

The facilitation and depression that occurs at the motoneuron synapses is also a feature of higher nervous systems, as is the alternate dorsal-ventral inhibitory intervention required to produce the swimming motion, controlled in this case by a pacemaker cell located in the creature's brain[262]. It is of interest that the results from the model that follows are to a very considerable extent independent of microstructural details. The cell membrane is taken to be a semi-permeable barrier separating the cytoplasm from the extracellular fluid, both of which are electrolytes differing in ionic composition and electrochemical potential. It follows from Debye theory that the densities of all ionic species should be continuous at the membrane surface though they may vary rapidly within a small distance on either side. The electric potential φ must also be continuous, even though the potential gradient will be discontinuous because of the change in dielectric constant that occurs at the surface.

In the equilibrium state, as a result of diffusion processes, a high concentration of sodium ions will be present within the membrane adjacent to the inner Debye layer, while a high concentration of potassium ions will exist next to the layer in the cytoplasm; and the outer Debye layer will remain closely attached to the exterior membrane surface because of the grounding provided by the extracellular fluid. But when an external electric field, such as might result from a propagating action potential, is applied, the inner Debye layer will be disrupted, oscillatory ion motions generated by the coupling of the ionic currents with the electrostatic field will result, and the injection of sodium ions followed by the efflux of potassium ions required to sustain the action potential will develop.

Normally, the relaxation times of these oscillations in an electrolyte are very short; but with the intervention of a membrane they may, due to its high resistance, extend to the millisecond range. Similarly in the dynamical situation the Debye layer, within which charge neutrality does not hold, may extend across the entire membrane. A transient current results which can grow many orders of magnitude greater than the normal ohmic current within the electrolyte. It was shown in Section 4.4 that this condition depends on the existence of appropriate solutions of the governing dispersion equation (4.4.9); in the present application, it is useful to note that the following prove to be controlling factors:

(1) The presence of calcium ions which, though not required as an energy source, possess properties allowing them to initiate a form of resonance that greatly increases the amplitude of the overall oscillations.

(2) The interchange of sodium and potassium ions at the inner membrane surface, which results from the wide difference in their chemical potentials (per unit charge) φ_a on opposite sides of the Debye layer and provides the major source of energy for the plasma oscillations.

Instead of relying on the detailed analysis of Chapter 4, we shall give a brief summary of the essential results and take the opportunity to introduce a somewhat more general treatment of the ionic dynamics that is relevant to our present purpose. Coulomb's law of electrostatics, already formulated in (4.3.6), may be written

$$\nabla^2 \varphi = -(4\pi/\kappa) \sum_a \epsilon_a), \tag{5.2.2}$$

where φ is the electric potential, ϵ_a is the charge density associated with ions of the a-th type, and κ is the dielectric constant. The ionic charge density can be written as $\epsilon_a = e_a n_a$, where e_a represents the charge of the ion and n_a is the corresponding number density. The equation of conservation of charge, as formulated in (4.3.12), can also be written

$$\frac{\partial n_a}{\partial t} + \nabla \cdot (n_a \mathbf{u_a}) = 0, \tag{5.2.3}$$

where $\mathbf{u}_a$ is the mean velocity of an ion of the a-th type. Finally, the chemical potentials are related to the number densities by (4.3.2), which can also be written

$$n_a = n_a^0 \exp(-\beta e_a \varphi_a). \tag{5.2.4}$$

To formulate the equation of conservation of momentum, we note that the electric force on an ion of the ath type is $-e_a \nabla \varphi$, and the mean force of resistance exerted by the solvent on the same ion is given by $-m_a \theta_a \mathbf{u_a}$, where m_a is the ionic mass and $m_a \theta_a$ is a coefficient of drag that is determined largely by its degree of hydration. The remaining force $-\nabla P_a$ is due to the gradient of the partial pressure $P_a = n_a/\beta$ where $\beta = 1/kT$ if k is Boltzmann's constant and T is the absolute temperature. Since $m_a \mathbf{u}_a$ is the mean momentum of an ion of the a-th type, we obtain

$$m_a \frac{\partial}{\partial t}(n_a \mathbf{u_a}) + \nabla P_a = -n_a(e_a \nabla \varphi + m_a \theta_a \mathbf{u_a}), \tag{5.2.5}$$

It follows with the help of (5.2.4) that the ionic current $\mathbf{j}_a = e_a n_a \mathbf{u}$ satisfies

$$\mathbf{j}_a = -\frac{e_a^2 n_a}{m_a \theta_a} \nabla(\varphi - \varphi_a) - \frac{1}{\theta_a} \frac{\partial \mathbf{j}_a}{\partial t}, \tag{5.2.6}$$

a generalized form of Ohm's law commonly used in plasma physics. On taking the divergence of (5.2.5), we obtain also a definitive set of non-linear equations for the interior of the membrane in the form

$$\gamma_a \frac{\partial \varphi_a}{\partial t} + \beta m_a \frac{\partial^2 \varphi_a}{\partial t^2} = \nabla^2 \varphi_a + \frac{4\pi}{\kappa} \sum_b e_b n_b^0 \exp(-\beta e_b \varphi_b) \tag{5.2.7}$$

where $\gamma_a = \beta_a m_a \theta_a$ is the inverse diffusion coefficient. This reduces to (4.6.1) if the second term on the left side is omitted, which is usually permissible because the coefficient βm_a is very small. However, when the potentials are varying rapidly, or in dealing with instabilities that may be encountered in the integration of the equations, the additional term may be important.

The above equation may be solved to determine the variations in the potentials near the membrane surface. We note first that in a linear approximation, analogous to that adopted in Section 4.4, the potentials satisfying these equations are functions of the time t and position $\mathbf{x}$ of the form

$$\varphi_a = \Re \sum_r \frac{f^{(r)} \exp(\lambda^{(r)} t - \mathbf{k}^{(\mathbf{r})} \cdot \mathbf{x})}{\mathbf{k}^{(r)2} - \lambda^{(r)}(\gamma_a + \lambda^{(r)} \beta m_a)}. \tag{5.2.8}$$

Here $\Re$ denotes the real part of the expression that follows, since the inverse time constants $\lambda^{(r)}$ and the wave vectors $\mathbf{k}^{(r)}$ are complex in general. In the following, we shall for the sake of simplicity consider the mode corresponding to a particular term under the summation in (5.2.8), and write $\lambda = \lambda^{(r)}$ and $q + \lambda p = \mathbf{k}^2$, where q and p are real constants. If we also write $C_b = 4\pi e_b^2 \beta_b n_b / \kappa$, it is easy to verify that the linearized form of (5.2.7) is satisfied, provided that the dispersion equation

$$\sum_b \frac{C_b}{q + \lambda(p - \gamma_b + \lambda \beta m_b)} = 1 \tag{5.2.9}$$

is satisfied. This is obviously a generalization of (4.4.9).

It can be seen from (5.2.8) that solutions for which $\Re\lambda$ is positive grow exponentially with time, and must be excluded as unphysical. On the other hand, $\Re\lambda < 0$ and $\Re\lambda = 0$ define irreversible damped and reversible oscillatory modes, respectively, of the various ions. For the oscillatory modes, $\lambda = i\omega$, where ω is the angular frequency of the oscillations, and in any event the separation of (5.2.9) into real and imaginary parts yields *two* equations that determine p and q in terms of λ. The constant q is necessarily positive, and $q^{-\frac{1}{2}}$ may be interpreted as the non-equilibrium thickness of the Debye layer at the membrane surface, while p is the effective mean resistance of the membrane.From Coulomb's law it follows that the electric potential can be expressed in terms of two of the chemical potentials, thus:

$$(\gamma_b - \gamma_a)(q^2 + \lambda^2 p^2)\varphi = \gamma_b[q^2 + \lambda^2(p - \gamma_a)^2]\varphi_a - \gamma_a[q^2 + \lambda^2(p - \gamma_b)]^2 \varphi_b, \tag{5.2.10}$$

Fluctuations of the potentials with amplitudes greater than ~ 20 mV are no longer even approximately periodic, and the linearized equations are no longer valid. However, solutions of the non-linear equations

(5.2.7) compatible with the above can be obtained with the help of the *anzatz* (4.4.15), and if we again consider just one value of r, we are led to the equations

$$(\gamma_a - p)\frac{\partial \varphi_a}{\partial t} + \beta m_a \frac{\partial^2 \varphi_a}{\partial t^2} = q\varphi_a + \sum_b C_b \exp(-\beta_b e_b \varphi_b) \qquad (5.2.11)$$

to determined the potentials at any point in the neighbourhood of the membrane.

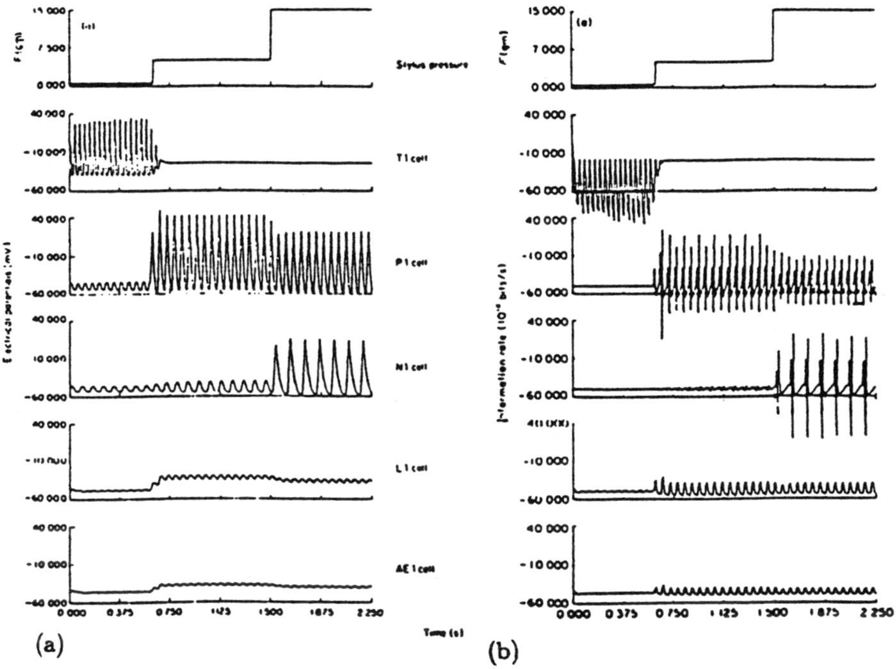

Fig. 5.5 (a) Computed frequencies and magnitudes of action potentials of the T, P, N, L and AE neurons in the circuit diagram of Fig. 5.4, subjected to various external pressures; and (b) the rate of information transfer associated with these action potential trains.

Using a modified Runge-Kutta method with a variable interval of integration, these equations may then be solved and a direct comparison made of the electrical potentials arising from stimulation of the 'neurons' in the circuit displayed in Figure 5.4 with those of Figure 5.3 measured experimentally. To produce the results presented in Figure 5.5(a) it is only necessary to distinguish the cells by their calcium concentration (which mediates the ionic resonances), to adjust the coupling constants so as to override inhibitions where necessary, and to introduce a small amount of damping to quell the natural excitability of the T cells.

It is apparent that all of the qualitative features and many of the quantitative aspects of the experimental measurements can be reproduced by the model. The firing sequences are nearly identical, the amplitudes and frequencies of the firing pulses are closely comparable and the basic features of the pulse shapes, including prominent differences in buildup rates and refractory phases, are much the same. The potential of the L neurons goes through an initial facilitation phase before firing commences in response to the firing of the P and N neurons, and remains in an elevated state thereafter, exhibiting distinct spikes which produce incremental increases in muscle tension up to some maximum value. The same is true of the potential in the AE neurons; but the facilitation phase is longer, and they do not begin to fire until after the P neurons since they are not connected to the T cells.

Interestingly, though not shown in the Figure, each firing pulse in a neuron on the stimulated side of the ganglion circuit elevates the potential by only a small amount in the corresponding neuron on the unstimulated side. Basically this is because of the non-linear character of the oscillatory systems involved. It is especially notable that, for the same reason, the complex sequence of events occurring on one side, including the sudden depression of the T cells when the P cells begin to fire, can be closely reproduced with no inhibitory connections in the network. The implication is that this primitive control mechanism may play a larger part in the functioning of higher nervous systems than has previously been recognized.

Under the conditions adopted the electrical potential is determined mainly by the potassium potential, but it was found that synaptic junctions could be changed from excitatory to inhibitory either by increasing the potassium potential or decreasing the chloride potential. The information transfer rate, on the other hand, depends primarily on the calcium potential and its derivative. This was calculated by applying the principles developed in the preceding Chapter.

The definitive equations. (5.2.1) to (5.2.7) are valid in both classical and quantum mechanics, and can be exhibited as the result of an averaging procedure applied to corresponding microscopic equations. We shall indicate briefly how this is done in a quantum mechanical context.

In quantum mechanics, [cf. (3.4.5)], the information in thermodynamical units is given by

$$I = -\beta \mathrm{tr}_N (P_N \log P_N), \tag{5.2.12}$$

where P_N is the statistical matrix of the neural system under consideration. According to the statistical mechanics of thermodynamical equilibrium, however, P_N can be expressed in terms of the Hamiltonian energy H, the thermodynamical free energy F, and $\beta = 1/kT$ as before:

$$P_N = \exp\{-\beta(H - F + pV - \sum_i e_i \varphi_{ai}\}, \tag{5.2.13}$$

where φ_{ai} indicates the chemical potential per unit charge of the i-th ion, supposed to be a-th kind, and

$$H = \sum_i (H_i + e_i \varphi_i), \tag{5.2.14}$$

where H_i is the energy of the i-th ion, disregarding the effect of the ambient electrical field, and φ_i is the electrical potential of this ion. Although a time-dependent perturbation is necessary to take the system from an equilibrium to a non-equilibrium state, the total energy including the perturbation energy is conserved, so that (5.2.12) reduces to

$$I = \beta \mathrm{tr}_N \{P_N [H_0 - F - \sum_i e_i (\varphi_{ai} - \varphi_i)]\} = \beta \langle H_0 - F - \sum_i e_i (\varphi_{ai} - \varphi_i) \rangle, \tag{5.2.15}$$

where the bracketing $\langle \cdots \rangle$ denotes the statistical average. Disregarding the unavailable thermal contribution $\langle H_0 + F \rangle$, this obviously reduces to the expression (4.4.30), from which (5.2.1) is derived.

As the values of φ_a and φ are known from above, and their significant variations are in the Debye layer in contact with the internal membrane boundary, this relation can be used to calculate the information flow displayed in Figure 5.5 (b). It is again evident from (5.2.15) that the total amount of information transferred to a given neuron consists of two distinct parts, one of which, coded in the first term, is entirely chemical in character, while the other, coded in the second term, is purely electrical. This division is reflected quite clearly in the differences between the two sets of plotted results.

The outstanding feature of the information rate transfer curves compared with the electrical potential curves is their bimodal character. Since $-dI/dt$ is being plotted, negative increments indicate increasing rates of information transferred to a given neuron, while positive increments indicate decreasing rates representing transmission states of the neuron. In the case of a T neuron the rate of information transferred inward as a result of the external stimulus being applied increases rapidly until the electrical potential reaches about half of its maximum value. The neuron then transmits a sharp fast burst of information outward, directly to the L neurons, indirectly to the rest of the system. This is followed by a second much slower transmission that contains a considerably larger amount of information. Much the same sequence of events occurs in the P and N neurons, though rather than proceeding continuously, the slow buildup of the secondary transmission occurs at two widely different rates, the sudden bursts being associated with electrical polarization effects, the slower transmission with ion motions representing the chemical component. Consistent with their early warning role, the T neurons operate dominantly in the receiving mode, while the P and N neurons emphasize transmission to the L and AE neurons, the latter assuming part of this function when they begin to fire; and the electrical character of the T-L synapse as opposed to the chemical character of the P-L and N-L synapses is reflected in the different shapes of the two types of curves. Synaptic sensitization and habituation are also in evidence, but appear more clearly in the mollusc studies of the following Section.

The foregoing relations may also be used to compute the changes of the neurons' total energy with time, allowing curves resembling those of Figure 5 (a) to be plotted[50]. Comparison of these with those of Figure 5 (b) further emphasizes the dominate role of internal ion motions in information transmission, for the sharp peaks of the latter fall entirely within the energy peaks (which coincide in turn with the firing pulses of the potential curves), while the secondary maxima of the information rate curves lie entirely outside these regions. However, the amounts of energy transferred are always less than 100 ergs, while the amounts of information transferred are normally greater than 10^{15} bits/sec. This is the essence of nervous system operation: minute energy transfers control massive information exchanges through highly non-linear relationships, such as those specified.

5.3 Mollusc Sensitization and Habituation

Many investigators have confirmed the critical role that fluctuating calcium concentrations play in the generation and propagation of transient neuron potentials, and in the release of neurotransmitter substances at synaptic junctions[153,264–268]; but of special interest in the present connection, Kandel, Kupfermann, Castellucci and their collaborators[269–274] have demonstrated that habituation and sensitization as observed in a behavioral reflex of the large marine mollusc *Aplysia Californica* (Figure 5.6) can be explained in the same terms.

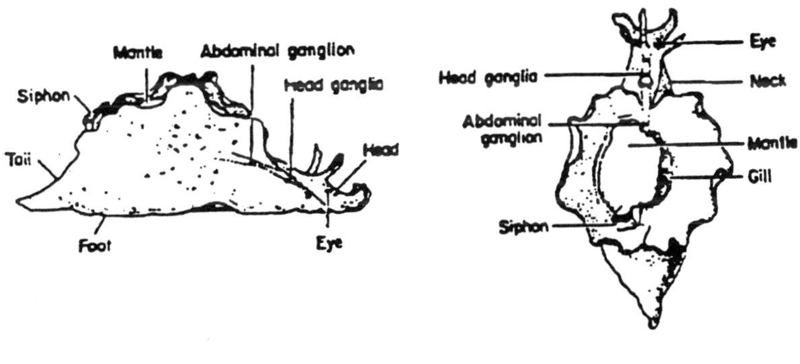

Fig. 5.6 Side and top views of the giant sea snail *Aplysia Californica* showing the locations of the ganglia, mantle, gill and syphon featured in the experiments.

In particular they have shown that the repetitive firing of a sensory neuron which forms a chemical synapse with a motoneuron results in a degradation of the potential pulse induced in the latter that is quantitatively related to the depletion of calcium in the former; and, further, that subsequent stimulation of an interneuron terminating on the presynaptic sensory bouton will rapidly restore the full response of the motoneuron by raising the calcium concentration there to its initial level. This work makes it possible to apply the definitive equations

$$\gamma_a \frac{\partial \varphi_a}{\partial t} + \beta m_a \frac{\partial^2 \varphi_a}{\partial t^2} = \nabla^2 \varphi_a + \frac{4\pi}{\kappa} \sum_b \epsilon_b^0 [\exp(-\beta e_b \varphi_b) - 1], \qquad (5.3.1)$$

equivalent to (5.2.7) of the preceding Section, where $\varphi_a$and φ_b represent ionic chemical potentials, γ_a is the mean resistance of the membrane and its associated Debye layer for the ath type of ion in the dynamical state, e_b is the ionic charge and $\epsilon_b^o = e_b n_b^0$ is the charge density at a fixed point of electrical neutrality; κ is the dielectric constant and $\beta = 1/(kT)$ is inversely proportional to the absolute temperature T. These equations can be used to account for potential variations proportional to those actually observed for both sensitization and habituation by one unified ion kinetic mechanism using the neuronal circuits established by these investigators. It will be seen that calcium depletion and replenishment in the sensory axon terminus under the conditions noted is precisely what the equations predict, and the actual magnitudes of the varying concentrations closely match those measured by others. Additionally, the resonant oscillations of the calcium ions prove to provide the necessary stimulus for the exchange of sodium and potassium ions long recognized to constitute the basis for the growth and propagation of the action potential (see ref. [50], and other references therein).

Aplysia has been used extensively in neurobiological experiments, partly because of the large size and easy accessibility of the neurons in its abdominal ganglion, but also because it possesses an interesting set of behaviors found in higher animals. These creatures, giant sea snails which can reach 1 metre in length and weigh 10 kg or more, normally crawl with a caterpillar-like motion. They will withdraw the gill illustrated in the Figure if touched on the mantle or siphon, and can perform more complex withdrawal maneuvers and release an inky substance if threatened, as well as participate in coordinated group matings, lay egg chains in an all-or-none action much like inking, locate variable seaweed food sources, and aerate the gill by pumping.

Also, when the gill of the creature is extended, a weak water jet applied to its siphon causes the gill to be withdrawn in a rapid reflex action. If, however, the jet is applied repeatedly at from 10 sec to 3 minute intervals this withdrawal will gradually decrease to less than 20% of its beginning value[275] and require 30 minutes or more to recover to the initial sensitized state after the stimulus ceases. Clearly this is an elementary form of habituation, or conditioning to ignore a non-threatening bodily pressure; but if a strong sustained jet is applied to the neck during deep habituation, resensitization occurs almost immediately.

There are actually at least 24 sensory neurons, all of which synapse on excitatory and inhibitory interneurons, and on the 20 or more motor neurons involved in gill-withdrawal. The habituation of this reflex, and possibly its sensitization as well[276], has been traced to the plastic properties of a particular synapse on L7 in the sophisticated series of experiments referenced initially. Moreover, the critical role that intracellular and extracellular calcium concentrations play in controlling impulse transmission at such chemical synapses has been extensively documented by others[170,277–278]. For these reasons the following discussion is limited to this particular behavior and the specific region indicated in Figure 5.7.

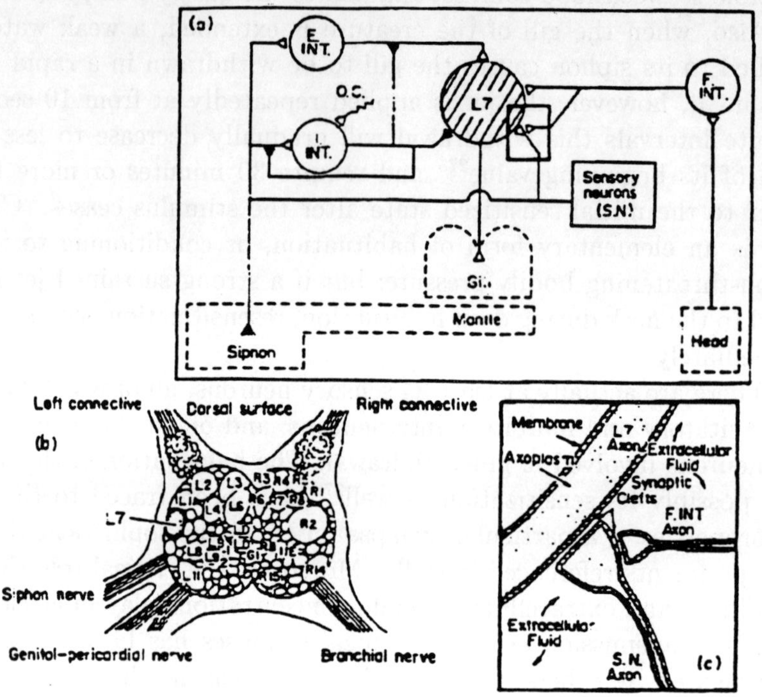

Fig. 5.7 (a) Test circuit used to study potential variations in the motor neuron illustrated in (b); and (c) the synaptic configuration simulated in the experiments.

In the preceding Section, concerned mainly with the transmission of energy and information across the neural membrane, solutions of (5.3.1) could be obtained by treating the non-equilibrium thickness of the Debye layer determined by q, as well as the effective mean resistance of the membrane p, as constants characteristic of the internal conducting Debye layer. Among these were stable oscillatory modes, periodic at small amplitudes, but also resonant states dominated by the oscillations associated with the calcium and sodium ions. To deal with the spatial variations of the potentials across and along the membrane, we need a non-linear generalization of the analysis given in Section 4.5. This suggests that q and p should be allowed to vary continuously across the membrane, but appropriate solutions can also be obtained by resolving potential differences in different layers into components associated with the two dominant resonances. Following earlier work by the authors[279], the potentials are expressed as in (4.6.5) and (5.3.1) and can then be written

$$\gamma_a \frac{\partial \varphi_a^{(r)}}{\partial t} + \beta m_a \frac{\partial^2 \varphi_a^{(r)}}{\partial t^2} = \nabla^2 \varphi_a^{(r)} +$$

$$+ \frac{4\pi}{\kappa} \sum_b \epsilon_b^o \exp(-\beta e_b \sum_{s=1}^{r} \varphi_b^{(s)})[\exp(-\beta e_b \varphi_b^{(r)}) - 1] \tag{5.3.2}$$

where the superscripts r and s indicate the different resonances. For the r-th resonance, we may use a generalization

$$\nabla^2 \varphi_a^{(r)} = \sum_s (p^{(rs)} \frac{\partial \varphi_a^{(s)}}{\partial t} + q^{(rs)} \varphi_a^{(s)}), \tag{5.3.3}$$

with the $p^{(rs)}$ representing partial resistance coefficients and the $q^{(rs)}$ partial inverse square Debye shielding distances. These partial parameters must be chosen so as to yield the same result as (4.4.15) after summation with respect to r. Then it is easy to verify that, in the linearized approximation, the parameters $p^{(r)}$ and $q^{(r)}$ of (4.4.15) must satisfy a dispersion equation of the form

$$\sum_b \frac{C_b}{q^{(r)} + \lambda^{(r)}(p^{(r)} - \gamma_b + \lambda^{(r)} \beta m_b)} = 1 \tag{5.3.4}$$

where $\lambda^{(r)}$ is the inverse time constant, usually complex, corresponding to $p^{(r)}$ and $q^{(r)}$, and $C_b = 4\pi\beta e_b^2 n_b^0/\kappa$, as usual.

Since in the development of an action or graded potential in a given layer principally affects only the next layer, the coefficients representing the coupling of the other layers become vanishingly small. Hence, attention may be restricted to two at a time; $r = 1$ and 2 can be associated with the calcium and sodium modes of the inner membrane layer, while $r = 3$ and 4 are associated with the corresponding modes of the outer membrane layer. As in Sections 4.4 to 4.6, it is natural to introduce a radial coordinate z normal to the surface of an axon, that takes values between z_o on the inner surface and z_s on the outer surface, and to designate the longitudinal cylindrical coordinate as x. In channels within the membrane, the concentrations vary with z, and solutions of the linearized equations can be obtained in the way discussed in Section 4.5. Here we shall indicate briefly how it possible to solve the non-linear equations for the potentials and hence obtain the current densities $\mathbf{j}_a$ from the formula

$$\mathbf{j}_a = -\sigma_a \nabla(\varphi - \varphi_a), \tag{5.3.6}$$

in which the conductivities σ_a are proportional to the concentrations and are given by

$$\sigma_a = \frac{\kappa C_a}{4\pi\gamma_a} \exp(-\beta e_a \varphi_a). \tag{5.3.7}$$

The coefficients C_b in the dispersion equation (5.3.4) are proportional to the ionic concentrations in the resting state and therefore depend on z. Separable solutions of (5.3.3) can be obtained that depend on the transverse coordinate z through the values of $q^{(r)}$ and $p^{(r)}$ and on the longitudinal coordinate x as a function of $x - vt$, where v is the velocity of propagation. But more generally it is possible to introduce an attenuation coefficient $f(x)$, so that $\varphi_a^{(r)}$ satisfies the differential equation

$$\frac{\partial \varphi_a^{(r)}}{\partial x} + \frac{1}{v}\frac{\partial \varphi_a^{(r)}}{\partial t} = f(x)\varphi_a^{(r)}. \tag{5.3.8}$$

This can be solved in the form

$$\varphi_a^{(r)} = \exp\{-f_o(x_m - x)\} \cosh[g(x_m - x)] \overline{\varphi}_a^{(r)}[t - (x - x_m)/v\}, \tag{5.3.9}$$

where x_m represents the constant of integration and the constant g depends on v, q and γ_a but not on x. From (5.3.6) we then obtain the longitudinal ionic currents in the form

$$j_{ax} = \frac{\kappa C_a}{4\pi\gamma_a} \exp(-\beta_a \varphi_a) \left[\frac{1}{v} \frac{\partial}{\partial t} (\varphi - \varphi_a) + f(\varphi - \varphi_a) \right] \tag{5.3.10}$$

which can be computed as a by-product of the numerical integration of (5.3.2).

As might be expected from the special conditions imposed to achieve these relations, the shape of a potential propagating in a given direction along the membrane depends strongly on the calcium concentration in that direction. But also, perhaps surprisingly, the passage of a potential peak causes the calcium current to flow in a direction opposite to the direction of propagation. If the resting state is well below the firing threshold and the excitation applied to the calcium ions of the inner Debye layer is sufficiently small, say a change in concentration less than 10^{-8} M over 10^{-2} sec, the only effect will be to modify the simple harmonic background oscillations of potential less than 1 mV characteristic of the nervous systems of all living creatures. But if the potential of the neuron is closer to threshold, the non-linearity of the governing equations becomes increasingly important and a local excitation greater than the above produces a much larger effect, as illustrated in Figure 5.8.

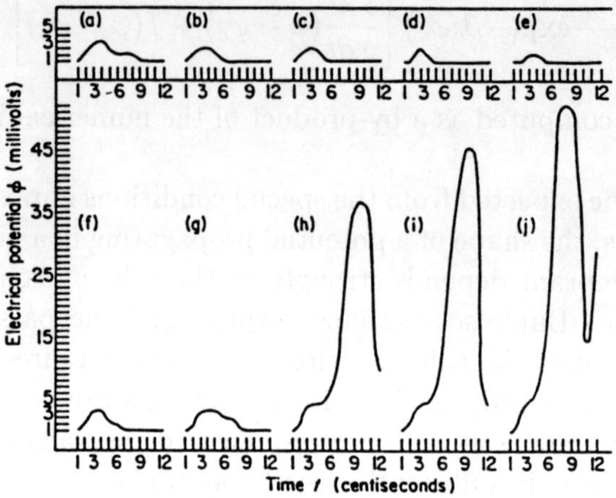

Fig. 5.8 Effects of increasing and decreasing calcium concentrations on the electrical potential of the inner Debye layer. For (a) through (j) within the figure, concentrations are 2.5, 2.25, 2.0, 1.75, 1.5, 2.75, 3.0, 3.25, 3.5 and 3.75 $\times 10^{-5}$ M.

The mechanism underlying these changes in potential is evident when the behavior of the ionic and currents are examined. Although the excitation noted affects only the calcium directly and these ions are the first to respond, even for graded potentials there is a substantial decrease in the sodium concentration of the inner Debye layer and, at the same time, a radial efflux of sodium to the intracellular fluid, joined with a much smaller influx from the channels in the membrane, though the longitudinal currents remain very small. But if the initial calcium concentration is somewhat higher or the excitation considerably greater, a preliminary threshold is reached (at about 5 mV in Figure 5.8), the potential of the inner membrane layer spreads to the outer layer, and the potential increases almost discontinuously by more than an order of magnitude. The same sequence of events at even higher levels of concentration and excitation account for the action potentials shown in Figure 5.9 below.

Though useful for the above purposes and for studying situations in which the mean resistances of the inner and outer membrane layers differ slightly, it is unnecessary to consider the outer layers separately. The effect of such a difference is illustrated in the Figure 5.9; a pair of action potentials of nearly ideal shape with amplitudes of approximately 75 mV is produced. Clearly the forward shoulders of these curves, always observed at expanded scale in experimental studies, are large graded potentials from which the action peak develops when the final threshold is exceeded.

In fact, action potentials up to 100 mV or more can be generated by the triggering action of the calcium resonance coupled to the sodium resonance. The maximum is determined by the relative values of the ionic resistances, but also by the concentrations c_K and c_{Cl} of the potassium and chloride ions, as shown by the formula[280],

$$\varphi_{\max} = \frac{(\gamma_{Na} - \gamma_K)\ln(c_K/c_{Cl})}{\beta e(2\gamma_{Na} - \gamma_K - \gamma_{Cl})}, \tag{5.3.11}$$

but it is worth stressing that the process of activation could not even begin if calcium were absent, and that its depletion at the inner membrane surface will restrict amplitudes to those characteristic of graded potentials. This is the chemical analogue to the electrical component of information transfer in the brain; and it is evident that in the last analysis the sensitivity of both depends on changes at the quantum level.

Additionally, Figure 5.9 shows that the longitudinal flux of calcium undergoes large variations during an action potential, and confirms that the flux is in the opposite direction to that of the action potential. There is therefore a depletion of calcium by diffusion at the bouton of an axon transmitting a potential, and it can be estimated[279] that after the arrival of no more than 12 action potentials, the calcium concentration in the bouton of the axon shown in Figure 5.7 (c) will be so reduced that no effective response is possible, thus accounting for the observed phenomenon of habituation. Of equal interest, however, is the fact that the same mechanism may also account for the sensitization established by Kandel and his colleagues, providing the bouton is stimulated from an outside source, as also illustrated in Figure 5.7 (c).

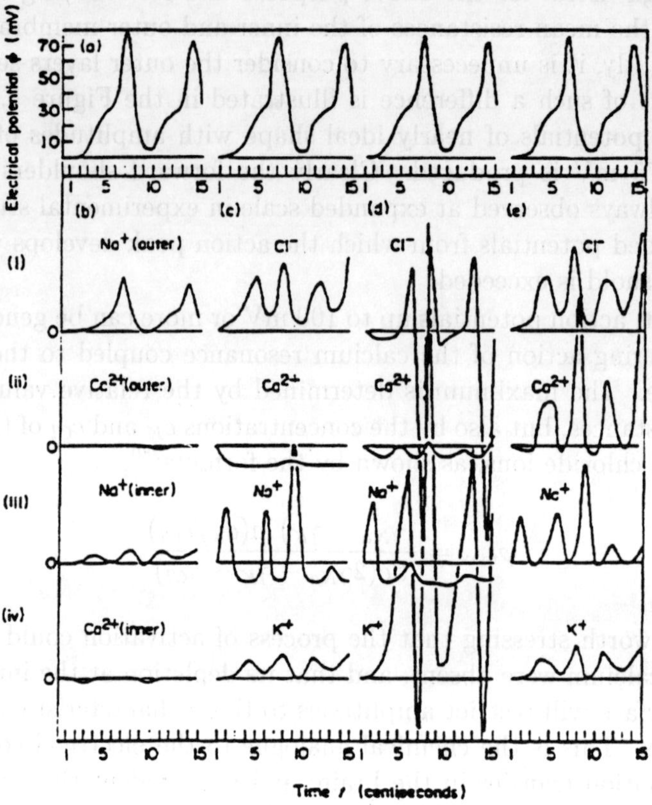

Fig. 5.9 Variations of potential and ionic variables for different resonances in the inner and outer Debye layers; (a) potentials, (b) ionic resonances, (c) ionic density factors, (d) radial currents, and (e) longitudinal currents; for i - iv, k = 4 - 1.

In this case the resulting large graded potentials would propagate up the axon in the direction of increasing calcium concentration, but by so doing produce a current of calcium ions flowing back into the bouton, effectively reversing the habituated state. Thus the analysis provides important insights into the mechanisms of habituation and learning in a primitive animal, under conditions where conscious intervention is necessarily minimal.

5.4 Insect Motor Control

Although the nervous systems of insects are very simple compared with those of most animals, they are remarkably well-adapted to their ecological niche; and strange as it may seem, within that niche their behaviour exhibits to some degree most of the attributes of intelligence. In pursuit of sustenance, self-preservation and reproduction, for example, they display a high degree of motivation, and do appear to possess some measure of awareness and volition. In this Section we shall discuss what is known about the motor activity of certain insects that guides the development of computer models to simulate their behaviour. Such simulations permit the electronic representation of a degree of intelligence and motivation approaching that of their biological counterparts, and help to clarify what could be required to invest an artificial insect with some measure of consciousness, in the sense that we have proposed in the Introduction to this volume.

Certain insects, such as cockroaches, crickets, locusts, and the stick insect are large enough to have allowed detailed investigations of the mechanisms controlling their motor functions. As might be expected, assuming them to have originated like vertebrates from creatures of the seas, these prove to be similar to those of the arthropods, including crustaceans such as shrimp, crayfish[281] and the crab[282]. *Pattern generators*, or small circuits that are autonomous in the sense that they are not necessarily activated by the central nervous system, play an important part in the motor activity of such insects. Those of the stick insects *cuniculina impigra* and *carausius morosus*, for instance, have been studied extensively by Bässler and his associates[283,284]. The six legs of the insect are controlled to a major extent by these generators, which appear to coordinate its movements.

The generator for each leg consists of a ganglion, which is located near the beginning of the leg, and is activated by a chorodontal organ that senses the velocity but also the relative position of the two main segments (tibia and fibula) of the leg. By a combination of excitation and inhibition, mediated by interneurons, the chorodontal organ in turn activates a set of motor neurons. The latter are finally responsible for the innervation of the flexor and extensor muscles that control the joint connecting the tibia and fibula. The contraction of the flexor muscle and extension of the extensor muscle is again sensed by the chorodontal organ; and the contraction and relaxation of the muscles of the leg are controlled directly by a combination of excitatory and inhibitory impulses that correspond appropriately to the sensory stimuli, thereby providing a highly effective feedback-based mechanism of control.

Burrows[285] has made a related study of the neural mechanism controlling the legs of the locust. There the sensory feedback appears to be provided to a large extent by tactile stimuli originating in hairs of the insect's leg, but the basic mechanism is similar in principle to that of the cockroach illustrated in Figure 5.10 below. An elaborate system for coordinating feedback cycles, such that as provided for the insect's legs, is clearly unnecessary for the movement of the wings of the locust; a central rhythm generator, belonging to the CNS, is all that is needed for flight.

Collectively, central pattern generators and localized feedback circuits fulfill a role similar to that of the cerebellum in the cortex of the higher animals: that is, to exercise autonomous control of refined motor action. Of course the circuitry is primitive compared with that of the cerebellum, and the control it exerts appears to be largely the result of genetic programming, whereas, as we shall see in the next Chapter, the control functions of the cerebellum are acquired primarily by trial-and-error learning. Nevertheless, it is likely that the synapses of the neurons involved in the control of the motor activity of insects are sensitized by use in the same way as those in more elaborate nervous systems, and thus satisfy the fundamental requirement of Hebb's rule of learning[101].

Substantial progress has been made towards the computer simulation of the behaviour of insects, partly because it is not only desirable but conducive to maximum efficiency to imitate the essential features of their nervous system, especially those concerned with motor activity. For example, the pattern generator of Bässler's experimental investigations includes spiking interneurons with an excitatory role similar to that of cerebellar granule cells; non-spiking interneurons with an inhibitory role similar to that of the Golgi, stellate and basket cells; and motor neurons with an action similar to that of the cerebellar Purkinje cells. Also included are intersegmental neurons that coordinate the activity of different segments.

Bässler[286] has also discussed the role of a neural network of the CNS of the stick insect which is responsible for providing the timing cues of a rhythmic motor output pattern. Pearson[287] proposed that a similar subsystem in the cockroach should be designated as a *central rhythm generator*, rather than a pattern generator, in recognition of the fact that it is free of responsibility for the detailed movements of the legs. If the insect may be considered to have some degree of volition, this should appear in the mode of action of the central rhythm generator.

Simulated and Artificial Insects

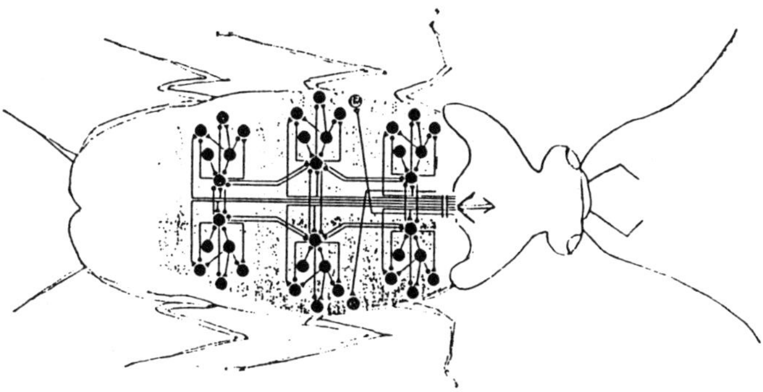

Fig. 5.10 Diagram of the circuitry controlling the legs of the Beer model of the American cockroach *Periplaneta Americana* with connections indicated to the circuits responsible for pacemaking, the sensing of obstacles by antennae, eating and the utilization of energy, located in the head ganglia.

As we have noted in the first Chapter, the requirements of artificial life, in the form of self-replicating automata, are relatively well understood, and a great deal of progress has been made towards the development of artificial intelligence. However, if artificial consciousness is ever achieved it is likely to be initially at a primitive level comparable with that of the insects. There is an important distinction between the simulation and the creation of consciousness; the first can be realized by the construction of a computer model, but the second requires the development of a physical device. Nevertheless, the construction of a computer model to simulate the effects of consciousness is a useful preliminary step to the development of such a device; and it is worthwhile to consider some features of computer programs that simulate the motor activity of insects. As an important step in this direction, Beer[288,289] developed a remarkable computer model to simulate the behaviour of the cockroach illustrated in Figure 5.10.

Animated by only 78 neurons with 156 connections, including not only the circuits shown for controlling each of the six legs but also those located in the head ganglia controlling higher functions, this artificial insect can simulate a number of the cockroach's basic behaviors, e.g., locomotion in three different gaits at various speeds, random wandering, edge-searching at obstacles to discover an unobstructed path, searching for food, and renewal of an initial energy supply by simulated eating.

A computer simulation of an insect with comparable capabilities, but based on a much simpler neural network of the type described in this volume, has been constructed [see Appendix A5.4]. In formulating this model we have simulated the action of a central rhythm generator to provide for alternate, and usually forward, movements of the legs of the insect, but also a pattern generator to provide for turning motions in response to tactile stimuli. Varying combinations of forward and turning motions are sufficient to produce changes of gait.

It is the combined action of the rhythm generator and the pattern generator that determines the overall motion of the insect. The motion is constrained by a tactile environment of blocks that can be put into any initial position and changed at any time. In spite of its simplicity, the model *simulates* features that satisfy the definitions of intelligence and motivation. However, for the more advanced manifestations of consciousness it would, of course, be necessary to simulate the behaviour of the higher animals.

In Section 1.1 we have suggested the following criteria for intelligence: (i) the ability to respond to external stimuli; (ii) the ability to form memories of experiences; (iii) the ability to perform tasks without supervision; (iv) the ability to adapt, or learn, as a result of experience; and (v) the ability to anticipate future developments, and make mistakes. To what extent do the artificial insects satisfy these criteria?

In our simulation, there are two insects, and each responds to two stimuli. It responds by avoidance to the tactile stimulus (pressure) provided by the environment, which can be altered at any time but always serves to confine the insect. It also responds, by attraction, to the sight of food, which can be replenished by the observer at any time. When the food is within sight but cannot be reached without encountering pressure, the response is complex. The program simulates the formation of a limited memory by the long-term potentiation and sensitization of a small set of neurons, which represent the central rhythm generator of the insect. The ability of the insects to explore their environment without supervision is demonstrated by the fact that each does so in a different manner, which is never repeated exactly, even when its initial position and orientation, and the environment are unchanged. The process of adaptation to the environment is commensurate with their learning capabilities and takes place during the period of formation of memory. Finally, there is some simulation of anticipation in their search for and pursuit of food. We conclude that the artificial insects simulated by the program possess a limited degree of intelligence.

The insects are also highly motivated in their motor activity, displaying a convincing aversion to the pressure exerted by blocks in their environment, and an unfailing attraction to food placed within their field of vision. To a certain extent, their response to tactile and visual stimuli is automatic and predictable, and certainly does not imply either awareness of their situation or volition. The model therefore illustrates the fact that a high degree of motivation or the appearance of goal fixation does not necessarily imply any degree of consciousness, in the sense of the definition that we have given in Section 1.2.

However, computer simulation of insect behaviour poses in a new form the question raised by Turing's invention of the 'imitation' game described in Section 1.5. Presumably Turing would have argued that if insects are conscious, and if there were no way to distinguish between a sufficiently lifelike simulation and the actual behaviour of an insect, then the simulated behaviour should be considered as a manifestation of consciousness. This is in fact a plausible corollary of his thesis that a deterministic computer may be developed in the future with all the mental attributes of a human being, but it is one which we find equally difficult to accept. Insects are a form of life displaying in a primitive form the elements of consciousness, in the sense of our definition. Some of their activities are clearly instinctive, but others display awareness, the acquisition of information, and volition, the creation of information. For example, bees have an instinctive sense of direction, which seems to depend partly on the direction of incidence and polarization of light and partly on an innate sense of the time of day; all this is capable of simulation. They do not display much intelligence in adaptation to a changed environment, such as may be occasioned by the displacement of their hive. However they are able to communicate and act on information transferred by various types of 'dance language'[290] and in doing so display both awareness and volition. We conclude that, as long as apparently spontaneous processes are *in principle* predictable, they cannot be attributed to conscious volition, and that under certain conditions the difference between simulation and reality may be extremely difficult to discern. However, a distinction can be made where there is objective evidence for the creation and observation of new information by the action of consciousness. The only way of creating new information, as far as we know, is by allowing the intervention of quantum-mechanical processes, such as will be described in the final Chapters of this book.

Chapter 6

Avenues to Artificial Intelligence

6.1 Expert, Genetic and Network Programs

Inspired by digital computing theory and fueled by the explosive development of its accompanying technology, the last half of the twentieth century witnessed remarkable progress toward achieving the ancient human dream of creating intelligent robotic systems[291]. Motivated largely by the desire to expand mental abilities, in the same way as the technologies of the Industrial Revolution expanded physical abilities, quite naturally this has been accompanied by corresponding progress in the brain sciences, each field profiting from discoveries of the other.

The symbiotic relationship between the two disciplines became apparent almost as soon as the concepts of the Turing machine[292], and von Neumann's stored program[293] were implemented. The general features of the Turing machine and its 'tape', which implements the program, have already been discussed in Section 1.5. In this Chapter we shall discuss the progress which has been made towards the simulation of various functions of the brain and its representation as a Turing machine.

One of the first computer models of the neural networks of the brain, in which the 'neurons' were small digital processing units converting input into output, was developed by McCullough and Pitts[294].

This was the precursor of the 'perceptron' models[295] which followed, stimulating other forms of research into neural circuitry and synaptic junctions, which led in turn to Hebbian refinement of weighting factors[101] for the simulation of learning, the incorporation of Wiener cycles[296] to represent feedback, and more realistic digital networks. Some of these models will be discussed in more detail in the following Section. Their remarkable functional properties suggested a wide range of new investigations in neurobiology, from direct applications to invertebrate nervous systems[164], to discoveries of analogous circuitry in mammalian cortical structures[100]. Meanwhile the cognitive sciences, aided both by these developments and computerized analytical equipment, have spread the findings to the fields of psychology[297], and even contemporary philosophy[298].

To date, however, the computing architectures available have, for the most part, limited practical applications to implementation in software; that is, to programs able to take advantage of the ever-larger memories and ever-faster retrieval and execution times of such machines to simulate simple cognitive functions, as well as elementary neural networks and their performance. The result has been the emergence of a form of intelligence which, though necessarily deviating from animal intelligence dependent on the interconnections and support systems of biological neurons, nevertheless expands human mental ability in several important ways.

The first of these forms of artificial intelligence to prove its worth was found in programs featuring *if-then* logical sequences and *trees*, or *frames,* constructed from rules provided by specialists in a given area, operating on a database compiled for that area. Typically, when some problem is to be solved within a given context, the program asks certain questions which the user must answer, then supplies a solution; as in the following questions asked and course of action recommended by the EMYCIN program to deal with a hazardous substance spill, illustrated in Table 6.1 on the next page. This is an example of what is commonly called an 'expert system'[299]. Today such systems are widely applied in a variety of contexts, enabling the retrieval of information from databases much larger, and at rates much faster than the human brain can accommodate. The rules can incorporate, and thereby preserve, the wisdom of many different experts, the database can grow, and both can even handle small amounts of uncertainty in definitions and at branch points by utilizing the principles of 'fuzzy logic'[300].

SPILL 100

1) What is the spilled substance? .... **Oil**
[Expected responses are Oil, Acid or Other; enter HELP for user options]
2) Where was the spill first spotted? .... **Along creek**
3) Is the liquid flowing? .... **Yes**
4) Please walk along the creek looking for the outfall from which the liquid is draining. If you find one, please enter the outfall number: . **Why?**
[i.e., why is it important to determine the outfall?]
[1.01] This will aid in determining the spill basin.
It has already been established that
  1.1 the location where the spill was first reported was along creek
Therefore, if
  1.2 the outfall from which the liquid is draining is known
then
  it is definite that the outfall from which the liquid is draining
  is the spill basin [RULE001]
.... **WOC6** [The answer to question 4]
5) Please inspect M6-1. Is the liquid flowing in this manhole? .... **Yes**
6) Is there flow from M6-1 from direction of P3513A? .... **No**
7) Please inspect M6-2. Is the liquid flowing in this manhole? ..... **Yes**
8) Please inspect M6-4. Is the liquid flowing in this manhole? ..... **Yes**
9) Please inspect M6-5. Is the liquid flowing in this manhole? ..... **Yes**
10) Please inspect M6-11 Is the liquid flowing in this manhole? ... **No**
11) Please inspect B3404A Is the liquid flowing in this manhole? . **No**
12) Please inspect M6-6 Is the liquid flowing in this manhole? ..... **Yes**
13) Please inspect M6-7 Is the liquid flowing in this manhole? ..... **No**
14) Are there any stationary sites listed in the inventory from which the observed volume of oil might have originated? .... **No**
The recommended emergency containment procedures are as follows:
  Locate the spill front, set up an absobent boom to stop futher flow.
  Suggestions for discovering the source of the spill are as follows:
    Check possible sources near, or that drain into M6-6.
    Consider possible mobile sources.
    Request chemical analysis to assist in identification.

Table 6.1: The trace generated by the EMCYN spill model. User input is shown in boldface type, explanations of the trace in square brackets.

Typical of such systems that are proven to exceed human performance are DENDRAL[301], which analyzes nuclear magnetic resonance, atomic bonding, and other chemical data to generate plausible molecular structures; and MACSYMA[302], which performs symbolic mathematics, including algebraic, differential and integral calculus operations. The development of both, the first at Stanford University, and the second at the Massachusetts Institute of Technology, has been ongoing for over twenty-five years; and both are widely used for research as well as commercial purposes.

Many other examples could be given, e.g., CADUCEUS, MYCIN, and PUFF are names of programs for diagnosing and treating internal, blood and respiratory diseases, HEARSAY for understanding speech, R1 for configuring complex computer systems, PROSPECTOR for locating deposits of specific minerals[303]. But because the success of such systems depends on the biologically unrealistic high-speed retrieval and sequential processing of conventional computers, it is not our intention to treat them in any greater detail.

From the present point of view neural network systems are more relevant, even though at present they must be implemented on linear or parallel versions of such machines. Despite their successful application in a number of areas, they can not yet claim to exceed human performance in most cases. But because they utilize simplified functional units ('neurons') and organizational principles (inter/intra connection in/of specialized groups) based on those of the nervous systems of living creatures, some at least offer not only the possibility of simulating a broader range of mental activities, but also the possibility of understanding the brain mechanisms underlying these activities[158].

There can be no question that the storage, retrieval and processing methods of ordinary computers and organic brains are widely different. The former systems, for example, possess distinct addressable memory banks, discrete arithmetical registers and, being entirely electrical, normally process sequentially on picosecond to nanosecond time scales; while the latter possess none of these structures and, being electrochemical in character, always operate in parallel on time scales of milliseconds to seconds.

And yet, by storing memories in available groups of neurons by altering the conductivity of their synaptic connections, and recalling them by chemically-mediated signals of specific frequencies from distributed sources, brain networks more than compensate for any such 'deficiencies'. Somehow, they acquire the ability to recognize objects and make decisions under conditions of great uncertainty, often based on severely incomplete information[157]. They can evaluate memories - allowing some to fade and organizing others for long-term retention, will action by self-stimulation, and create an internal workspace for continuous modification of a world model[304]. Indeed, nearly all of the higher mental processes we associate with animal intelligence must arise from these very properties. Nevertheless, software simulations of neural networks on conventional machines constitute a promising starting point for attempting to understand such processes.

This is not to say that all such systems are equally valuable for the purpose. Many concentrate on exploiting only the expanded decision-making capabilities of simplified networks, primarily for commercial applications. In general these utilize a relatively small number of pseudo-neuron nodes connected in various ways between input and output layers through one or more 'hidden' layers, and rely on the high speed of modern computers to iterate weighting factors associated with the nodes by recirculating image output errors until some resolution criterion is satisfied[305–309].

Several, such as the *Neuralworks Professional* developed by Neural Ware, Inc. and Klimasauskas and Guiver[306], allow substantial increases in the number of nodes and supply a variety of popular configurations varying in the specific pattern of connections and the method of back-propagation (Figure 6.1).

Some of these have been quite successful in the marketplace (e.g., those based on the system developed by Hopfield[307,85]) but because of their highly simplified character, can shed little light on the nature of higher brain processes. The same is true for the genetic algorithms developed in the course of artificial life studies[308]. They are capable of tracing random evolutionary pathways of flora and fauna by self-reproduction, perhaps even of adding an additional dimension to the creation of artificial thought. But their restriction of signal propagation to nearest neighbors and, like expert systems, the elementary rules applied to govern the process, amount to still greater simplifications of biological conditions.

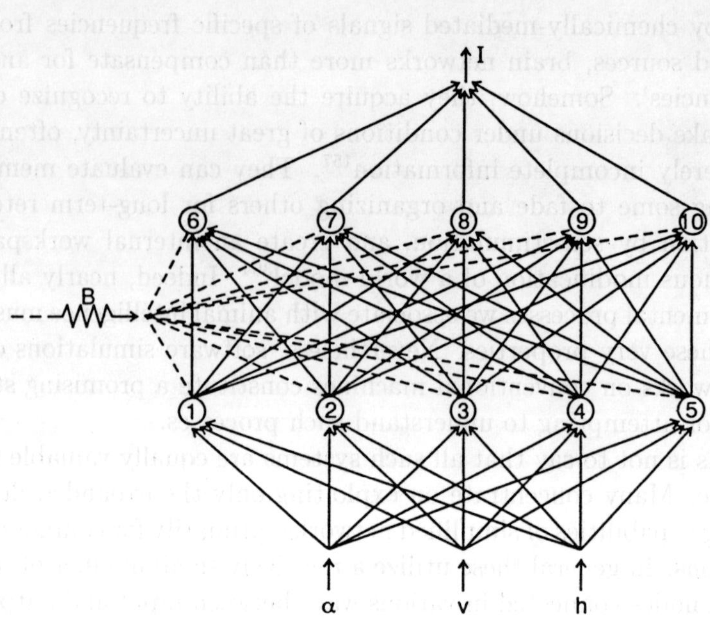

Fig. 6.1 A neural network for solving ballistic problems; the network is trained to calculate the horizontal distance to the impact point I of a missile fired with a specific velocity v at an angle α above ground level and a height h above I by biasing (B) the connections to the processing elements of two hidden layers (1 through 5 and 6 through 10).

Other approaches, however, believing the governing 'algorithms' of living brains to depend critically on the environment, synaptic connections and properties of real neurons, have focussed on achieving greater neurobiological fidelity. Notable examples are the evolving models of Grossberg[8], Kohonen[11], Anderson[309] and the present authors [310,311], all of which incorporate more realistic neural functions and structures with applications to nervous systems of increasing complexity. These are discussed in more detail in the following sections of this chapter.

6.2 Neurobiological Networks

The various attempts to model neurobiological networks are distinguished by the way in which the output of individual 'neurons' is related to their input, and by their interconnections. In the original McCulloch-Pitts model an activation level u_j, with a continuous spectrum of real values, was introduced to represent the state of the j-th neuron. The *output* of the i-th neuron was a function $v_i = f(u_i)$ of its activation level; but this was assumed to be a step function, so that v_i had the value 0 or 1 depending on whether u_i was negative or positive. The *input* from the j-th neuron to the i-th neuron was then of the form $w_{ij}v_j$, with the *weight* w_{ij} regarded as a measure of the strength of the synapse responsible for this particular input. The activation level u_i could therefore be expressed in the form

$$u_i = \sum_j w_{ij}v_j + \theta_i, \tag{6.2.1}$$

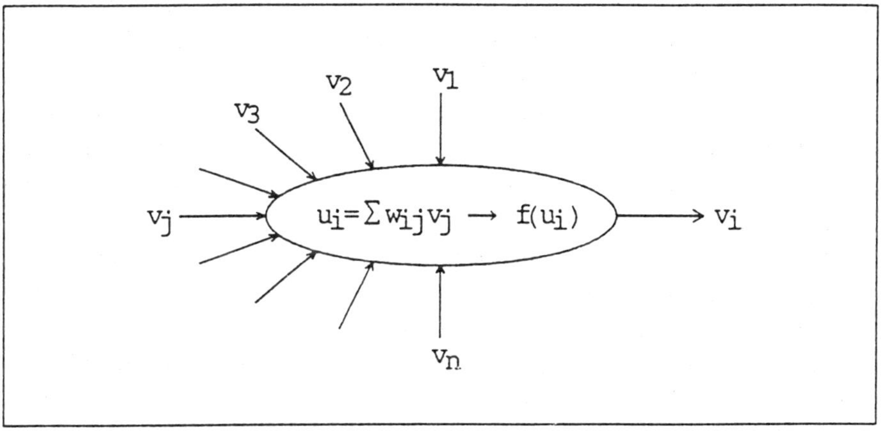

Fig. 6.2 Diagrammatic representation of Eq. (6.2.1), showing the processing element featured in many current neural network applications. Multiple synaptic inputs v_j are assigned weights w_{ij}, summed within the element, and transformed by a function f to produce a digital output v_i.

where θ_i was intended to take account of non-synaptic input, including perhaps inhibitory effects.

In the neurobiological context, a typical neuron often receives input from many others, varying in magnitude and sometimes in sign. The weight w_{ij} in (6.2.1) associated with synaptic input v_j from the j-th element to the focal i-th element must therefore be allowed to vary in magnitude and have either a negative inhibitory or a positive excitatory effect. Also, the neuron may receive input from another at more than one synapse and with varying strengths so as to produce different internal effects. It must therefore be assumed that it is the potential at the axon hillock of the i-th cell that determines the step-function output $v_i = f(u_i)$ of the cell. The inputs to a particular cell from other cells are assumed to be simply additive, and it is these considerations that determine in principle the individual terms under the summation of (6.2.1)

The McCulloch-Pitts model initiated various efforts to achieve greater realism in the representation of the action of the brain. The Rosenblatt perceptron[295], which in one of its forms attempted to represent sensory, association and response functions, was a significant early development; but it was less to the point for the present purpose since it introduced a statistical approach as a means to avoid neurobiological detail. On the other hand, the Hebbian synapse[101] and Widrow's Adeline and Madaline[312] proved immensely influential in stimulating further neurobiologically oriented developments.

The question of how synaptic functions could be approximated was among the first to be addressed by early investigators. As mentioned in Section 3.3, Hebb made a valuable contribution to the understanding of this question by suggesting a general mechanism for learning in the brain, through the progressive sensitization of neural circuits with use. Inspired, possibly, by Pavlov's experiments with sound and food linked to salivation in dogs, he stated the following principle:

"When an axon of cell A is near enough to excite a cell B and repeatedly or persistently takes part in firing it, some growth process or metabolic change takes place in one or both cells such that A's efficiency, as one of the cells firing B, is increased."

Not only did this statement lend itself to rules of increasing sophistication for treating synapse facilitation by programming methods, it established a firm connection with neurobiology and assured that these rules would reflect the results of related research in that science. Today Hebb's Rule enters virtually every advanced treatment of neural networks in one form or another, and increasingly concentrates attention on the synaptic junction as an essential seat of learning. In the context of the McCulloch-Pitts model, this would imply that a representative weight w_{ij} in (6.2.1) is not a constant, but has a tendency to increase, up to a certain limiting value, whenever there is input from the j-th to the i-th neuron.

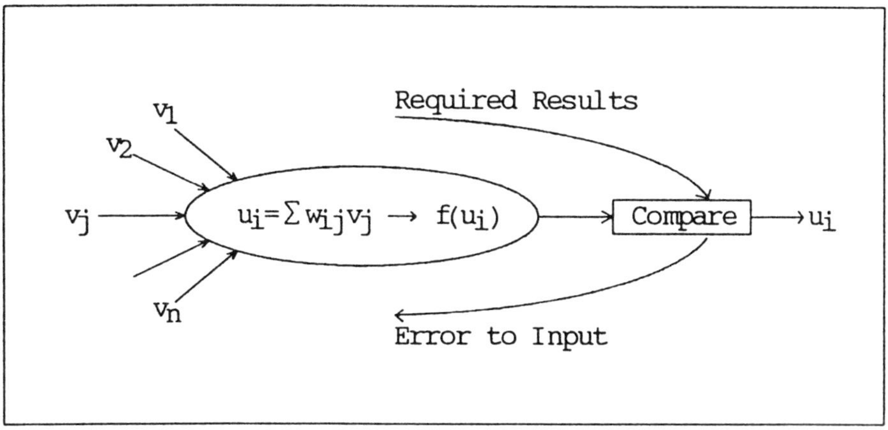

Fig. 6.3 The Widrow Adeline. Weighted inputs v_j D, summed and biased, generate a digital output u_i which is compared with a desired output, allowing feedback of error for modification of the weights w_j and a corrected output. Learning can be accelerated and the output enhanced by interconnecting a hierarchy of Adelines, called a Madeline, in such a way that their outputs converge to yield a single digital result.

The Adeline (adaptive linear network) was originally intended only as a device to filter noise from telephone circuits (Figure 6.3). It consisted of a biased linear signal combiner with variable resistance input weights and a bipolar output, but proved to be another vital component of progress, especially since many of these could be interconnected to form a Madeline (many-Adeline) capable of performing certain signal processing tasks, including the identification of patterns it had been trained to recognize. Thus the weights w_{ij} in this application of (6.2.1) needed to be modified in a systematic manner, so that the 'activation levels' u_i converged on predetermined values b_i. The implementation of this adaptive capability was done by a computation designed to minimize the mean square 'error' $\sum_i(u_i - b_i)^2$. This procedure required the location of the minimum of a weight-surface function which, assuming (6.2.1), has the form

$$\sum_i(\sum_j w_{ij}v_j + \theta_i - b_i)^2,$$

and was accomplished for the device by an application of the method of steepest descent[313].

For extended networks the higher dimensional weight-surfaces often contain many minima, and it was evident that other methods would be required to achieve analogous results; but the essential concepts were now in place and new developments soon followed. One of the most important of these was the analytical method advanced by Hopfield[307], both because it incorporated several additional neural system functions, and because it lent itself to implementation in electrical circuitry and semiconductor miniaturization. An autoassociative linear array of processing nodes with backward propagation of error was proposed for a memory unit; but external input to each node was allowed, and feedback loops characteristic of neural systems were introduced [as shown in Figure 6.4 (a)]. The outputs of the neurons, or *nodes*, were also treated more realistically by permitting them to have any value between 0 and 1 determined by the function

$$v_i = \tfrac{1}{2}\,[\tanh(\lambda u_i) + 1], \qquad (6.2.2)$$

where, as before, u_i represents the net input to the i-th node and the specific sigmoid function is determined by the gain parameter λ, as shown in Figure 6.4 (b), – which amounts to defining a transfer function, *i.e.* a relation between input and output, more general than the step-function suggested for (6.2.1).

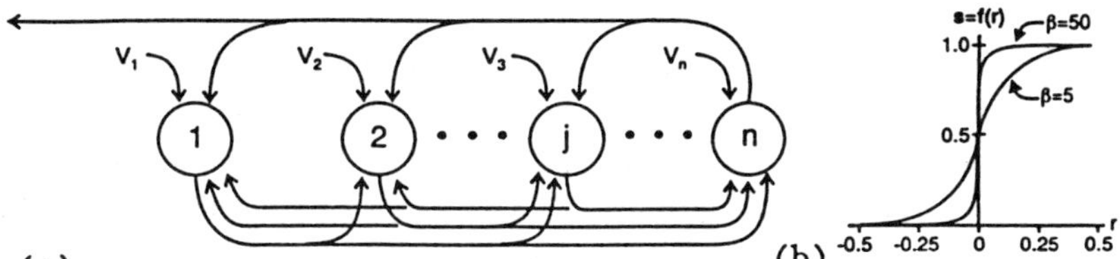

(a) (b)

Fig. 6.4 (a) A Hopfield autoassociative linear processing array, with external input (v_j) to the elements, internal feedback loops and backward propagation of error; and (b) transfer functions varying from a step function to a straight line through various sigmoid functions depending on the value of λ in (6.2.2).

In effect it was still necessary to locate the minimum of a complex functional surface, or at least some value close to it, but it proved possible to bring more powerful mathematical methods to bear on this problem by mapping the multi-weight surface to a Lyapunov energy surface

$$E = -\tfrac{1}{2}\sum_i [\sum_{j \neq i} v_i w_{ij} v_j - (I_i - U_i) v_i], \tag{6.2.3}$$

where the I_i denote input values and the U_i threshold conditions derived from some relation such as the above.

Nevertheless, it is notoriously difficult to obtain exact solutions for optimization problems of this type analytically, while iterative approximations require termination heuristics as well as exponentially increasing amounts of machine time as the number of units to be processed increases. Though a number of methods different from steepest descent – such as simulated annealing with and without Boltzmann statistics[314] – were proposed, and applied with varying degrees of success, others returned to neurobiology in search of principles to circumvent such difficulties.

Just below the surface of the Hebbian principle lay a number of fruitful questions. For example, the concept of long-term potentiation, so dependent on synapse electrochemistry, arose from attempting to explain the suggested facilitation. For example, the question of what would happen when many of 'cell A', as opposed to a single one, were allowed to excite 'cell B' simultaneously led to the concept of competition, as formulated by Kohonen[11], and to further improvements in modelling. By making the inputs to given cells compete and, in effect, select a single winner – perhaps by equilibrating excitatory and inhibitory v_j's – the matrices of the governing equations can be thinned and both analytical and numerical methods considerably simplified. Normally, instead of systems of linear algebraic equations, sets of linear first-order ordinary differential equations of the form

$$\frac{dv_i}{dt} = -A_i v_i + B_i + v_i \sum_j I_j \qquad (A_i > 0,\ B_i > 0) \tag{6.2.4}$$

must be solved, with $v_i = 0$ for equilibrium; but this poses little additional difficulty.

The adaptive resonance theory (ART) formulated by Grossberg with Carpenter and others[315] expands on these ideas to simulate such notable mental feats as ignoring irrelevant input, abandoning short-term memories, and storing similar long-term memories in such a way that they may be uniquely recalled. Since this theory is a particularly instructive example of recent psychologically-oriented developments, we shall discuss it briefly below; but, of course, others have contributed important ideas, and in some cases developed related, equally valuable approaches with similar or somewhat different psychological ends in view, *e.g.*, Hecht-Nielsen's counterpropagation pattern recognition[316], Kohonen's self- organizing and associative memory[11], and the parallel distributed processing of Rumelhart and McClelland[9]. Rapid progress, approaching ever closer to true neurobiological structure and function, is now being made throughout this research community[317,61].

ART networks are layered hierarchical systems made up of units resembling the one illustrated in Figure 6.5:

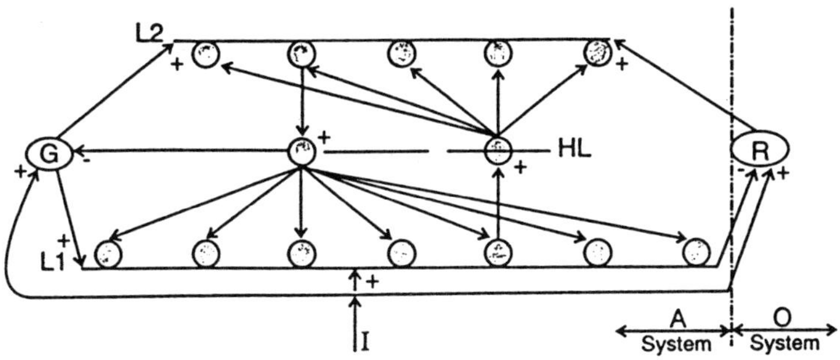

Fig. 6.5 Components of an ART neural network, with gain control (G) included in the attentional subsystem (A) and a reset signal (R) emanating from the orienting subsystem (O). As in the single examples illustrated for clarity, signals from a number of elements in the L_1 layer provide input to individual elements in an intermediate hidden layer (HL) that transmits signals to various elements in the L_2 layer (Instars), which in turn feed signals back through elements in HL to those in L_1(Outstars).

To simplify the diagram only one processing element in the L_1 and L_2 layers is shown connected to a processing element in the HL layer, though every element in both is actually connected in this way, as well as to gain and reset circuits, and may therefore form feedback loops with others in the same layer. Instars and Outstars may be treated as processing units on which many inputs v_j converge and whose output v_i declines exponentially from its equilibrium value at time t_0:

$$v_i = v_{i0} \exp\{-A_i(t - t_0)\}, \tag{6.2.5}$$

with v_{i0} and the positive constant A_i determined by the governing differential equations:

$$\frac{dv_i}{dt} = -A_i v_i + B_i \sum_{j \neq i} w_{ij} v_j, \tag{6.2.6}$$

where the B_i are also positive constants, and all other quantities vary with time. They may be assembled in competitive networks with a single winning output, determined perhaps by the largest net input of a v_j. Because of the built-in damping effect, they possess a short-term memory that can be reinforced to recognize a specific pattern, thereby simulating one requirement for the awareness component of consciousness. When training signals are received, the output of the network is determined by similar equations except for the addition of terms $C_i x_i$, where $C_i > 0$, due to these signals, which enhance the competitive thinning of forward propagating signals in the hidden layer.

$$\frac{dv_i}{dt} = -A_i v_i + B_i \sum_{j \neq i} w_{ij} v_j + C_i x_i \tag{6.2.7}$$

Because of these properties ART networks can support a form of Hebbian facilitation and long-term potentiation, and may be regarded as a kind of minimal neural unit circuit analogous to those observed in microanatomical studies of the mammalian cortex[318], other types of which will be discussed in the following sections. When an input pattern vector is applied to the circuit, signals circulate among the two layers, constituting a short-term memory trace; but repeated applications of the vector cause these to tend toward an adaptive resonant state, which then alters the weights w_{ij} and produces a long-term memory of the pattern that allows it to be recognized and recalled quickly without recourse to the process if presented again, thereby simulating one requirement for the volitional component of consciousness.

Elaborations of this circuit, together with the development of the above and other equations to model the various processes, have enabled Grossberg and Carpenter to make impressive progress toward understanding the actual neural mechanisms underlying such cognitive phenomena as pattern recognition and discrimination, the time-dependence of memory, the plasticity of learning, and the direction of attention[315].

But inspired by somewhat different aspects of the rapidly expanding state of knowledge in the cognitive and neurosciences, a number of other investigators have developed alternate methodologies which remain close to actual neurons and neural architecture. The Neocognitron, a multi-layered sequential convergence circuit for feature extraction and character recognition developed by Fukushima[319], is representative of such methods. Though inspired by Hubel and Wiesel's discovery of columnar neural structures in the visual cortex entirely devoted to identifying straight line and corner segments oriented in different directions[318], this model also features simplified versions of the optical pathways and pattern compression demonstrated to occur in intermediate brain structures, such as the lateral geniculate nuclei.

The general scheme is illustrated in Figure 6.6, showing how such features extracted from the letter Y by the processing elements of the first layer converge on specific elements of the next layer, which in turn converge on an element in the final layer to identify that particular letter.

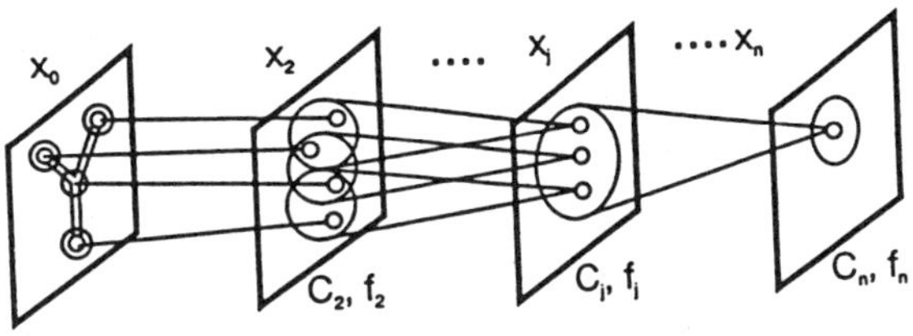

Fig. 6.6 Successively convergent stages of feature extraction performed by the Neocognitron.

Inputs to the elements are weighted and designated either excitatory or inhibitory. They can be biased in the usual way and the elements of the different layers can be connected electrically. But they can also be interconnected optically as pixels in a light-sensitive array, which makes the neocognitron a leading candidate for implementation on the optical computing systems currently under development by a number of university and industrial organizations[320].

Still other investigators have mounted frontal attacks on the higher brain functions revealed by neuroscience and cognitive science research, deviating further from microstructural detail, but bringing to bear powerful methods from the engineering, physical and mathematical sciences, such as those of systems theory and signal processing, the theory of collective phenomena, quantum mechanics and, more recently, chaos and complexity theory[57,201,321–324]. Concepts evolved in this way, as well as in the foregoing manner, will appear in subsequent sections and will be fully explained and referenced in context.

6.3 Electrochemical Neurons and Networks

Though great progress has been made in artificial intelligence during the last decade by implementing logical processes on conventional computing machines[325], it is widely recognized that this development is only loosely connected with neurobiology[157]. For some applications this lack of correspondence with the neural structures utilized by living creatures does not seem to matter, and may in fact represent an improvement on the systems nature has evolved. Expert system technology, for example, seems capable of more efficient rule-based searches of very large databases than the human brain[299], and properly trained neural networks can excel human operators in certain types of pattern recognition, such as signal processing[8].

In other cases, however, the limitations imposed by existing computer components and architectures may make it extremely difficult if not impossible to reproduce the functions of animal brains, especially those involving the various aspects of consciousness. The most advanced connectionist and other types of neural networks require unrealistic training times, parallel systems offer small, but perhaps some hope of achieving the degree of associative coordination required for creative thought[9], and computer consciousness is limited at present to the realm of science fiction. While the desirability of even attempting to achieve the latter for computers may be questionable, there seems little doubt that it could be controlled should it arise as an emergent property of increasing complexity[326]; and certainly the efficient simulation of human learning, goal-directed and associative capabilities are accepted as important goals of the computing and brain sciences[327].

For these reasons it is worthwhile to ask what characteristics of neurobiological systems, as opposed to digital computing systems, might be responsible for the above limitations, and several candidates immediately become apparent. The most obvious is that digital computers function entirely electrically, while brains function mainly electrochemically, primarily because neurons are analog/digital devices driven by this means. But their overall function, simplified in various ways, can be simulated in software on conventional computers, as the examples discussed in the two preceding Sections should establish; and integrated circuit 'neuron' chips intended for more realistic computer architectures are even now being fabricated and tested[328,329].

The latter, however, remain entirely electrical in character, featuring 'neural' junctions addressed at matrix nodal points with complex supplemental circuitry to provide for variable weights and delay times. But much of the performance of real neurobiological networks depends on the metabolic processes of the neurons, as well as their supporting cells, and on the electrochemical functions of their synaptic connections. Simulation of these is another matter.

In particular, the refractory period of a neuron, including its firing frequency under continuing stimulation, is controlled by metabolic delays from about 5 to 50 msec; and all synaptic connections to and from other neurons operate by the transmission of potentials across a synaptic cleft, a gap from a few to several hundred angstroms wide filled with extracellular fluid. Those with the wider gaps (200-300 A) pass no current directly but rely on the diffusion of neurotransmitter substances, such as acetylcholine (ACh) and gamma aminobutyric acid (GABA), to generate graded potentials at the postsynaptic membrane by altering its permeability. These may greatly outnumber the tight electrical connections with narrow gaps (20-30 A) in mammalian nervous systems[69].

Synapses of this type further slow execution times, requiring an average of 0.5 msec to function. Together with the refractory behavior of the neuron, this imposes a time scale widely different from the nano/picosecond scale of purely electronic systems. Equally important, they allow the organic changes at the junctions required for the adjustment of weights and the establishment of long term memories; and, by allowing the differing chemical reactions of a wide variety of neurotransmitters to influence transmission, they provide a vital link to the hormonal systems of the brain, on which emotional and other components of its function critically depend.

There are, of course, other basic properties of neural systems that affect their performance in possibly critical ways, such as their organization in unit circuits containing internal feedback loops, information transfer by global and localized electromagnetic waves, the probabilistic firing and variable response of neurons, their post-firing refractory behavior and their diffusion-limited communication. All of these established properties have been studied and the results presented in earlier publications[158], in part by the authors[311,330].

All of these characteristics imply a fundamental dependence on electrolytic chemistry. It is this fact that suggested the attempt summarized below to illustrate some of the issues[331,332] involved in developing a device capable of simulating neural functions more directly by incorporating electrochemical processes. But developed further, fully miniaturized and connected in integrated circuits, such 'electrochemical transistor' chips could open a new era in biocomputing.

An Artificial Neuron

Initially, the synapse of the neuron was greatly simplified, retaining little but its electrolytic character. Based on the exploratory 'memistor' work of Widrow[128], a series of experiments was performed with a junction consisting of small copper wire embedded in an insulating block and separated from a flat copper plate by a thin layer of copper sulphate solution. Though exhibiting desirable current vs.time characteristics, in particular a well-defined 'gating' pulse, corrosion proved to be a serious problem. Dendritic growths soon formed on the active electrode surface causing shorting of the device. However, when an aqueous potassium ferro/ferric cyanide electrolyte, containing Fe^{2+}/Fe^{3+} instead of Cu^{2+} ions, was used to fill the synaptic gap, no corrosion occurred for either cyclic testing or prolonged current flow. Similar results were obtained when, to simplify eventual packaging of the device and possibly increase its lifetime, the mobile ions were dispersed in an inert gel.

Subsequently, guided by a comprehensive physical/chemical model developed concurrently[6], several sets of wafers featuring Pd/Au integrated circuits with photoresist insulation were fabricated and used for all of the remaining tests. These miniaturized junctions, approximately two-dimensional but otherwise configured much the same as the above, yielded current spikes two orders of magnitude greater than the following steady-state current. Although corroding in the same way when aqueous $PdSO^4$ was the electrolyte, they showed no signs of dendritic growth when the Fe^{2+}/Fe^{3+}-rich potassium ferro/ferric cyanide solution was substituted[49,332].

These preliminary studies defined the objectives of the experimental work: (1) conversion of the 'action potential' arriving at the 'presynaptic' electrode of the device to a 'graded potential' at the receiving 'postsynaptic' electrode, (2) introduction of a 'synaptic' delay time of approximately 0.5 msec and a refractory period between 5 and 50 msec characteristic of neurobiological responses, and (3) the creation of electrochemical methods to simulate the neurochemical interactions underlying 'excitatory' and 'inhibitory' responses, 'weight' changes, 'long-term potentiation', and the permanent organic changes of long-term memory. Procedures by which these objectives might be achieved are outlined below.

Devising a practical method to control the properties of the electrolyte to simulate such neural functions is a critical requirement. Interpreting the layer separating the electrodes as the control 'wire' of a triode junction, an obvious possibility is to initiate chemical activity electrically by applying a separate voltage to the region. Ideally, however, to simplify the circuitry required, the device should be self-contained; that is, ionic and molecular activity subsequent to the arrival of a stimulating potential should be controlled entirely by reactions induced in the electrolyte. Two approaches are suggested: reconfiguring the original device and sol-gel coating the electrodes; or introducing electrochromic electrolyte technology [333–335,127].

In both cases, rather than using uniform plane electrodes, metal could be patterned on the glass substrates to provide a large number of junctions for supplying incremental pulses of potential. Delay times are, of course, a function of the thickness of the electrolytic layer; and in a simple two electrode-plus-electrolyte junction the refractory period is similar to the delay time, corresponding to the time taken for ion gradients to relax. But with the addition of an electrochromic layer or another reactive gel layer acting as a reservoir, the field-off relaxation time could no doubt be extended beyond the field-on response time to approximate a refractory period of at least 50 msec, with further improvement possible.

The graded potential could possibly be achieved by optical read-out of the electrochromic layer, since a series of short pulses will build up color density. It might also be possible to exploit other gel layers to produce a graded effect. A chargeable electrode, such as polypyrrole or polyaniline, subjected to a series of pulses will convert from a semiconducting to a conducting state capable of supporting a current.

Reversible and irreversible weight changes associated with long-term potentiation or permanent organic change will require electrodynamic modification of the junctions; but this could be accomplished by applying higher potentials to allow temporary or permanent chemical deposition on one or other electrode, or by modifying the optical readout system.

Excitatory and inhibitory responses could be produced by changing the position of the gel layer with respect to the current. With an optical readout, an inhibitory junction would have ions driven out of the layer, resulting in a color decrease. Similarly, with an electrochemical readout the removal of ions would decrease the conductivity of the gel. The simplest way to achieve these effects would be to reverse the pulse direction for one particular junction, which could easily be accomplished since the readout circuit would be separate from the input pulse circuit. Alternatively, it might prove preferable to produce two different types of devices, either with different electrolyte compositions, or with junctions having the gel layer on opposite faces of the cell.

Concurrently with such experimental work, the mathematical model developed earlier[6] must be modified and extended, both in order to guide device design and to facilitate comparison with neuron and neural network functions. But when devices developed in the manner described, or by some alternative approach, are available and fully characterized they can then be interconnected to form several of the common neural networks described in the preceding Sections. Then, with the help of this model their performance could be compared with that of these software systems and their additional capabilities documented.

6.4 Some Simple Networks in the Brain

In recent years results achieved by a number of skilled investigators have revealed that each of the three main divisions of the human cortex may be subdivided into interconnecting columns or zones based on the primary pyramidal or Purkinje output cells they contain[100,304,75,93]. Further, there is evidence that the columns of the cerebrum and zones of the allocortex and cerebellum are composed of sub-networks, commonly called unit circuits[310], each of which consists of a single pyramidal or

Purkinje cell linked to an adjacent group of excitatory and inhibitory cells in such a way that internal feedback loops are formed. From the smaller numbers of cortical layers in lower animals, the reduced neuron densities within these layers, and the known evolutionary strategy of multiplying successful forms, it seems reasonable to suppose that the brain has evolved in part by discovering such a circuit, reproducing and interconnecting it within an existing layer of the cortex, then with suitable modifications, in and between new layers as they were added.

Accordingly, considerable interest attaches to the functional properties of unit circuits and their assemblies, for these may so condition the operation of the brain that mental processes can not be properly understood without them. Indeed, to the extent that the model summarized below, which was created to explore these properties[311], eliminates the need for such operational procedures as back-propagation in neural network applications, and facilitates the incorporation of quantum statistical effects and non-synaptic extracellular communication by means of global potential waves, such a conjecture seems well justified.

As an effective means of simplification, the activity of every neuron in the unit circuits that follow is restricted to a set of discrete levels, its state at any time being represented by an activation level a which takes 10 integral values, and may be regarded as a nonlinear function of the membrane potential V in or near the axon hillock. The values of a may be chosen to describe the normal course of an action potential as accurately as required using, for example, a formula of the type

$$V = V_o \exp(Ka) \tag{6.4.1}$$

V_o and K being selected as suitable constants. The lowest level ($a = 0$) is reached immediately following an action potential ($a = 10$). Then the neuron enters a series of refractory states in which there is an automatic ascent from one level to the next above at subsequent time intervals (τ). In a refractory state the neuron is insensitive to external stimuli of any kind, until the lowest resting level ($a = 7$) is attained. Thereafter the level may be changed by synaptic or extracellular transmission, by a positive integer if the transmission is excitatory or by a negative integer if it is inhibitory. The effect is that the activation level a_j $(t + \tau)$ of the j-th neuron at time $t + \tau$ is related to $a_j(t)$ and the levels $a_k(t)$ of other neurons that form synapses with the j-th neuron by the equation

$$a_j(t+\tau) = a_j(t)+d_j(t)+x_j(t)\, i_j(t)+\sum_k i_j(t)\, w_{jk} o_k(t+\tau_k) \pmod{10} \tag{6.4.2}$$

wherein:

(i) The term $d_j(t)$ is 0 if $a_j(t) = 7$, 8 or 9 for the resting states, but is 1 if $a_j(t)$ has any of the values 0 - 6 of the refractory states., thereby taking account of the automatic changes of level resulting from an action potential. By treating the right side of the equation (mod 10) we ensure that only integral values between 0 and 9 will result from the computation. In the same way as level 10 is immediately reduced to level 0, the lowest refractory level, for any excitation exceeding level 10 by an integer a, the neuron is immediately transferred to a level a that is correspondingly higher in the refractory range.

(ii) The variable $x_j(t)$ is an integer varying with the amplitude of any component of the extracellular field to which the j-th cell may be sensitive, positive if the component is excitatory, or negative if it is inhibitory. The input variable $i_j(t)$ has the value 1 if the j-th neuron is in a resting state, or 0 otherwise; this ensures that only the automatic changes of level are effective, since it multiplies all of the remaining terms.

(iii) The summation of the last term takes account of excitations and inhibitions of the j-th neuron by the k neurons that synapse on it, that is, those for which the weighting factor w_{jk} is not 0. The value of w_{jk} is some integer that measures the intensity of excitation, positive if the synapse formed by the k-th neuron is excitatory but negative if it is inhibitory; and though taken to be independent of time during normal computational cycles, it can be changed discretely by learning processes to accommodate synaptic plasticity.

(iv) As a matter of computational convenience for sequential processing by conventional computers, the output variable $o_k(t)$ is defined to be 1 if the k-th neuron passes through the firing state at time t but 0 otherwise. The time interval τ_k is chosen so that the value $o_k(t+\tau_k)$ corresponds to the time at which the activation level a_k was last calculated from (6.4.2) by substituting the successive values of j required. In this case the order of enumeration of the neurons within the circuit being processed is not arbitrary but must be chosen in such a way as to satisfy this requirement. These restrictions could be relaxed, however, by adapting the model for parallel processing.

This notation agrees as closely as possible with that in common use for neural network research[9], but the given equations represent significant generalizations in several respects. Usually only two activation levels are considered; but with efficient programming the increase in the number of levels does not unduly restrict the size of the network that can be processed, nor greatly increase the time required to do so; and introduction of the input variable $i_j\,(t)$ obviously contributes to the realism of the simulation. Also, we have shown[311] that (6.4.2) may be derived by techniques borrowed from quantum field theory and statistical mechanics, which is useful for analyzing some of the more obscure neural network functions and for quantitative treatment of extracellular field effects.

As suggested above, global potential waves arising from extracellular field effects also fall within the scope of the model. The energy of these fields is assumed to be derived ultimately from the ongoing metabolic activity of the neural cells, stored in electrostatic form in their membranes, and released from time to time in the course of action potentials, graded potentials, and extracellular transmissions. Since the last component is itself produced by intracellular potentials, periodic extracellular potentials independent of synaptic transmission will be generated, resulting perhaps in synaptic processes of the same frequency which can be recognized by the presence of periodic spikes in extracellular records. Experimental evidence indicates that much spike activity is clearly synchronized with rhythmic potentials of this type[336,95]. To evaluate their effects on the functioning of the networks considered, the coefficients $x_j\,(t)$ in (6.4.2) are assumed to be of the form

$$x_j\,(t) = \mathrm{int}[p_j \sin(\omega_j t + \delta_j)] \tag{6.4.3}$$

where 'int' denotes the integral part of the expression that follows. More generally, a sum of such terms may be used, and the amplitudes p_j and phases δ_j are in principle to be determined from the position and geometry of the cells.

A great deal of evidence consistent with theoretical expectations exists that bears on the propagation of periodic potentials through the cortex and the sensitivity of individual neurons to them[100,337,95]. There are, among other possible modes, natural paths of conduction along the parallel fibers of the molecular layer and other long fibers responsible for axonal transmission between different regions of the brain, such as those terminating in the granular layers of the cerebellum and allocortex, and in Layer IV of the sensory cortex containing the spiny stellate cells. And since much of the space between neurons is occupied by glial cells, whose surfaces are roughly parallel to and normally less than 200 A from the surfaces of the neurons, it is also possible for potentials to be transmitted over shorter distances by polarization and conduction over their outer surfaces. This means that the granule and spiny stellate cells, which may be the principal repositories of memory, can easily be affected by such periodic potentials and must be modeled accordingly.

Cerebellar Functions

In this Section discussion will be confined to a typical zone of the cerebellum, each one of which serves some special purpose for muscular control and is made up of interconnecting unit circuits of the kind illustrated in Figure 6.7. This configuration was derived from descriptions given by Eccles, Palay and Chan Palay, Ito, Szentagothai, and others [100,64,60,338]. However, similar information is available for the cerebrum and allocortex and corresponding results have been obtained for these, as well as for simplified networks consisting of combinations of all three types of unit circuits[311].

Each cerebellar unit is based on a single Purkinje cell; but it should be stressed that, though all other common types of cerebellar neurons are included together with their known synaptic connections, the number of each type – especially of granule cells – is much less than actually observed. Those shown must be regarded only as representative and their connections as only partly proven. But it is well established that the Purkinje cells (P) provide the essential output of such units and exercise an important degree of control over motor activity initiated in the cerebral cortex, constituting thereby a form of operational memory for the repetition of specific patterns of muscular motions. operational memory for the repetition of specific patterns of muscular motions.

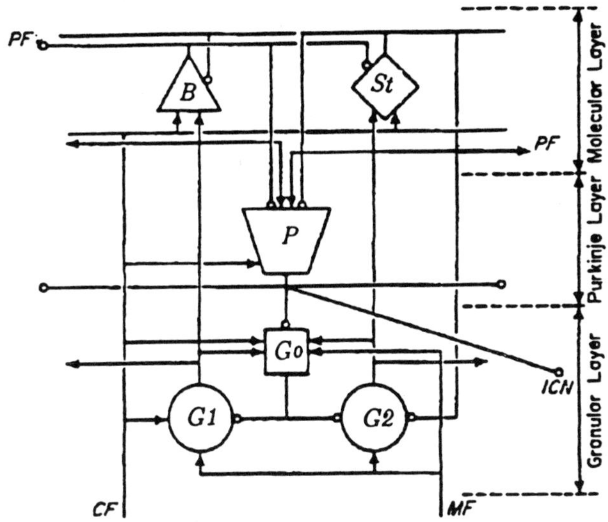

Fig. 6.7 Diagram for the unit circuit of the cerebellum, showing the climbing and mossy input fibres (CF, MF) and connecting parallel fibres (PF), the excitatory granule cells ($G1$, $G2$) and stellate cells (St), the inhibitory Golgi cells and Basket cells (B), and the Purkinje cell (P) with its output to the intercerebellar nuclei (ICN). Arrowheads and small circles indicate excitatory and inhibitory junctions and fibres.

Thus, the possibility of long-term potentiation and modification of certain synaptic junctions in the units must be included, and is provided in the model by the multiplicity of resting levels and the modifiable weights w_{jk}. There are many synapses in the cerebellum that exhibit modifications as the brain ages, perhaps the most striking of which are those formed by the climbing fiber (CF) on the Purkinje cell, and the rosettes formed by the mossy fiber (MF) at its synapses with the granule cells ($G1$ and $G2$).

If a neuron is repeatedly left in a potentiated state above the lowest resting level as a result of an external stimulus, the weights responsible are increased by an amount proportional to the difference between the two levels, making it more likely for the neuron to fire due to any synaptic or extracellular stimulus of the same type; that is, both w_{jk}

and x_j are treated as subject to modification. Evidently, this is an adaptation of Hebb's Rule[101], which is made even more explicit by requiring quantum indeterminacy to govern the final firing. The results shown below, derived by means of the learning process described for the circuit of Fig. 6.7, and produced by a computer program [see Appendix A6.4] based on the model, clearly demonstrate the importance of the synaptic plasticity associated with this Rule:

	CF	MF	G1	G2	B	St	Go	P	Ex	Input	Program
CF	0	0	0	0	0	0	0	0	3	(a)	CF,G1,B,St,Go
MF	0	0	0	0	0	0	0	0	3	(b)	MF,Go
G1	5	2	0	0	0	0	-3	0	2	(c+)	St
G2	0	2	0	0	0	-1	-3	0	2	(d+)	Go
B	1	0	3	0	0	-1	0	0	0	(a,c+)	CF,G1,B,St,Go,P
St	4	0	0	1	-1	0	0	0	3	(a,c−)	CF,G1,B,Go
Go	0	3	3	1	0	0	0	-2	3	(b,d+)	MF,G1,G2,B,Go,P
P	5	0	4	4	-5	-4	0	0	4	(b,d−)	MF

Table 6.2 On the left, synaptic weights and extracellular input for a trained cerebellar unit circuit. Source of the input in the topmost row (Ex for extracellular source), destination of each input in the leftmost column. On the right, the program executed by the circuit for various types of input.

The matrix w contains values of w_{jk} resulting from the synaptic input from cells shown above the matrix to those listed on the left, while the vector shown to the right contains the values of x_j representing input to the CF and MF fibres and maximum extracellular input to various cells. The values displayed are the final stabilized result of a simulated course of training during which the cerebellar unit circuit was subjected to a predetermined combination of external stimuli associated with a specific muscular action. Initially the matrix elements were all either 0 (where there would be no synaptic input from the k-th to the j-th neuron), 1 (where the input would be excitatory) or -1 (where the input would be inhibitory), as determined by the neurons and the circuit configuration.

Of special interest is the fact that on reaching the stable state after repeated cycling, the unit becomes capable of executing a number of different but definite firing sequences. By analogy with computing terminology these may be thought of as programs, since for stable values of the weights of the matrix w and excitations of the vector x they are completely determined by the type of ordered external input. Some of these programs are listed in Table 6.2 above, which shows the neurons that fire in response to the external inputs, and certain combinations of them, labeled as follows: (a) synaptic from CF, (b) synaptic from MF, (c) extracellular to St, B and P cells in the molecular layer, (d) extracellular to Go, $G1$ and $G2$ cells in the granular layer. Of course all cells begin and end in their lowest unpotentiated states.

Clearly the granule cells are the primary excitatory cells of the unit and their sensitization can be seen to play a key role in the development of the programs affecting the Purkinje cells. Additionally, as indicated in Figure 6.7, the longitudinal fibers formed by their axons make synaptic contacts with other unit circuits of the zone — in particular, with their Purkinje cells — and thus affect its overall pattern of activity. These observations, together with the great numerical preponderance of the granule cells, strongly suggest that they may be the principal repository of cerebellar memory. It is notable, however, that even though prior to training pure extracellular input has no effect on a Purkinje cell, afterward it will fire only if both synaptic and excitatory extracellular inputs are present. This is largely because of the inhibitory effects of the Golgi, stellate and basket cells, the last of which also synapse on the Purkinje cells of adjacent units and tend to inhibit their firing. Considered in isolation, it might seem that the cerebellar unit circuit is unnecessarily complicated; but when a zonal circuit such as the one to be described in Section 6.5 is formed, it becomes apparent that every neuron has an important and distinctive role to play in the programs the zone is capable of executing because of its particular type and the internal and external connections it makes.

The model can easily be applied to an assembly of 16 such circuits, for example, with synaptic weights of -5 for the basket cells and $+3$ for the granule cells connecting to the Purkinje cells of adjacent units. Then if processed in the order and manner shown below, with external inputs of the foregoing type, programs analogous to those of Table 6.2 evolve; two of these are displayed simply as patterns of output from the Purkinje cells of the units indicated in Table 6.3:

Number of circuit								Pattern of input							
1	3	5	7	9	11	13	15	0	+	0	−	0	+	0	−
2	4	6	8	10	12	14	16	0	+	0	−	0	+	0	−

Input	Output
(a),(c)	3,11
(b),(d)	3,5,6,11,13,14,1,2,9,10

Table 6.3 Above left, the numbering of the unit circuits in the cerebellar zone, and right, the assumed pattern of extracellular input. Below, the representative firing sequences, or programs, executed by the stabilized system.

Again no Purkinje cell fires if the input is purely synaptic of type (a) or (b), or purely extracellular of type (c) or (d), the additional excitatory effect of the granule cells on units in the same row being counteracted by the inhibitory effect of basket cells in the same column. This makes it easy to infer the effects of the interaction of an extracellular potential wave within the zone; as the wave advances from left to right, the extracellular input pattern on the right side will also advance, causing the output pattern to change in a corresponding manner, and creating a dynamical pattern of inhibition and facilitation in the accompanying electromagnetic field.

Circuits and Programs of the Cerebrum and Allocortex

As might be expected from evolutionary considerations, the mammalian cerebral cortex is more complex than the cerebellum, not only because of the greater number and variety of neurons present in a typical column, but also on account of variations in the organization of regions responsible for sensory, motor and related association functions. The allocortex has less neural variety and a simpler structure, though mediating most of the higher brain processes by its special functions. It is possible, nevertheless, to develop simple models for both based on characteristic unit circuits derived from the neurobiological data in the literature[100,338]. These circuits, together with descriptions of the neurons they contain (Figures 6.8 and 6.9) and some of the programs they are capable of executing, after stabilization in response to certain combinations of the external inputs (Tables 6.4 and 6.5) are discussed briefly below.

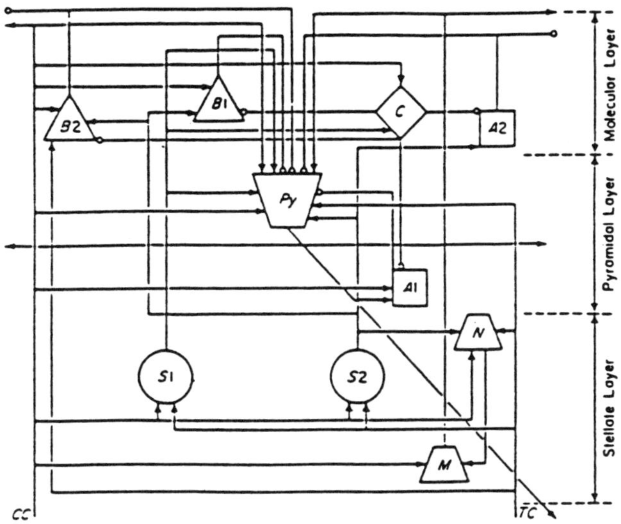

Fig. 6.8 Diagram of a model unit circuit of the cerebrum, showing the corticortical (CC) and thalmocortical (TC) input fibres, the excitatory spiny stellate cells ($S1$, $S2$), Martinotti cells (M) and neurogliaform cells (N), the inhibitory basket cells ($B1$, $B2$), double bouquet cells (C), and axoaxonic and axonal cells ($A1$,$A2$). The excitatory pyramidal cell (Py) transmits the output of the circuit to other circuits.

The pyramidal neuron (Py), the primary focal cell of this unit circuit, differs from the Purkinje neuron of the cerebellar circuit by having an excitatory rather than an inhibitory output; and the external synaptic input to the unit is from the corticocortical (CC) and thalamocortical (TC) fibers instead of climbing and mossy fibers. The small excitatory spiny stellate neurons, ($S1$) and ($S2$), clearly have the same role in this unit as the granule cells of the cerebellum; and the inhibitory axoaxonic and axonal tuft cells, ($A1$) and ($A2$), are well placed to play the same parts as the Golgi and stellate cells. However, two basket cells, ($B1$) and ($B2$), are required instead of one; and the excitatory Marinotti (M) and neurogliaform (N) cells, together with an inhibitory double bouquet neuron (C) have no apparent cerebellar analogues. A few of the more instructive programs resulting from the following types of inputs are listed in Table 6.4: (a) synaptic to CC, (b) synaptic to TC, (c) extracellular to Py and $A2$, (d) extracellular to $S1$, $S2$ and $A1$.

It is evident that because a potential wave will act on inhibitory as well as excitatory neurons in the same layer, a purely extracellular input has no effect on the pyramidal cell; but inhibition resulting from such input is necessary to allow it to fire when the excitatory Marinotti and neurogliaform cells fire in response to stimulation of the cortico-cortical and thalamocortical fibers. The semicolon in each of the last two programs denotes an increment τ in the processing time t, which will be seen in the following Section to have significant implications for the ability of the model to simulate sequential and recursive activity. It is important to note that when columns are formed of circuits of this type, each one, though still capable of suppressing the activity of adjacent columns, seems to act more independently than the zones of the cerebellum.

Input	Program
(a)	CC,S1,S2,M,N,A1,B1,B2,C,P
(b)	TC,S1,S2,N,B2,C,P,M
(c+)	A2
(d+)	S1,S2,N,A1,B2,C,M
(a,c+)	CC,S1,S2,M,N,A1,A2,B1,B2,C,P
(a,c−)	CC,S1,S2,M,N,A1,B1,B2,C
(b,d+)	TC,S1,S2,N,A1,B2,C;M,P
(b,d−)	TC,N,B2;M,P

Table 6.4 Programs executed by the cerebral circuit, for different inputs as described in text.

The process of sensitization of a set of 12 typical cells forming a unit circuit of the cerebrum is modelled in the second of a complete set of three computer programs [see Appendix A6.4]. When this program is run, the initial values (-1, 0, and 1) of the synaptic weights are progressively changed to the values attained in the programs representing the final function of the unit. After a complete cycle of activation and firing, each cell of the circuit returns to its lowest resting state.

The third of the programs mentioned is similar, but relates to the training of an analogous (hippocampal) unit of the allocortex shown below. The perforant pathway (PP) from a sensory region of the cerebral cortex features fibers analogous to the above thalamocortical fibers, and the commissural pathway (CP) from the septum introduces fibers analogous to those called corticocortical. The granule cells, of which only one, (Gr), is included, are adjacent to the molecular layer and provide an important excitatory input to the nearest and largest of a chain of pyramidal cells, ($P1$) and ($P2$); however, three of the basket cells, ($B1$, $B2$ and $B3$), are also included to provide the required inhibitory constraints. The illustrative programs generated by combinations of external inputs: (a) to CP, (b) to PP, (c) to Gr and $B1$, (d) to $P1$ and $B3$ are listed in Table 6.5; but in this case, since it is known that stimulation of the commissural pathway activates excitatory and inhibitory cells in both layers [95], the extracellular θ-rhythm is included and appropriate sequences applied, e.g, (a); (b); (a,c+); (a,c-):

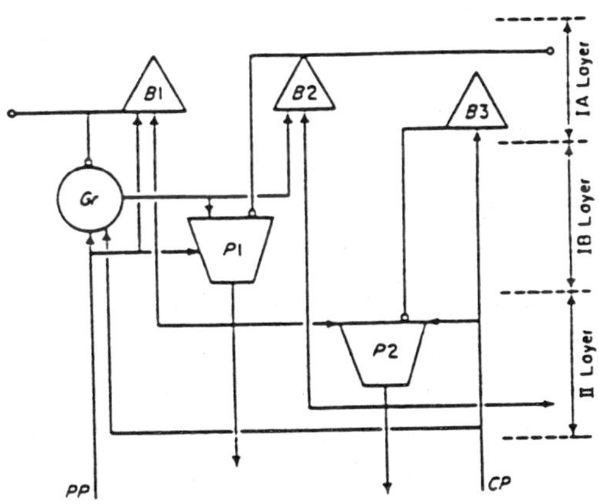

Fig. 6.9 Diagram of the unit circuit for the allocortex showing the input fibres of the perforant pathway (PP) and commissural pathway (CP), the excitatory granule cell (Gr), the inhibitory basket cells ($B1$, $B2$, $B3$), and the pyramidal cells ($P1$, $P2$) with their internal and external outputs.

Input	Program
(a)	CP, Gr, B2, B3
(b)	PP, Gr, B1, B2, P1,P2
(c+)	B3
(d−)	Gr, B1, B2
(a,c−)	CP, Gr, B2
(a,c+)	CP, Gr, B2, B3, P2
(b,d−)	PP, P1, P2, B1, B2
(b,d+)	PP, Gr, B1, B2, P1, P2

Table 6.5 Programs executed by a circuit of the allocortex following various types of input.

Experience gained in the formation of these programs suggests that while synaptic input from the perforant pathway to a unit circuit is required for the firing of the pyramidal neurons, the basket cells also play an important part in inhibiting not only their own but neighbouring units. The formation of memory is modelled in the early stages of running the program, when neurons are frequently left in a potentiated states in which the synaptic weights progressively increase in magnitude. When the synaptic weights have reached their final values, an entire program is repeated automatically whenever the unit receives the same external stimulus, and this is obviously one of the fundamental requirements for the reactivation of memory that has already been formed. In these respects the allocortical circuits do not differ essentially from those in other parts of the brain. However, it is essential that elements of memory should be activated in sequential order, and it is likely that one of the most important functions of the allocortex, in particular of the hippocampus, is to achieve the synchronization of firings with the θ-rhythm through gradually recruiting more and more cells by the processes of sensitization and long-term potentiation[86,87,92,339,340]. In the next Section it will be seen that cells recruited in this way are able to initiate a well-ordered train of activity in other regions of the cortex, and thus contribute significantly to the formation of sequential memory.

6.5 Modelling Cortical Circuits

The transfer equation (6.4.2) of the preceding Section can also be used to model the internal behavior and consequent motor action of a cortical system containing zones of cerebellar, cerebral and allocortical unit circuits as it responds to some sensory stimulus. This is the type of neurobiological activity which has been investigated extensively, primarily by means of EEG techniques[190,341]; and it has been found that the stimulus initiates a complex series of extracellular potentials. The first of these is a 'readiness potential' extending throughout the cortex, which includes a more localized component of the θ-rhythm and has the essential features of wave propagation in the lower frequencies[342,195]. Then, about 50 msec before the motor action is initiated, a contralateral potential localized in the motor cortex appears, as well as complementary activity in the cerebellum. Finally, widespread activity associated with evaluation of the intended motor action develops, which also contains a θ-component.

To highlight the main features of the model, since this can easily be generalized to incorporate the other types of unit circuits, a zonal cerebellar model will be discussed in some detail below. First, however, it is important to note that when a composite system is constructed and subjected to such sensory stimuli, stable programs result from appropriate training resembling those listed earlier for the different types of zonal circuits (Tables 6.2, 6.4 and 6.5, of the previous Section). As will be seen, these lead to rapid identification of a wide variety of input patterns without requiring iterative error correction.

A computer program has been constructed [see Appendix A6.5] that models the action of 256 interconnected cells contained in 28 unit circuits: a set of 4 independent sensory association cerebral type (A_s), a set of 4 independent motor association cerebral type (A_m), a set of 4 independent allocortical type (B), and a set of 16 interconnected cerebellar circuits forming a typical zone (C). Initially the weights w_{jk} of the internal connections within a unit circuit are assumed to be those specified for the cerebellar, allocortical and cerebral circuits in the preceding Section. But to allow individual variations of these matrix elements to develop, connections between different sets are chosen so that when any one of the cerebral set A_s receives a sensory stimulus, its pyramidal 'neuron' Py (Figure 6.8) provides the essential input to a corresponding circuit of B by the perforant pathway PP (Figure 6.9). Next, the pyramid $P2$ of this allocortical circuit of B projects to a corresponding circuit of A_m by way of the thalamocortical fibers TC. The pyramid of this circuit then projects to four of the neighboring cerebellar circuits of C by way of the mossy fibers MF (Figure 6.7).

The resultant motor activity is controlled by the output of the Purkinje cells P of these unit circuits of C; but in addition to the direct connections, a separate feedback connection from each circuit of B to another of A_s is required to provide for sequential and recursive processing. This completes the 'circuit of Papez' and implements the interconnection of all 256 cells. Distant connections of this kind are actually made through various relay nuclei[80,343], but such connections can be replaced by direct connections in the model without affecting the outcome.

After making these connections, the values that have been attained following a course of training are assigned to the non-vanishing weights $w(PP_k, Py_k)$, $w(TC_{k+4}, P2_k)$, $w(MF_{4k-3}, Py_{k+4})$, $w(MF_{4k-2}, Py_{k+4})$, $w(MF_{4k-1}, Py_{k+4})$, $w(MF_{4k}, Py_{k+4})$, and $w(TC_k, P2_{k-1})$; and by allowing the subscript k to vary from 1 to 4, it becomes possible to investigate the relation between the synaptic input to fibers leading to the sensory association set A_s (when $k = 1$) and the pattern of output from the Purkinje neurons of the cerebellar zone C.

As noted earlier, because of the balance between excitatory and inhibitory synaptic input, individual unit circuits remain largely inactive in the absence of extracellular stimuli. The same turns out to be true for the composite system, and even in the presence of synaptic input, the output of the system is strongly influenced by the way the extracellular input varies with time. If the input to the mossy fibers MF of the cerebellar zone C is not well synchronized its output is irregular, but it can be regularized by applying an extracellular stimulus to pivotal cells of the network at intervals exceeding the longest refractory time.

In particular, simulation of a θ-rhythm with a frequency of 5-10 Hz applied to the granular layer of the allocortex circuits evokes a response of the same frequency from those units which have been trained as described in the preceding Section. Since in a lengthy processing sequence a neuron activated more than once must return to its lowest resting state before it is able to function correctly again, this implies a critical need for periodic stimulation in the formation of sequential memory, and suggests an essential role for the hippocampus of the allocortex, which has been observed to generate a θ-rhythm[86,87].

When such a processing sequence is executed by the computer program, in order to train this composite cellular system[311], it becomes apparent that at successive stages various Purkinje and other neurons of the cerebellar units are left in potentiated states and must be further stimulated by an appropriate periodic potential for the system as a whole to reach a minimal resting state analogous to the states described for the separate unit circuits, wherein all four of the $w(TC_k, P2_{k-1})$ have reached the defined training value and all neurons of the cerebellar zone are fully sensitized:

$$TC_1; Py_1, PP_1, P2_1, TC_5; TC_2, Py_5, MF_1, P_1, MF_2, MF_3, P_3, MF_4, P_5, P_6; Py_2, PP_2, P2_2, TC_6; TC_3, Py_6, MF_5, MF_6, MF_7, P_7, MF_8, P_9, P_{10}; Py_3, PP_3, P2_3, TC_7, P_4; TC_4, Py_7, MF_9, MF_{10}, MF_{11}, P_{11}, MF_{12}, P_{13}, P_{14}; Py_4, PP_4, P2_4, TC_8, P_8; Py_8, MF_{13}, MF_{14}, MF_{15}, P_{15}, MF_{16}, P_{16}; P_{12},$$

where the semicolons designate cycle time increments τ, and only those neurons or fibers that receive or transmit impulses between the unit circuits indicated by the subscripts are shown. To attain this stable state it was only necessary to apply an external synaptic input to the first unit of the sensory set A_s a few times, provided an excitatory extracellular stimulus arrived at all of the units affected at the same time.

As this suggests, the activity of the entire system can be visualized as a moving pattern of facilitation which follows the crest of an extracellular excitation wave. Once established by the learning process, such a pattern can be reproduced indefinitely by repetition of the external stimulus in synchrony with this wave, and may therefore be considered a sequence 'memorized' without supervision, though directed toward no specific goal. Moreover, when the program has been learned with participation of the allocortex, the same pattern of Purkinje output can be produced by a suitable input to the motor units of A_m without intervention by the allocortex, which is consistent with the suggestion that the allocortex is essential for the formation but not the retention of memory[93]. It is also clear that, since zones and columns may be defined dynamically and different neuron weights selected by global waves of various frequencies arriving in sequence, the system possesses the capability to store and recall a very large number of such patterns.

The zonal cerebellar network (Figure 6.10), is restricted to a single macrozone containing minizones consisting entirely of cerebellar unit circuits, but has the advantage of allowing the unsupervised learning process to be goal-directed, and thus to learn specified patterns, such as the one provided later in Figure 6.11. The program embodying the model, discussed below, requires only 8 unit circuits in each minizone and 12 such macrozones to function properly; but it is important to emphasize that both of these numbers can easily be increased by one or more orders of magnitude, and may, in fact, be extended to the limit of available machine memory [330]. This flexibility is indicated by the non-terminating lines in the Figure, and by the neuron numbers which increase sequentially for each additional unit circuit.

Of course the model simplifies the actual biological unit in several ways, perhaps most significantly in the numbers of other types of neurons associated with each Purkinje; the two granule cells, for example, are merely representative of a much larger number. Also, its overall operation depends on the particular interconnections shown for the unit circuits, minizones and macrozone. However, both the structure of the unit cerebellar circuit and its extended connections are based on experimental results documented in the literature[100,338]. No doubt additional microanatomical research will be required to confirm and expand these results; but the existence of such self-contained computational neural units containing inhibitory feedback loops and interacting by means of distant connections is well established, and thus sufficient for present purposes.

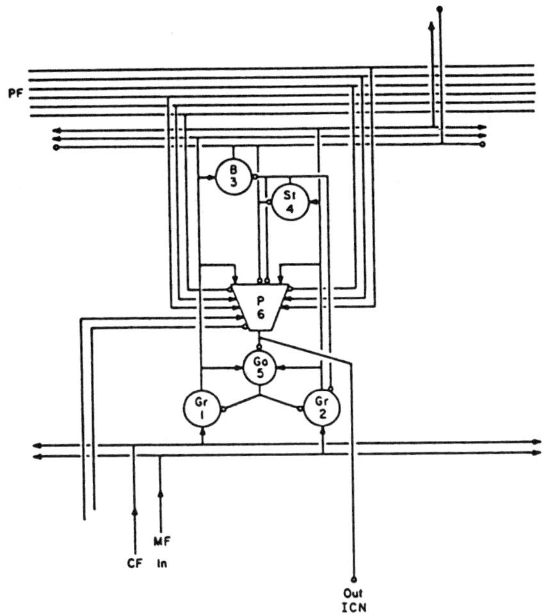

Fig. 6.10 An element of a macrozone network in the cerebellum. Internal connections of the unit circuit are as shown in Fig. 6.7, while long-range connections are suggested by non-terminating lines, non-intersecting crossings by line-breaks, excitatory and inhibitory junctions or fibres by arrowheads or small circles as before.

Depending on the frequency of the synaptic input and, of course, the phase and amplitude of the extracellular component, the number of action potentials delivered in unit time by each of the input fibers CF and MF may be increased from a value just sufficient to cause firing, representing a single pulse, to values producing trains of pulses. Since information is encoded in the frequency of such pulse trains, this is an especially important quantity, and treated as one of the variable parameters of the model . It will be evident in the computer program that processing satisfies the basic equations of the preceding Section, rewritten as the sequence:

$$a_j(t+\tau_o) = a_j(t) + x_j(t),$$
$$a_j(t+\tau_{k+1}) = a_j(t+\tau_k) + i_j(t)w_{jk}o_k(t+\tau_k), (k=0,...,n),$$
$$a_j(t+\tau) = a_j(t+\tau_n) + d_j(t), \tag{6.5.1}$$

where the neuron response obeys the discrete mod 10 activation level function, described earlier and illustrated below. The times $t+\tau_k$ may be regarded as ordering the operations required between the times t and $t+\tau$; but, being cycle times, they do not appear explicitly.

1	2	3	4	5	6	7	8	9	10	11	$\longrightarrow$	1
−9	−8	−7	−6	−5	−4	−3	−2	−1	0	1	$\longrightarrow$	−9

$\longleftarrow$ Refractory $\longrightarrow$ $\leftarrow$Resting$\rightarrow$ $\leftarrow$ Firing

Fig. 6.11 The refractory, resting and firing levels of a neuron. The activation levels may be numbered from 1 to 10 or, equivalently, from -9 to 0. On firing the level is immediately reduced to an equivalent lower level consistent with the mod 10 requirement.

The matrix w_{jk} does not appear explicitly in the program, primarily because in some applications j and k may take values from 1 to 10,000 or more; instead a sparse matrix technique is adopted in which only non-vanishing elements are read from data statements, and repetitions are avoided as far as possible. Hence, data listings are restricted to those for the first unit circuit and automatically indexed upward to include the others. While this means that all unit circuits, like their minizones and connections with others, are identical, the input to different units is generally different, and the weights of all synaptic connections receive individual treatment. Networks composed of different types of circuits can readily be treated by substituting data descriptive of their structure.

The sparse matrix technique has the added advantage that it allows the simulation of parallel processing by any sequential processor. All that is necessary is to list the matrix elements in the temporal order in which the processes they represent are supposed to occur, with excitatory interactions generally preceding inhibitory ones. The arithmetic is further simplified by normalizing $i_j(t)$ and $o_k(t+\tau_k)$ to 1; this eliminates the matrix multiplication implicit in the above equations.

The transfer function identified in the program reflects the conditions established by (6.5.1), while the learning rule represents a modified and more specific form of Hebb's Rule which makes possible a unit change in the weight w_{jk} associated with a particular synapse whenever it transmits a potential that leaves the targeted neuron in a potentiated state. However, this change is not invariable, but occurs with a probability proportional to the difference between the possible potentiated and lowest resting levels, thereby allowing quantum indeterminacy to influence long-term potentiation. The implication is that neither the exact course of learning nor its final result can be predicted with certainty, resulting in the variations of motor action which characterize animal behavior.

The process required for the network to complete its internal adjustments is controlled by the number of iterations needed, which depends in turn on the number of refractory levels the neuron potentials must ascend to reach a resting state, and must be continued until a state of equilibrium is achieved with all connection weights modified to produce a unique output pattern. During this process 'good' features are preserved and 'bad' features allowed to change, judged by whether they are or are not in accord with the numbers representing the original intention; and training is judged to be complete when no further changes in the w_{jk} are possible because no neuron in an active unit is left in a potentiated state.

Unsupervised learning by the program, which is available to the reader as described in the Foreword, is motivated to reproduce the letter 'B', is illustrated in Figure 6.12. In this case the learning rate was set at 30 on a scale from 0 to 100, and the pattern, a graphical substitute for a pattern of intended motor action, was accurately reproduced after 20 iterations, each taking less than a second on an IBM 486-class machine. At the end of the learning process the neurons in all active units were left in their lowest resting states; but some of the inhibitory neurons in other units remained in potentiated states, which is entirely consistent with experimental findings that both presynaptic and postsynaptic stimulation are required for sustained synaptic development, and that long-term potentiation is unlikely to be effective in the absence

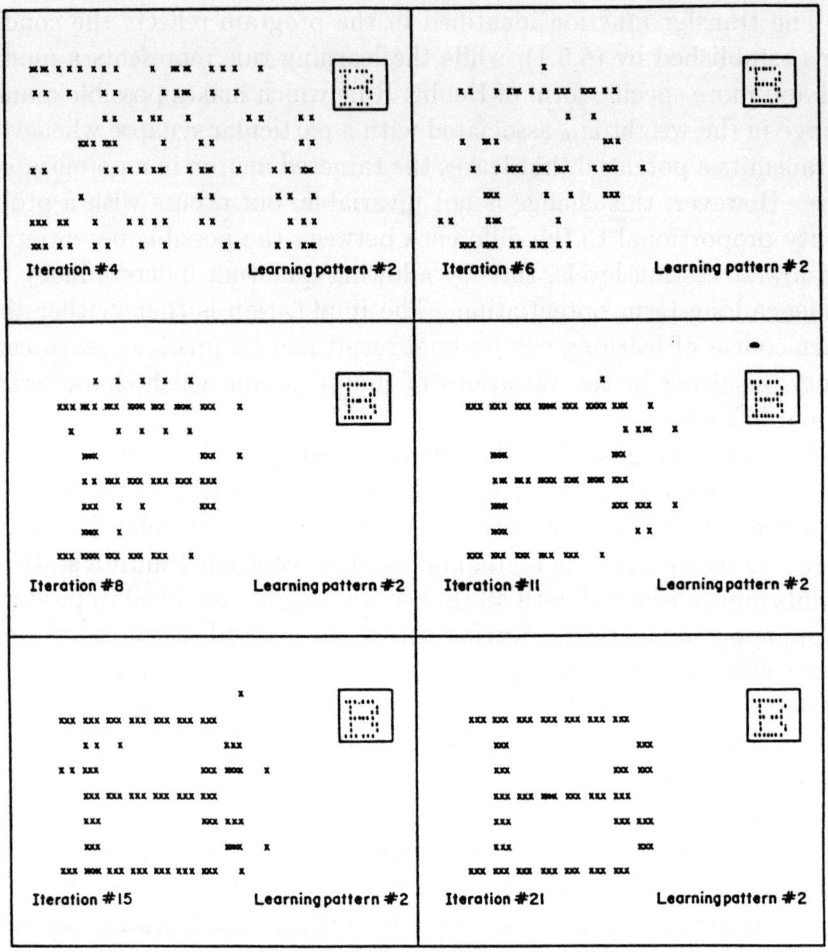

Fig. 6.12 Iteration stages in the simulated learning of the B pattern shown in the top right corner of the panels shown on the computer screen.

of activation[101,344].

It is of interest that, with more rapid rates of learning mistakes are occasionally made, resulting in the omission of one or more points from the pattern to be learned. However, such omissions can almost always be corrected by a second attempt to learn the pattern with a different random input, faithfully reproducing this characteristic of analogous biological systems. The ability of the human brain to assess the value of unintentional mistakes seems to be an essential prerequisite for creativity in nearly all fields of endeavour. Typical frequencies of the weights acquired by the neurons in a representative cerebellar unit circuit in the process of learning a pattern (a) similar to the above, and two others, differing only in having rows of two dots (b) and three dots (c) in the top left-hand corner of the input pattern, are shown in Table 6.6.

Weights	G1	G2	B	St	Go	P		G1	G2	B	St	Go	P
2	31	31	27	19	71	118		26	26	25	29	74	107
-2	6	8	5	9	18	24		15	13	14	13	33	49
3	36	12	12	8	15	39		36	39	8	10	11	32
-3	0	0	0	2	0	2		0	0	3	4	0	6
4	1	2	18	18	21	33		3	2	19	19	22	41

[Pattern (a)] [Pattern (b)]

Weights	G1	G2	B	St	Go	P
2	27	31	24	29	75	130
-2	26	23	19	18	51	76
3	42	37	16	8	16	22
-3	0	0	5	5	2	9
4	1	1	20	20	21	35

[Pattern (c)]

Table 6.6 Frequencies of weights found after cerebellar learning of patterns differing by only one dot.

It may be seen from the Table that the weights of the Purkinje neurons undergo the largest development, followed by those of the Golgi neurons, which supports the contention that the Purkinjes and their associated interneurons constitute the principal locus of memory in the cerebellum. But the frequencies of the granule neurons are also significant, and in view of their overwhelming numbers, they could prove to be even more important[66,99]. Additionally, the frequencies associated with the weights of the Golgi, basket and stellate neurons show a significant increase when the extra dots are included. This suggests that the importance of inhibitory synapses increases with the complexity of the pattern to be learned.

To study the mechanisms of memory in more detail, however, it is preferable to return to the composite system discussed in the beginning and apply the program in a different way. The operation of the sensory association cells A_s and allocortical/hippocampal cells B in matching a pattern such as that shown in Figure 6.12 can be isolated and examined by forming the interconnections illustrated in Figure 6.13 between only the stellate, granule and pyramidal neurons of the appropriate unit circuits.

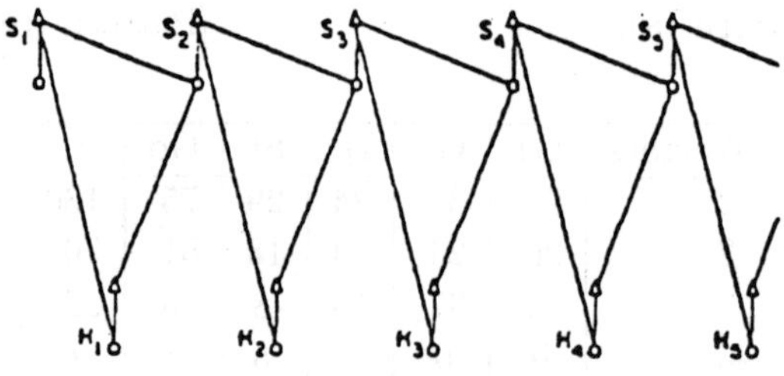

Fig. 6.13 Interconnection of sensory association circuits (S_i) and hippocampal circuits (H_i) with stellate neurons of the former and granule neurons of the latter indicated by small circles. Pyramidal neurons of all circuits are represented by small triangles, and excitatory activation flows from left to right.

The unit circuits S_j are selected to belong to the set of sensitized cells of the association cortex containing pyramidal neurons that are excited to a firing level at the times t_j in the course of processing; and these times are separated by intervals approximating the period of the θ-rhythm generated by the hippocampus, not by the shorter fundamental period τ governing changes in neural activation levels. The unit circuits H_j are selected from the hippocampal projections of the sensory association cells S_j and belong to the subset of circuits in the hippocampus containing granule neurons potentiated as a result of the firing of the cerebral pyramidal neurons. But as shown in the Figure, each of the S_j must also belong to a projection of H_{j-1} back to the cerebrum. In actuality, though they need not be considered in this simplified analysis, these interconnections are made by way of complex systems of nuclei involving the stellate neurons[345].

A sensory impression may be imposed on the system by activating granule neurons of the A_s which have been sensitized enough to insure the firing of their pyramidal neurons and potentiation of their corresponding hippocampal granule neurons. The latter requires a coincidence of this synaptic excitation with the extracellular stimulus provided by the θ-rhythm, as noted above; but it is known[93] that such neurons may remain potentiated for many hours following a combined stimulus of this kind.

If then, assuming the flow of activation to be excitatory and from left to right in the Figure, the sensitized sensory cell S_1 receives a stimulus unrelated to the imposed impression, the potentiated granule cell of H_1 will be raised to a firing level with a probability proportional to its level of potentiation. Simultaneously the cerebral cell S_2 will be activated by S_1 and H_1, and its pyramidal neurons will be raised to a firing level even if, due to inhibitory constraints within the cell, they can not fire in response to a single excitation.

By continuing this process the entire sequence of firings which resulted from the original impression can be recreated without repetition of that impression, merely by activating S_1, constituting thereby a medium-term memory. It also follows that S_1 could be activated by random mental processes, evoking the same impression below the level of consciousness, further increasing the weights of the synapses of the stellate and other neurons of the S_j, and enhancing the probability that their pyramidal neurons will fire in sequence without the necessity of intervention by the hippocampus, thereby constituting a long-term memory. But as will now be evident, no such memory could have been formed if for any reason the action of the hippocampal cells had been impaired, a result in full accord with the findings of neurophysiological investigations[346] and clinical observations[347].

In fact, the computer program simulates the action of a zone in the cerebellum made up of C interconnected minizones (matrix columns), each of which consists of R interconnected unit circuits (matrix rows). The output of the zone is the firing pattern of the Purkinje neurons of the unit circuits, which is progressively modified by a learning process. Climbing fiber and/or mossy fiber input to the minizones is initially random, but is changed in the course of processing if the output pattern does not match a pre-recorded pattern. Minimum weights for specified synapses are modified progressively during learning, and are stored for automatic recall as sparse matrices in sequentially numbered files when learning is complete.

Chapter 7

From Quanta to Consciousness

7.1 Indeterminism in Physics and Biology

Even today there is no generally accepted resolution of the problem of free will, but it is possible to distinguish between various 'idealistic' or deterministic solutions that regard the future as predetermined, and a 'realistic' or indeterministic quantum mechanical solution that assumes no more than our present knowledge can justify.

For a detailed factual account of the genesis of quantum mechanics the reader is referred to the review of van der Waerden[348]. Until 1926 the generally accepted scientific view of the physical world was essentially deterministic, based on Newton's classical laws of mechanics and Faraday and Maxwell's formulation of the laws of electromagnetism. To Maxwell we also owe the idea that light and other forms of radiation that propagate with the velocity of light consist of electromagnetic waves. But this idea was hard to reconcile with Planck's theory of black body radiation, and Bohr's theory of atomic energy levels, according to which electromagnetic radiation was absorbed and emitted in *quanta*. In 1925 this difficulty was resolved in principle when Born and Jordan[34] published the first correct formulation of quantum mechanics. They made use of a proposal by Heisenberg[349] that only observable quantities should play a role in physics, but implemented this by representing all observables as operators (matrices) instead of numerical variables. The energy of an atomic system, for instance, was an operator defined as the agent of changes in time. Their theory was subsequently developed by Born, Jordan, Heisenberg, Pauli and Dirac into what should be regarded as the logical successor of Newton's classical theory, at least in the microscopic domain.

But in 1926, Schrödinger introduced a new and very influential form of quantum theory known as wave mechanics. It was Schrödinger's view that not only light, but atoms and indeed all other forms of matter, consist of waves, and that the fact that they appear in discrete quanta was a consequence of the mathematical properties of his wave equation. He believed in a *universal wave function* that determines the past, present and future, and is therefore consistent with determinism. This interpretation of quantum mechanics has some problematic consequences, including the necessity of action at a distance. Although Schrödinger was able to show that wave mechanics was in many contexts computationally equivalent to quantum mechanics, the deterministic view was contested by Bohr and other protagonists of the 'Copenhagen interpretation' of quantum mechanics which included the founders of the subject mentioned above. They advocated a more subtle dualistic principle, according to which matter has both wave-like and particle-like properties either of which may predominate, depending on the way it is observed. In the following years, many physicists have been happy to make use of wave mechanics as an effective computational tool, unperturbed by any implications concerning the ultimate nature of matter.

The Copenhagen interpretation of quantum mechanics was essentially determined by the theory of measurement propounded by Born in 1926[22]. According to this theory, the result of any measurement made on a microscopic system such as an atom cannot be predicted, in general, and it is possible to determine only the probability that any particular result will be obtained. It was therefore necessary to abandon the determinism of the classical theories of Newton and his followers.

Schrödinger would not agree with Born's interpretation of quantum mechanics, and proposed a theory in which the future was completely determined by the universal wave function. Other theoretical physicists of great distinction, Einstein in particular, maintained that quantum mechanics was an incomplete theory, and would eventually be superseded by a theory in which the future could be predicted in detail, given sufficient information concerning the present and past. Bohm's theory of *hidden variables*[16] may be regarded as another attempt to develop a deterministic interpretation of wave mechanics, in terms of particles moving, as in Newton's theory, in accordance with deterministic laws. To implement this idea it is necessary to introduce quantum mechanical forces of unlimited strength acting instantaneously over unlimited distances. This did not satisfy Einstein or many other physicists.

The third deterministic interpretation of quantum mechanics, called the *many worlds* interpretation, was elaborated by Everett III[20]. This assumes that every possibility consistent with quantum mechanics is actually realized, so that at every moment an unlimited number of copies of the world as we know it, all differing in minor respects, is brought into existence. This suggestion is particularly interesting because of suggestions that some of these other worlds might be accessible from the one we know. There are some paradoxes associated with travel in time, which is permitted to some extent by the theory of relativity. We accept as non-controversial the possibility of accelerated travel into the future, since there is very good experimental evidence that the apparent life of unstable particles such as mesons can be extended indefinitely by acceleration. There is no reason to doubt that human beings would be likewise affected: that, after an excursion into space lasting a few years but reaching velocities approaching the velocity of light, the traveller could return to find the earth as it would be perhaps centuries later. On the other hand, there have also been suggestions, inspired by the general theory of relativity, that it might be possible to travel through wormholes in space into the past; and return to the present, where new *choices* might be made in response to new *perceptions* in another of the worlds postulated by the many worlds interpretation of quantum mechanics. It has to said that there is no credible experimental evidence encouraging this possibility: it may make good science fiction, but not good science!

But also, even more than the Newtonian theory that they seek to emulate, *the deterministic theories imply that there are countless physical processes that reproduce without error or effort the results of calculations beyond the power of any classical Turing machine.* They all postulate the existence of an unobservable substratum of events of immense complexity. No theory of this or any other type has yet led to more detailed predictions than Born's quantum theory of measurement allows, and even if they are accepted, the deterministic theories do not affect the unpredictability of the world as we know it. Some of the reasons for such departures from common sense have been suggested earlier; but in what follows our task is to show in some detail how they can be avoided, and how the indeterministic view of quantum mechanics is relevant to the incontrovertible fact of consciousness[39].

An important step in the clarification of Born's original formulation was Heisenberg's discovery of the 'uncertainty' relations[350]. It is a consequence of these relations, a general proof of which will be given in Section 7.3, that information concerning a microscopic system can never be complete, in the sense of the classical theories. Thus, if as the result of measurement, the distance of a particle from some reference point were known to be between Q and $Q + \Delta Q$, so that the 'uncertainty' in its position was ΔQ, then the 'uncertainty' ΔP in momentum in the same direction would necessarily satisfy the inequality $\Delta Q \Delta P \geq \frac{1}{2}\hbar$, where $\hbar = 1.054588 \times 10^{-27}$ erg sec. will be referred to as Planck's constant. (though $h = 2\pi\hbar$ was the constant, with the dimensions of action, appearing in Planck's theory of the black-body radiation). The word *Unbestimmtheit* used by Heisenberg to describe his relations would be better translated as 'indeterminacy' than as 'uncertainty'. The latter is misleading in this context, since it could imply that there are two numerical quantities Q and P that could, in principle, be measured in the same experiment. On the contrary, it follows from the indeterminacy relations that it is impossible, even in principle, to obtain the information necessary to integrate the Newtonian equations of motion and so predict the future motion of a microscopic system, irrespective of whether those equations, or others like them, are valid. As the logo of this volume proclaims, an uncertainty relation between information and action exists which forbids it!

The development of quantum mechanics was accompanied by a parallel development of quantized field theory. The first steps towards the quantization of the electromagnetic field were taken by Born, Jordan, Heisenberg and Dirac from 1925 to 1927, and culminated in the relativistic formulations of quantum electrodynamics by Tomonaga, Feynman, Schwinger and Dyson[351]. In a sense, quantized field theory supersedes quantum mechanics, since it shows not only how the electromagnetic field can be regarded as made up of quanta or particles, called photons, but how the appearance of electrons and other elementary particles can be derived from corresponding field theories. However, many of the details of field quantization are irrelevant to our present purpose; in the following we shall be concerned only with the electromagnetic fields and potentials generated by ions in the electrolytic fluid of the animal cortex.

It will now be evident that the theory of observation is the area of quantum mechanics where the issue of determinism cannot be avoided. Most attempts to grapple with this theory have assumed that demonstration by Schrödinger of the mathematical equivalence of his wave mechanics to the matrix mechanics of Born, Jordan and Heisenberg in the treatment of microscopic problems could be extended to the treatment of the interaction of a microscopic system with a macroscopic detector, by means of which the microsystem is rendered observable. Usually such attempts, following Dirac[32] and von Neumann[33], have also assumed that the microsystem can be represented by a wave function; or, when this assumption is proved to be untenable, that the system consisting of microsystem, detector and possibly the observer can be represented by a wave function. Examples of the paradoxes that flow from this have been given in the Introduction, and in Sections 7.3 and 8.1 we shall discuss others, due essentially to Einstein and de Broglie. There has been a curious reluctance to admit what is quite obvious from the following easily proven theorem:

There is no system in nature (with the dubious exception of the entire universe) that can be represented by a single wave function.

This theorem has no serious consequences for applications of wave mechanics to microscopic physics, where it can still be used as a powerful computational system in excellent agreement with observation. However, the same results can be obtained in that context by the use of the theory of the *statistical matrix* (the *density matrix*, in Dirac's terminology, or the *statistical operator*, in the sense of von Neumann). Unlike the wave function, the elements of the statistical matrix are all probabilities that can be measured, so that its existence is never in doubt.

If a physical system could be represented by a wave function, it would be in what is called a *pure state*, but the statistical matrix can also represent a system in an impure state. The distinction between pure and impure states can be most easily understood in terms of information theory. If a system is in a pure state, no further information can be gained concerning the system by observation; if it is in an impure state, however, there is information to be gained. So long as the system does not interact with any other system, the information to be gained by observing it does not change. But no information can be gained concerning any system until it interacts with a second system and the result of the interaction is observed. Furthermore, while the interaction is in progress with the other system, the result is unpredictable; therefore, in the course of interaction, some part of the information concerning each of the two systems is lost. This may be compensated, to some extent, by a gain of information concerning the state of the system *before the interaction took place*. But, since information is gained, and no information can be gained from a system in a pure state, it cannot have been known to be in a pure state to begin with. That is the content of the above theorem.

Another way of stating this is to say that, as a result of the interaction of two systems, the total entropy, defined as a non-negative additive quantity, always increases. This would not be possible if the entropy of the first system were zero, as it certainly would be in a pure state.

The increase of entropy in irreversible processes is actually a corollary of the second law of thermodynamics, which does not necessarily have anything to do with quantum mechanics. Statistical thermodynamics had its beginnings in the eighteenth century, when it was developed by Maxwell, Boltzmann and Gibbs to circumvent the obvious difficulty in measuring all the microscopic variables necessary to define the state of a macrosopic body. It did not suppose that there was any limit to the information that could be gained in principle by sufficiently accurate measurements. But, as explained above, the Copenhagen interpretation of quantum mechanics introduced fundamental limitations on the acquisition of information, in particular the information that can be gained by measurement and observation on systems in the microscopic domain. In quantum mechanics, moreover, the role of the observer in the process of observation is no longer immaterial. In our view, this is not, as Wigner appears to have thought, because the observer is subject to laws different from the ordinary laws of physics, but because biological memory is the ultimate repository of information of which the observer becomes aware.

Real and Artificial Consciousness

Even when the indeterministic interpretation of quantum mechanics is accepted, there remains the vital question of whether the behaviour of a macroscopic system, the nervous system of an animal in particular, might not be predictable in principle. Calculations made on the basis of Newtonian mechanics are very successful in predicting the motions of the planets and other heavenly bodies, and also in a wide variety of terrestrial applications; similarly, Maxwell's equations are very successful in predicting a wide range of electromagnetic phenomena. But these classical theories have their limitations, even at the macroscopic level. The accuracy to which they are verified cannot validate their application to phenomena where Planck's constant is significant; and such phenomena are more universal in the macroscopic domain than is generally realized.

A wide variety of macroscopic devices exists that are activated by events at the microscopic level, including Geiger counters, photo-emulsions, cloud chambers, wire chambers, and other devices used to detect elementary particles. A common feature of these devices is that they incorporate some form of matter in a metastable state, so that even the smallest perturbation is sufficient to precipitate a transition to the corresponding stable state, accompanied by an increase in entropy and a loss of information concerning the device.

Further, apart from such man-made devices, various forms of matter in a metastable state are of frequent occurrence in nature. Supercooled vapour is common in the atmosphere, and there is no doubt that cosmic ray particles produce tracks consisting of water droplets in the vapour, that are similar to those found in a cloud chamber, even though they escape observation. The study of turbulence provides another example. It is impossible to predict the details of turbulent motion in a fluid on the basis of Newtonian mechanics; the only successful theories of turbulence are statistical in character. Though it is usually not possible to trace the origin of a particular turbulent eddy, it is quite likely to have arisen from fluctuations at the microscopic level. Similar considerations apply to hydromagnetic instabilities and other chaotic phenomena.

Most naturally occurring phenomena are non-linear, and as Poincaré pointed out long ago, an arbitrarily small perturbation of a non-linear system at a particular time will have a very perceptible effect on the observed behaviour of the system at sufficiently later times. It follows that the influence of individual quanta on the behaviour of such a system will, sooner or later, become apparent at the macroscopic level. Moreover, the greater the non-linearity, the more rapid the escalation of events from the microscopic to the macroscopic level. We conclude that nearly all natural phenomena, microscopic or macroscopic, are unpredictable *on a characteristic time scale*, and that this time scale may be very short for matter in an metastable state. It seems likely that metastability is a necessary, though obviously not a sufficient characteristic of an artificial consciousness operating on the same time scale as our own.

Because of the large gradient in the electrochemical potentials of calcium and sodium across the cellular membrane, all equilibrated cells are in fact in a metastable state. The graded and action potentials of the nervous system have been shown in previous Chapters to be a consequence of this metastability. But in the cortex the columnar or zonal organization, with systems of excitatory and inhibitory cells in close association, serves to enhance the metastability and secure the synchronization of many graded and action potentials with small fluctuations in the extracellular field. Theory and experiment converge in suggesting that the activity of a particular cell or group of cells depends not on these fluctuations as a whole but on the amplification by the membrane of even smaller components of the field corresponding to particular frequencies. Although these field components in an electrolytic fluid are generated by ions and are very different in character from the components of an electromagnetic field in a vacuum, they are quantized and subject to the same indeterminism as all quantum mechanical phenomena.

Thus, the special configuration of the nervous system fulfils all the requirements for the rapid escalation of events from the microscopic to the macroscopic level. Some of the detailed macroscopic behaviour of the nervous system is, therefore, indeterministic and influenced by events (ionic movements) subject to the laws of quantum rather than classical mechanics.

Most indeterministic events do not appear to be the result of conscious intervention, however. Much of the activity of the biological nervous system, though also unpredictable in detail, is in fact unconscious. Ordinary language provides for demarcation between conscious and unconscious activity in many different ways: in the distinctions made between looking and seeing, listening and hearing, feeling and contact, and between voluntary and involuntary motor action. These distinctions are not merely subjective, but correspond to different patterns of extracellular nervous activity that can be recognized in EEG records. As described in more detail in Section 3.2, the specific patterns associated with conscious activity have been studied experimentally[191], especially in the course of evoked potentials, where a human subject responds to a sensory stimulus with a prearranged motor action. The classic example[193] concerns the observations made in diffuse scalp recording preceding the movement of a finger. There is first a bilateral readiness potential widespread over precentral and parietal regions, then a second potential 90-80 msec before the movement, also bilateral and widespread. A third potential, 50 msec before the movement of the finger, is limited to the hand area of the contralateral motor cortex.

More recent experimental work[82] has shown that distinctive extracellular potentials in a narrow frequency range are evoked in conscious activity such as that required to do arithmetical calculations or to trace a maze. The associated theta waves (in the 4-9 Hz frequency range) have been found to trace circular or elliptical trajectories on either side of the frontal midline of the cortex, in a clockwise direction in the left hemisphere and in an anti-clockwise direction in the right hemisphere. We have seen in Section 3.2 that, even where fluctuations in extracellular potential are apparently random, careful analysis[28] has revealed the underlying presence of characteristic frequencies associated with particular types of conscious activity. Given that individual cells and groups of cells of the cortex are responsive to particular frequencies, there can be no reason to doubt the importance of extremely small rhythmic components of the extracellular field for some types of conscious activity.

Given that such components are quantized, the avenue for the intervention of indeterministic quantum mechanical effects is clear. Of course, even under experimental conditions, the crucial quantum mechanical indeterministic events underlying such patterns of conscious activity are undetected and only their macroscopic consequences are accessible to experimental observation.

In our foregoing and subsequent account, we have emphasized the 'realistic' view that quantum mechanics is essentially a form of information theory. The awareness underlying the attention given to sensory stimuli corresponds to the acquisition of information, and the volition underlying the initiation of a voluntary motor action has the effect of generating new information. But consciousness requires not only the continual acquisition and generation of information, but also its storage and retrieval, supported by the formation and reading of sequential memory.

We have identified the attributes of consciousness that any artificial consciousness should possess: awareness with the formation of memory, and volition with access to memory. One of the objects of the following Sections will be to define awareness and volition more precisely, and connect these attributes with the quantum mechanics of detection and decision-making respectively, as well as the processing of information that they require. However, readers wishing to escape the mathematical details may proceed to the summary at the end of this Chapter.

7.2 Modern Quantum Mechanics

Observables and Matrices

It is only since the development of relativistic quantized field theories that the importance of the observer and the process of observation in quantum mechanics has been generally accepted. Apart from this, there has been an increasing interest[352] in hitherto unresolved questions relating to the theory of measurement and observation in terms of information theory. On the mathematical side, applications and extensions of the theory of Lie groups and algebras are now a very important part of the literature, and there is a wider appreciation[353] of their physical implications. It is not the purpose of this book to provide a detailed account of quantum mechanics, but we shall discuss in simple contemporary terms the topics that are important in understanding the theory of measurement and observation. This discussion is based in part on two recent papers of the authors[39,354].

In the following we shall consider the detection of a system S, usually of atomic dimensions which can only be detected by means of its interaction with a macroscopic device, such as a cloud chamber. From the present point of view, the essential result of the detection of the system is an exchange of information. The device must have some component that is initially in a metastable state; this will be understood to mean that its entropy is below that of a corresponding stable state. In the process of its interaction with S, there is an increase of entropy which, if it is sufficiently large, results in a transition from the metastable to the stable state, and consequently in the detection of the system. According to Section 4.2, the increase of entropy is equivalent to a loss of thermodynamic information, which in this instance is compensated in part by the gain of information concerning the microscopic system. The meaning of 'information' here is compatible with its previous use in a classical context though, as we shall see, most quantities, including information, acquire an extra dimension in quantum mechanics.

In some applications, such as in the use of a Geiger counter, the detection of a microscopic system does no more than provide an observer with evidence of its existence. By a suitable experimental arrangement, usually involving the placement of apertures and electromagnetic guides, it can be ensured that a suitably chosen detector will interact with systems having only a certain value or values of some *selected* observable or set of observables, such as momentum or wavelength, energy or frequency, and helicity. By the use of a composite detector with several independently functioning components, it may also be possible to distinguish between different values of any selected observable, though obviously the experimental arrangement determines the type of information obtained. In the following discussion we shall show how to quantify this type of information, and in the process shall confirm that the biological cell has all the features required to detect certain microscopic events.

We have noted that according to Heisenberg's uncertainty principle there are pairs of observables, called *complementary* observables by Bohr, associated with any system, such that an experimental arrangement to measure one of them accurately precludes the possibility of measuring the other. In Born and Jordan's quantum mechanics this was provided for by representing any microscopic observable by a matrix operator O, whose eigenvalues o_r are the possible values that may result from measurement. In mathematical terms, this means that the matrix O can be expressed in terms of a set of matrices g_r, with numerical coefficients o_r, thus:

$$O = \sum_r o_r g_r, \tag{7.2.1}$$

where the summation extends over all values of r. If the system has n degrees of freedom, where $n > 1$, it is often convenient to regard the subscript r as a vector $(r_1, r_2, ...r_n)$, in which any component r_c may take an infinite number of values. The g_r are minimal idempotents, *i.e.*, projective matrices satisfying

$$g_r g_s = \delta_{rs} g_s, \qquad \mathrm{tr}(g_r) = 1, \qquad \sum_r g_r = 1, \tag{7.2.2}$$

so that $o_r = \mathrm{tr}(O g_r)$. Here and in the following, 'tr' denotes the *trace*, or the sum of the diagonal elements, of the matrix which follows and, in a relation between matrices, 1 denotes the unit matrix. It is convenient to assume that all the matrices are *hermitean*, so that if $(g_r)_{ij}$ is the element of the matrix g_r in the i-th row and the j-th column, this may be a complex number in general, but it is the complex conjugate $(g_r)^*_{ji}$ of the element $(g_r)_{ji}$ in the j-th row and the i-th column.

If O is a diagonal matrix, its diagonal elements are the eigenvalues $o_1, o_2, ...$, and g_r is the matrix with just one non-zero element, $(g_r)_{rr} = 1$. But it is not necessary that a matrix should be diagonal to be expressed in the above way. If O and $\widehat{O}$ represent two observables that are complementary and cannot be measured by the same detector, then they do not commute: if $\widehat{O} = \sum_s \widehat{o}_s \widehat{g}_s$, then $O\widehat{O} \neq \widehat{O}O$ and $g_r \widehat{g}_s - \widehat{g}_s g_r \neq 0$ in general, so that at least one of the matrices O and $\widehat{O}$ is not diagonal. Any matrix m of the system S can be expressed in terms of products $g_r \widehat{g}_s$ of the idempotents of complementary observables:

$$m = \sum_{r,s} m_{rs} g_r \widehat{g}_s, \qquad m_{rs} = \mathrm{tr}(m \widehat{g}_s g_r). \tag{7.2.3}$$

The coefficients m_{rs} are *skew* matrix elements of m corresponding to the idempotents $(g_r, \widehat{g}_s)$. If m^*_{rs} denotes the complex conjugate of m_{rs}, the hermitean conjugate m^* of the matrix m is defined by

$$m^* = \sum_{r,s} m^*_{rs}\widehat{g}_s g_r, \tag{7.2.4}$$

and the product mm^* is *positive definite*, meaning that (as is obvious when m is a diagonal matrix) all its eigenvalues are non-negative. If m is hermitean it is also possible to write $m = \sum_{s,r} m^*_{rs}\widehat{g}_s g_r$.

The Statistical Matrix

There is a special observable P, the statistical matrix (or the statistical operator in von Neumann's terminology[33]), that plays a central part in quantum-mechanical information theory. This matrix is related to what we have called the *selected* observables. In fact, a selected observable $\tilde{O}$ can be found such that any eigenvalue $\tilde{p}_s$ of P is the probability that the measurement of $\tilde{O}$, with a suitably chosen detector D, will yield the value $\tilde{o}_s$. If $\tilde{O} = \sum_s \tilde{o}_s\tilde{g}_s$,then the statistical matrix may be defined by

$$P = \sum_s \tilde{p}_s\tilde{g}_s, \tag{7.2.5}$$

and since $\sum_s \tilde{p}_s = 1$, $\mathrm{tr}(P) = 1$. It will be noticed that P commutes with the selected observable $\tilde{O}$, but not, in general, with another observable O. The nature of the selected observable is sometimes determined by an experimental arrangement designed to ensure that only the value $\tilde{o}_r$ of the selected observable $\tilde{O}$ will be detected by a particular component of the detector. However, where there is no such experimental arrangement, in the absence of other information the selected observable is simply the energy, as defined below. In any event, according to Born's theory of measurement, the probability p_r that the measurement of *any* observable $O = \sum_r o_r g_r$ by a suitable detector D will yield the value o_r is

$$p_r = \mathrm{tr}(g_r P). \tag{7.2.6}$$

It is easily verified from (7.2.1), (7.2.2) and (7.2.4) that this is true if O and $\tilde{O}$ are the same, or commuting observables, but it is also true if O and $\tilde{O}$ do not commute.

In general, it follows from (7.2.6) that the expectation value of O is

$$<O>=\sum_r o_r p_r = \mathrm{tr}(OP) \tag{7.2.7}$$

and from (7.2.5) and (7.2.6) that

$$p_r = \sum_s p_{rs}\tilde{p}_s, \qquad p_{rs} = \mathrm{tr}(g_r\tilde{g}_s), . \tag{7.2.8}$$

where, since $\sum_r p_{rs} = 1$, p_{rs} can be interpreted as a *transition* probability, or the conditional probability that a measurement of O would yield the value o_r if the value of the selected observable were $\tilde{o}_s$.

We shall next discuss the determination of the matrices representing fundamental observables, such as the position, momentum, angular momentum and energy of a system S, possibly an ion, atom or molecule, in the microscopic domain. The matrices that we shall use to represent these observables are defined independently of the conditions under which they are measured, or indeed whether they are measured at all. However, in general the probabilities p_r, and therefore the statistical matrix P, obviously depend on the time, the spatial configuration and the state of motion of the detector D. Assuming that the latter is a rigid unaccelerated body, a sufficient specification includes the position $\mathbf{x}$ of the centre of mass of the detector at any time t, its orientation $\mathbf{u}$, and its velocity $\mathbf{v}$ relative to some other rigid unaccelerated body D_0. If the detector of the microscopic system is D, we denote the density matrix of the microscopic system by $P = P(t, \mathbf{x}, \mathbf{u}, \mathbf{v})$; if, in particular, the detector is D_0, the statistical matrix is $P_0 = P(0, \mathbf{0}, \mathbf{0}, \mathbf{0})$. Because of the interpretation of the eigenvalues as probabilities, these two statistical matrices must be related by a *similarity* transformation:

$$P(t, \mathbf{x}, \mathbf{u}, \mathbf{v}) = U(t, \mathbf{x}, \mathbf{u}, \mathbf{v}) P_0 \overline{U}(t, \mathbf{x}, \mathbf{u}, \mathbf{v}),$$
$$\overline{U}(t, \mathbf{x}, \mathbf{u}, \mathbf{v}) U(t, \mathbf{x}, \mathbf{u}, \mathbf{v}) = 1, \tag{7.2.9}$$

where 1 again stands for the unit matrix. In fact, as both density matrices are hermitean, this is also a *unitary* transformation: $\overline{U}$ is the hermitean conjugate U^* of U and also its inverse U^{-1}: any matrix element $\overline{U}_{rs}$ of $\overline{U}$ is the complex conjugate of the corresponding element U_{rs} of U.

The above equations imply that we are adopting the *Schrödinger representation*, in which the statistical matrix usually varies with time, but the matrices representing other fundamental observables, such as the total energy and momentum of the system, are independent of time.

The Fundamental Observables

If we consider a small change δt in the time t at which the measurement is made, we may write

$$U(t+\delta t, \mathbf{x}, \mathbf{u}, \mathbf{v}) = (1 - iH\delta t/\hbar)U(t, \mathbf{x}, \mathbf{u}, \mathbf{v}), \qquad (7.2.10)$$

where $\hbar$ is Planck's constant and H is an hermitean matrix. It then follows, with the use of (7.2.9), that

$$i\hbar\frac{\partial U}{\partial t} = HU, \qquad i\hbar\frac{\partial P}{\partial t} = HP - PH. \qquad (7.2.11)$$

Adopting Heisenberg's definition of the energy as the agent of change with time (in suitable units with Planck's constant equal to 1), we conclude that the observable H is the energy of the microscopic system.

So long as a microscopic system is free of external interactions, all probabilities, and therefore the statistical matrix of the system, are independent of the time. Then it follows that $HP = PH$, and the energy is a selected observable, as defined above. Under these conditions, the matrix U satisfies the same equation as the wave function in Schrödinger's wave mechanics, and can be regarded as a set of wave functions. *The solution of Schrödinger's equation is essentially a method of evaluation of the elements of the U-matrix.*.

There are similar definitions, analogous to Heisenberg's definition of the energy, for the momentum $\mathbf{P}$, the angular momentum $\mathbf{J}$, and the central vector $\mathbf{K}$ ($= M\mathbf{Q}$, where M is the mass and $\mathbf{Q}$ the position of the mass centre) of a microscopic system, as the agents of change with position, orientation and velocity, respectively. In consequence of these definitions, we have

$$-i\hbar\frac{\partial U}{\partial \mathbf{x}} = \mathbf{P}U, \qquad -i\hbar\frac{\partial U}{\partial \mathbf{u}} = \mathbf{J}U, \qquad i\hbar\frac{\partial U}{\partial \mathbf{v}} = \mathbf{K}U = M\mathbf{Q}U. \qquad (7.2.12)$$

The above equations determine the way in which the outcome of any measurement made with the device D will depend on the set of ten parameters (t, x_1, x_2, x_3, u_1, u_2, u_3, v_1, v_2, v_3), where the subscripts denote cartesian components of the vectors. The parameters are those of what is known as the Galilei group, a Lie group that plays a fundamental role in non-relativistic quantum mechanics. The matrix U is an element of the group, and the observables H, P_1, P_2, P_3, J_1, J_2, J_3, K_1, K_2 and K_3 are the elements of the corresponding Lie algebra, for which we have adopted a matrix representation. The mass M can be regarded as an additional fundamental observable and an element of the Lie group, associated with the parameter $\mathbf{x} \cdot \mathbf{v}$; however, as it commutes with all the other matrices we shall treat it as a numerical multiple of the unit matrix. The fundamental observables must satisfy the *commutation relations*

$$K_\lambda H - HK_\lambda = ihP_\lambda, \qquad K_\lambda P_\mu - P_\mu K_\lambda = i\hbar M\delta_{lm},$$
$$J_\lambda K_\mu - K_\mu J_\lambda = i\hbar\epsilon_{\lambda\mu\nu}K_\nu, \qquad J_\lambda P_\mu - P_\mu J_\lambda = i\hbar\epsilon_{\lambda\mu\nu}P_\nu,$$
$$J_\lambda J_\mu - J_\mu J_\lambda = i\hbar\epsilon_{\lambda\mu\nu}J_\nu, \tag{7.2.13}$$

where $\epsilon_{\lambda\mu\nu}$ is the permutation symbol, which has the value 1 when (λ, μ,ν) is a cyclic permutation of $(1,2,3)$, -1 if it is a cyclic permutation of $(1,3,2)$, and 0 otherwise. Other commutators, such as $P_\lambda H - HP_\lambda$ and $J_\lambda H - HJ_\lambda$, are zero. From the second of the above relations, the important result

$$Q_\lambda P_\mu - P_\mu Q_\lambda = i\hbar\delta_{\lambda\mu} \tag{7.2.14}$$

of Born and Jordan immediately follows.

The necessity of the above commutation relations can be proved in various ways, for instance by considering two successive unitary transformations $U = U(t, \mathbf{x}, \mathbf{u}, \mathbf{v})$ and $U' = U(t', \mathbf{x}', \mathbf{u}', \mathbf{v}')$, where the parameters $(t', \mathbf{x}', \mathbf{u}', \mathbf{v}')$ determine the configuration and motion of a new detector D′ relative to D. For this purpose it can be supposed that all the parameters are small. The result of the successive transformations U and U' must be another unitary transformation $\widetilde{U} = U(\widetilde{t}, \widetilde{\mathbf{x}}, \widetilde{\mathbf{u}}, \widetilde{\mathbf{v}})$, where it is easy to verify that

$$\widetilde{t} = t + t', \qquad \widetilde{x}_\lambda = x_\lambda + x'_\lambda + \epsilon_{\lambda\mu\nu}u_\mu x'_\nu + v_\lambda t',$$

$$\widetilde{u}_\lambda = u_\lambda + u'_\lambda + \tfrac{1}{2}\,\epsilon_{\lambda\mu\nu} u_\mu u'_\nu, \qquad \widetilde{v}_\lambda = v_\lambda + v'_\lambda + \epsilon_{\lambda\mu\nu} u_\mu v'_\nu, \tag{7.2.15}$$

correct to terms involving products of the small parameters. The commutation relations are obtained by equating products of parameters in the relation $\widetilde{U} = UU'$, after writing

$$U = \exp(-iA) \approx 1 - iA - \tfrac{1}{2}\,A^2, \qquad A = Ht - \mathbf{P}\cdot\mathbf{x} - \mathbf{J}\cdot\mathbf{u} + \mathbf{K}\cdot\mathbf{v}. \tag{7.2.16}$$

The last equations, together with (7.2.12), show how the statistical matrix, and all the fundamental observables of a microscopic system, are completely determined by the *action* A, regarded as a function $A(t, \mathbf{x}, \mathbf{u}, \mathbf{v})$ of the set of parameters introduced above. In the Lagrangian formulation of Newtonian mechanics, the parameters are regarded as specifying the system adopted by a particular observer O relative to that of some other observer O_0, and the interpretation given above in terms of detectors is entirely consistent with this idea. In quantum mechanics the action associated with a microscopic system is treated as an observable and, for reasons already discussed, represented by a matrix; but the derivation of the observables is unchanged. It is clear from (7.2.9) that the statistical matrix P is completely determined by its value P_0 for $t = 0$ and $\mathbf{x} = \mathbf{u} = \mathbf{v} = \mathbf{0}$, and the action A.

The commutation relations given in (7.2.13) can be used to determine the form of the matrices representing the observables unambiguously, apart from a similarity transformation; and all of the properties that are needed here can be derived directly from the commutation relations.

Composite Systems

We conclude this Section with a discussion of composite systems. It is sufficient to consider a system S consisting of two subsystems S$'$ and S$''$. We assume that these systems are disjoint, without any parts in common, and denote observables of the two systems separately by O' and O''. When these are regarded as matrices of the composite system, however, they are expressed as direct (outer) products of the form $O^{(1)} = O'\otimes 1$ and $O^{(2)} = 1\otimes O''$ with idempotents $g_r^{(1)} = g_r\otimes 1$ and $g_v^{(2)} = 1\otimes g_v$. Like ordinary matrix multiplication, direct multiplication is distributive, but direct products satisfy the coproduct rule: $(g_r \otimes$

$g_u)(g_s \otimes g_v) = g_r g_s \otimes g_v g_w$, so that $g_r^{(1)}$ commutes with $g_v^{(2)}$. The trace of a direct product of two matrices is the ordinary product of their traces, so that $\mathrm{tr}(g_r^{(1)} g_v^{(2)}) = \mathrm{tr}(g_r \otimes g_v) = \mathrm{tr}'(g_r)\mathrm{tr}''(g_v) = 1$. By a generalization of (7.2.3), all matrices of the composite system, can be expressed in terms of the direct products

$$m = \sum_{r,s.v,w} m_{rs,vw} g_r \widehat{g}_s \otimes g_v \widehat{g}_w, \qquad m_{rs,vw} = \mathrm{tr}[m(\widehat{g}_s g_r \otimes \widehat{g}_w g_v)]. \quad (7.2.17)$$

of matrices $g_r \widehat{g}_s$ and $g_v \widehat{g}_w$ of the subsystems.

Of course there is a statistical matrix P for the composite system, but it is also always possible to define density matrices P' and P'' for the separate subsystems as partial traces of P, thus:

$$P' = \sum_{r,s} g_r \widehat{g}_s \mathrm{tr}[P(\widehat{g}_s g_r \otimes 1)], \qquad P'' = \sum_{v,w} g_v \widehat{g}_w \mathrm{tr}[P(1 \otimes \widehat{g}_w g_v)]. \quad (7.2.18)$$

If $O' = \sum_v o'_u g_u$ is an observable of the first subsystem, the probability p'_u that a measurement of O' will yield the value o'_u, according to (7.2.6), is $\mathrm{tr}'(P' g_u) = \mathrm{tr}'(g_u P')$, and as $\mathrm{tr}\,'(g_u g_r) = \delta_{ur}$, this is the same as $\mathrm{tr}(P g_u^{(1)}) = \mathrm{tr}(g_u^{(1)} P)$, as required.

If the two subsystems of the composite system are not interacting and have not interacted, directly or indirectly, in the recent past, they are statistically independent of one another, and the joint probability that the measurement of observables $O' = \sum_r o'_r g_r$ and $O'' = \sum_v o''_v g''_v$ of the subsystems will yield the values o'_r and o''_v respectively must be the product $p_{rv} = p'_r p''_v$ of the separate probabilities. From (7.2.5) it can be seen that this condition for independence implies that the statistical matrix P of the composite systems is the direct product of the density matrices P' and P'' of the subsystems:

$$P = P' \otimes P'', \quad (7.2.19)$$

From (7.2.9) it follows that, subject to the same restriction, a unitary transformation U of the type considered there must also be a direct product: $U = U' \otimes U''$. From (7.2.16) it is then obvious that the action observable A is additive in the sense that $A = A^{(1)} + A^{(2)}$, and the same is true for all the fundamental observables:

$$H = H^{(1)} + H^{(2)}, \qquad \mathbf{P} = \mathbf{P}^{(1)} + \mathbf{P}^{(2)}, \qquad \mathbf{J} = \mathbf{J}^{(1)} + \mathbf{J}^{(2)},$$

$$\mathbf{K} = \mathbf{K}^{(1)} + \mathbf{K}^{(2)}, \qquad M = M^{(1)} + M^{(2)}. \tag{7.2.20}$$

However, (7.2.19) and (7.2.20) hold only as long as the systems have had no interaction, and with interaction we must write

$$H = H^{(1)} + H^{(2)} + V, \tag{7.2.21}$$

where V is the interaction energy. For simple subsystems, each consisting of a single particle, V is a usually a scalar function of the relative position $\mathbf{Q}^{(2)} - \mathbf{Q}^{(1)}$, and the observables $\mathbf{P}$, $\mathbf{J}$, $\mathbf{K}$ and M are still simply additive.

In the following Sections, we shall develop a quantum-mechanical theory of measurement and observation based on information theory and the principles summarized above.

7.3 Quantal Information and Uncertainty

Our discussion of the principles of quantum mechanics in the previous Section differs from many others in the literature, firstly, by the prominence given to the role of the detector in the theory of microscopic observables, and secondly by the avoidance of mathematical constructs that are not directly related to observable quantities. In a theory of observation, there is no role for Schrödinger's wave function, or for the vectors introduced by Dirac[32] and von Neumann[33] to represent the state of a microscopic system, except as components of the unitary matrix U. These constructs may be used for computational purposes; but, according to the theorem of Section 7.1, there is no single wave function or vector that can represent the state of a microscopic system in interaction with any other system, and without interaction it is not possible to perform measurements or to observe such a system. As is evident from the literature, any discussion of the theory of measurement and observation in terms of wave functions or state vectors is an invitation to confusion; while the theory of the statistical matrix and information theory provide a useful basis for rational discussion of these topics.

Quantal Information

In quantum mechanics the definition of information in (4.2.4) can be generalized. We follow the general rule that observables are represented by matrices, and that the extensive (additive) quantities of classical physics are expectation values of their quantal analogues. The classical information to be gained from the measurement of an observable $O = \sum_r o_r g_r$ of a system S is additive; also, it is the expectation value of $-\log p_r$ where, according to (7.2.6), $p_r = \mathrm{tr}(Pg_r)$ is the probability that the measured value will be o_r. We therefore define the quantal information to be gained from the measurement of O by

$$I = -\sum_r \log(p_r) g_r, \tag{7.3.1}$$

The summation is over all possible values, so that *impossible* values, with $p_r = 0$, need not be considered. Even so, their inclusion would not affect the classical information, defined as the expectation value

$$< I >= -\mathrm{tr}[\sum_r \log(p_r) g_r P] = -\sum_r p_r \log p_r. \tag{7.3.2}$$

Here, for convenience, we are choosing $k = \log 2$ as the unit of information. A classical 'bit' can have only two values, usually chosen to be 0 and 1, and the information to be gained from reading the bit is k. A quantal bit is defined as an observable n with just two *eigenvalues* 0 and 1, which therefore has an irreducible two-dimensional representation of the general type

$$n = \begin{pmatrix} \frac{1}{2}(1-\cos\theta) & \frac{1}{2}e^{i\varphi}\sin\theta \\ \frac{1}{2}e^{-i\varphi}\sin\theta & \frac{1}{2}(1+\cos\theta) \end{pmatrix}. \tag{7.3.3}$$

This matrix satisfies the conditions $n^2 = n$ and $\mathrm{tr}(n) = 1$, so for this particular observable we can take $g_0 = 1-n$ and $g_1 = n$. If p_0 and p_1 are the probabilities that a measurement of B will yield the values 0 and 1, respectively, the statistical matrix P_n and the quantal information I_n to be gained from the measurement are given by

$$P_n = p_0(1-n) + p_1 n, \quad I_n = -\log p_0(1-n) - \log p_1 \cdot n. \tag{7.3.4}$$

If $\theta = 0$, both of the above matrices are diagonal. But, even then, there are elements of I_n that can be arbitrarily large if one of the probabilities is sufficiently small, though $< I_n >$ is near to zero. This is not surprising; the chance that a monkey using a word processor will fortuitously type one of Shakespeare's sonnets is very small, but the information to be gained if it does so is correspondingly large! The differences between classical and quantal information theory arise when the value of the bit is not selected for observation. For instance, if θ depends on the time, as it does in some applications, the observed value of the bit will fluctuate with time.

There are important physical observables that can be represented as quantal 'bits'. If s_i is some component of the spin angular momentum of an electron or of any particle with spin $\frac{1}{2}$, $s_i + \frac{1}{2}$ is a quantal bit. The number of electrons or fermions of any type with specified properties, such as spin and momentum, is also a quantal bit. For a composite system S formed from two bits n' and n'', a four-dimensional representation is needed, and when considered as part of S, the individual bits are most conveniently expressed as direct products of the type $n^{(1)} = n' \otimes 1$ and $n^{(2)} = 1 \otimes n''$, where the two-dimensional matrices n' and n'' are of the type shown in (7.3.3), though possibly with different values of θ and φ, and where 1 denotes the the two-dimensional unit matrix. More generally, the i-th bit $n^{(i)}$ in a composite system of N bits forming a *quantal 'tape'* can be expressed as a direct product of N matrix factors, of which the i-th factor is like n in (7.3.3) and the others are two-dimensional unit matrices. In the next Section we shall show that periodic components of the extracellular potential in the brain can be regarded as bits, in precisely this sense, so that the extracellular fluid can be thought of as a quantal tape.

In the most general context, it is easy to see that quantal information depends on the selected observable. If $\tilde{O} = \sum_r \tilde{o}_r \tilde{g}_r$ is selected, then $\tilde{O}$ commutes with P, so that $P = \sum_r \tilde{p}_r \tilde{g}_r$, where $\tilde{p}_r$ is the probability that a measurement of $\tilde{O}$ will yield the value $\tilde{o}_r$, and the information to be gained by measuring $\tilde{O}$ is $\tilde{I} = -\sum_r \log(\tilde{p}_r)\tilde{g}_r$, or $-\log P$, which commutes with P. *The information gained from the measurement of a* selected *observable is therefore not different in kind from the information gained from the observation of a macroscopic event.* But the information I defined in (7.3.1) is in general different from $\tilde{I}$, and by using

(7.2.8) it can be shown that the expectation value $< I - \tilde{I} >$ of the difference is never negative. For this reason, when an observable other than a selected observable is being measured it is appropriate to consider some of the information as missing, or even non-existent, before the measurement, and *created* by the process of measurement. The classical information created in such circumstances is $< I - \tilde{I} >$ and it can, of course, be gained by an observer only *after* it has been created.

This is a quite unexpected result, from the point of view of classical information theory. As an extreme example, let us suppose it is possible for the measurement of the selected observable $\tilde{O}$ of a system to yield only the value $\tilde{o}_u$, or equivalently, for $\tilde{p}_r$ to have the value 1 if $r = u$, and zero otherwise ($\tilde{p}_r = \delta_{ru}$). The statistical matrix P then reduces to the single idempotent $\tilde{g}_u$, the microscopic system is in a pure state, and the information $\tilde{I}$ to be gained by measuring the selected observable is zero. This is what is implied if the actual state of the system is represented by a wave function or a state vector. The pure state is a mathematical construct from hypothetical information concerning the result of the measurement of selected observables. Such information may never become available though it can be made the basis of valid statistical predictions; it is, of course, distinct from the information to be gained from an actual measurement. The theorem of Section 7.1 shows that a pure state of a particular system, in which the *current* values of all its selected observables are known, is actually an idealization that cannot be realized in any experiment. But where particular values of the selected observables of a system are observed, it is possible to conclude that the system *was* in a pure state only after the observation has been made.

At the other extreme, suppose that O is the observable $\widehat{O}$ complementary to the one selected. Then, if the system is in a pure state, the information I to be gained concerning O is defined by (7.3.1) and has its maximum value. When a measurement is made of O, the information I is created in the process, since it was not previously available.

We shall present a general theory of measurement in Section 7.5. From this it will be clear that it is possible under controlled experimental conditions to construct a new statistical matrix P_i for a system at a time before a measurement was made on the basis of the information actually gained from the measurement. Since, in general, the content of the information cannot be predicted in advance, P_i differs from P in a way that can only be known to an observer following the measurement, and therefore has a retrospective element. Nevertheless, information should not be regarded as subjective; the same value of P_i will be constructed by any observer acquainted with the result of the measurement, because the information is derived from the measuring apparatus. This is the explanation given by orthodox quantum mechanics for the paradoxes (of Schrödinger's cat and Wigner's friend) that were related in the Introduction.

The statistical matrix P_i is related to its value P_{i0} at time $t = 0$ by the same equation (7.2.9) that connects P with P_0. The replacement of P by P_i is often referred to in the literature as the 'collapse of the wave packet', as though it were a physical event; but we shall call it the 'revision of the statistical matrix', which better suggests its dependence on information already gained by the measurement of an observable. The revision of the statistical matrix is a classical procedure that does not differ essentially from what occurs when the outcome of a horse race, or any other uncertain event, becomes known.

Uncertainty Relations

If O and $\widehat{O}$ are complementary observables and

$$[O, \widehat{O}] \equiv O\widehat{O} - \widehat{O}O = iC, . \tag{7.3.5}$$

then the commutator iC of O and $\widehat{O}$ is an non-vanishing matrix and C is hermitean. The mean value of the observable $\delta O = O - < O >$ is zero, and the *variances* or *uncertainties* ΔO and $\Delta\widehat{O}$ in measurements of the observables O and $\widehat{O}$, respectively, under similar experimental conditions are defined by

$$\Delta O = < \delta O^2 >^{\frac{1}{2}}, \quad \Delta\widehat{O} = < \delta\widehat{O}^2 >^{\frac{1}{2}} . \tag{7.3.6}$$

Further, for any real value of λ, the matrix

$$(\delta O - i\lambda\delta\widehat{O})(\delta O + i\lambda\delta\widehat{O}) = \delta O^2 + \lambda^2\delta\widehat{O}^2 - \lambda C$$

is the product of a matrix $(\delta O - i\lambda\delta\widehat{O})$ with its hermitean conjugate, and is therefore positive definite. It follows that the expectation value cannot be negative:

$$\Delta O^2 + \lambda^2 \Delta\widehat{O}^2 - \lambda\langle C\rangle \geq 0$$

To make the most of this result, we give the left side its minimum value by setting $\lambda = \frac{1}{2}\langle C\rangle/\Delta\widehat{O}^2$ and thus obtain the uncertainty relation

$$\Delta O \Delta\widehat{O} \geq \tfrac{1}{2}\,|\langle C\rangle|\,. \tag{7.3.7}$$

The general implications of (7.3.7) are clear; in an experiment designed to measure the microscopic observable O with great precision, so that ΔO is small, the precision with which it is possible to measure the complementary observable $\widehat{O}$ becomes correspondingly poor. Later we shall apply this analysis to obtain a very fundamental result: an uncertainty relation connecting information and action. The best known application of the above result, however, is to a component Q_λ of the position vector $\mathbf{Q}$ and the corresponding component P_λ of the momentum $\mathbf{P}$ of a particle, where Heisenberg's relation $\Delta Q_\lambda \Delta P_\lambda \geq \frac{1}{2}\hbar$ follows from the commutation relations $Q_\lambda P_\lambda - P_\lambda Q_\lambda = i\hbar$. Using this as an example, we now consider the implications for the theory of measurement in more detail.

Assume, then, that the complementary observables are the momentum $\mathbf{P}$ and the position $\mathbf{Q}$ of the centre of mass of a microscopic system S. When information is first gained concerning the system, it is localized in the detector or detectors, where it may possibly be recorded and transmitted elsewhere by electromagnetic or some other physical means. However, the detection is usually distributed over an extended region of space. The momentum of the system, in particular, can only be measured approximately by the detection of wave-like properties of the system over an extended region, and the information gained in this way is extensively non-local. The position may be measured approximately by the observation of particle-like properties, for instance by placing a detector immediately behind a small aperture through which the system must pass; and the information gained in this way is localized at the detector. Bohr's discussion of complementary measurements[23] made the point that one of these measurements excludes the other. But his 'principle of complementarity' should not be interpreted to mean that the wave-like and particle-like properties of matter are mutually exclusive. Recently there has been interest in experiments in which both are evident[355,356]; and in such experiments the information concerning the wave-like properties, gained by detecting coincidences or anti-coincidences, is at least partly non-local.

The EPR Paradox

Information theory is helpful in clarifying not only the paradoxes already mentioned, but others that were probably formulated in the first instance with the intention of raising doubts concerning the indeterministic (Copenhagen) interpretation of quantum mechanics. One of these, the EPR paradox, was due to Einstein, Podolsky and Rosen[357]. It concerns a composite system S that is supposed to be in a pure state, so that the statistical matrix P_i (constructed from information available only *after* a measurement) may be approximated by an idempotent. It is supposed that the system consists of two microscopic subsystems S′ and S″ that are not in interaction but have interacted previously, so that the statistical matrix P for the composite system is not simply a direct product of the density matrices P' and P'' of the separate subsystems, and these density matrices are certainly not idempotents. Let us suppose, for simplicity, that the resultant momentum $\mathbf{P} = \mathbf{P}^{(1)} + \mathbf{P}^{(2)}$ and the relative position $\mathbf{R} = \mathbf{Q}^{(2)} - \mathbf{Q}^{(1)}$ are the selected observables, with given eigenvalues $\mathbf{p}$ and $\mathbf{r}$. In such circumstances, a measurement performed on S′ to determine the value $\mathbf{p}^{(1)}$ of $\mathbf{P}^{(1)}$ also determines the momentum $\mathbf{p}^{(2)} = \mathbf{p} - \mathbf{p}^{(1)}$ of the distant system S″, and a measurement performed on S″ to determine the value $\mathbf{q}^{(2)}$ of $\mathbf{Q}^{(2)}$ also determines the position $\mathbf{q}^{(1)} = \mathbf{r} + \mathbf{q}^{(2)}$ of S′. Since quantum mechanics does not allow the accurate determination of the position and momentum of the same particle, this was interpreted by Einstein as showing that quantum mechanics was an incomplete theory.

All actual experiments relevant to the EPR paradox have so far confirmed the validity of the predictions of quantum mechanics. A measurement of $\mathbf{P}^{(1)}$ cannot be made without affecting the status of $\mathbf{R}$ as a selected observable, so that a subsequent measurement of $\mathbf{Q}^{(2)}$ leaves $\mathbf{Q}^{(1)}$ indeterminate, while a measurement of $\mathbf{Q}^{(2)}$ cannot be made without affecting the status of $\mathbf{P}$ as a selected observable, so that a subsequent measurement of $\mathbf{P}^{(1)}$ leaves $\mathbf{P}^{(2)}$ indeterminate. Moreover, the experimental results are of course not affected by any 'complete' (deterministic) theory so far proposed.

However, another suggestion to be found in the literature[14,358] is that there is some form of action at a distance that allows a measurement made in one place to affect a distant system. This, in fact, seems inevitable if quantum mechanics is interpreted either in terms of a universal wave function or in terms of hidden variables. But when the EPR and similar quantum mechanical paradoxes are interpreted in the light of indeterministic information theory, the problematic concept of action at a distance will be found unnecessary.

The first point to be made is that it should be no surprise that measurements made in different places should be correlated. Consider again a composite system for which the selected observables are $\mathbf{P}$ and $\mathbf{R}$, with eigenvalues $\mathbf{p}$ and $\mathbf{r}$. It is not surprising that if the measurement of $\mathbf{P}^{(1)}$ yields the value $\mathbf{p}^{(1)}$, a distant measurement of $\mathbf{P}^{(2)}$ should yield the value $\mathbf{p} - \mathbf{p}^{(1)}$, or that if *alternatively*, the measurement of $\mathbf{Q}^{(1)}$ yields the value $\mathbf{q}^{(1)}$, a distant measurement of $\mathbf{Q}^{(2)}$ should yield the value $\mathbf{r} + \mathbf{q}^{(1)}$. As we have pointed out above, the measurements of the complementary observables $\mathbf{P}^{(1)}$ and $\mathbf{Q}^{(1)}$ are mutually exclusive and yield different information. It is important to avoid the assumption that a suitable experiment could yield precise information concerning the values of both $\mathbf{p} - \mathbf{p}^{(1)}$ and $\mathbf{r} + \mathbf{q}^{(1)}$, or that either was already determinate, in some sense, before any measurement was made.

The second essential point is that the information gained from the idealized measurement of the momentum $\mathbf{P}$ is associated with an extended region of space; furthermore, the information gained from the idealized measurement of the relative position $\mathbf{R}$ is also non-local. Whatever its nature, it is not necessary to suppose that information is transmitted by action at a distance from point to point. The conservation laws satisfied by the fundamental observables are sufficient to ensure that no surprising discrepancies should be found between information concerning the same system, acquired in different ways. There are certainly serious problems if the information obtained from a measurement on a microscopic system is supposed to be predetermined; but, viewed from the point of view of indeterministic information theory, quantum mechanics offers no affront to common sense.

Eigenvalues by Factorization

The outcome of an experiment to measure an observable must be one of its eigenvalues. It is therefore a recurrent problem to determine the eigenvalues of an observable related to the fundamental or other observables in a specified way. In Schrödinger's wave mechanics this is usually done by a study of the solutions of a differential equation to discover which of these satisfies a physically plausible set of boundary conditions. In the matrix formulation of quantum mechanics, however, essentially the same results can be obtained by intrinsically simpler though less familiar methods[359]. Eigenvalues are obtained by the factorization of a closely related observable, and we shall conclude this Section by giving a few examples of the procedure.

Consider first the simplest instance, where there are just two eigenvalues. Then the observable must be expressible as some function $F(n)$ of the matrix n representing a quantal bit in (7.3.3). Since $n^2 = n$, the eigenvalues are obviously $f_0 = F(0)$ and $f_1 = F(1)$; but we shall find it useful to make use of the factors of n:

$$n = c^* c, \qquad c = \begin{pmatrix} \frac{1}{2}\sin\theta & \frac{1}{2}(1+\cos\theta)e^{i\varphi} \\ -\frac{1}{2}(1-\cos\theta)e^{-i\varphi} & -\frac{1}{2}\sin\theta \end{pmatrix}, \tag{7.3.8}$$

where c^*, as usual, denotes the hermitean conjugate of c. It is easy to verify that

$$c^2 = c^{*2} = 0, \qquad cc^* + c^*c = 1, \tag{7.3.9}$$

so that $cn = c = (1-n)c$. Since c changes the eigenvalue of n from 1 to 0, it is called an *annihilation operator* in applications to particle physics, where n is the number of fermions of some kind, while c^* is the corresponding *creation operator*. We note that the factorization

$$F(n) - f_0 = (f_1 - f_0)c^*c \tag{7.3.10}$$

can be made for any two-dimensional matrix $F(n)$, and that the existence of a relation of this type identifies f_0 as an eigenvalue of the matrix. There is a similar result for matrices of any finite dimension, but here we shall proceed at once to an analogous result for observables represented by infinite dimensional matrices.

A matrix observable H, such as the energy of a system, with a countably infinite set of eigenvalues must of course be infinite-dimensional. We shall suppose, as must be true for the energy, that the eigenvalues have a lower bound, but possibly no upper bound. The eigenvalues may then be determined by a series of factorizations of the same form as (7.3.10), beginning with

$$H - h_0 = c_0^* c_0, \tag{7.3.11}$$

There are in general two or more factorizations of this type, with different values of h_0; and it is important to choose the one with the least value of h_0. Then H_r, h_r and c_r are defined successively for $r = 1, 2, ...$ by

$$H_r = h_{r-1} + c_{r-1} c_{r-1}^* = h_r + c_r^* c_r, \tag{7.3.12}$$

where $h_r > h_{r-1}$. The numbers $h_0, h_1, h_2, ...$ generated in this way are the only possible eigenvalues of H less than their upper bound h_∞ if there is one, or ∞ otherwise, for from (7.3.11) and (7.3.12) it follows that $H_r c_{r-1} = c_{r-1} H_{r-1}$ and

$$c_0^* c_1^* ... c_r^* c_r ... c_1 c_0 = (H - h_0)(H - h_1) ... (H - h_r). \tag{7.3.13}$$

But the left hand side is the product of the matrix $c_r ... c_1 c_0$ and its hermitean conjugate, and is therefore positive definite; thus, for each value of r, any eigenvalue of the right side is either zero or positive, as required.

There are many applications of this result[359], but the simplest is to the energy levels of a harmonic oscillator of mass $\hbar\omega$ (in suitable units) and frequency ω. In terms of the position Q and the momentum P, the energy is given by

$$H = (P^2 + \omega^2 Q^2)/(2\hbar\omega) \tag{7.3.14}$$

with the commutation relation $QP - PQ = i\hbar$. The time derivative of P is given by $\dot{P} = (PH - HP)/(i\hbar) = -\omega Q/\hbar$, as in classical mechanics. The 'factors' of H are obviously $c_0 = (P - i\omega Q)/\sqrt{2\omega\hbar}$ and $c_0^* = (P + i\omega Q)/\sqrt{2\omega\hbar}$, and (7.3.14) reduces to $H = \frac{1}{2} + c_0^* c_0$. For all values of r, $h_{r+1} = h_r + 1$, and

$$c_r = (P - i\omega Q)/\sqrt{2\omega h}, \qquad c_r^* = (P + i\omega Q)/\sqrt{2\omega h}, \qquad h_r = (r+\tfrac{1}{2}). \tag{7.3.15}$$

The lowest energy level, $h_0 = \frac{1}{2}$, is the 'zero-point energy' of the harmonic oscillator, and it is evident that if we write

$$H = (N+\tfrac{1}{2}), \tag{7.3.16}$$

then the matrix N has non-negative integral eigenvalues, and the relations between the matrices can be summarized by

$$c_0^* c_0 = N = c c_0^* - 1, \quad cN = (N+1)c, \quad c^*(N+1) = Nc^*. \tag{7.3.17}$$

The 'commutation relation' $c_0 c_0^* - c_0^* c_0 = 1$ may be compared with the relation (7.3.9) satisfied by annihilation and creation operators for fermions. In quantized field theory, relations of the type shown in (7.3.17) are satisfied by the annihilation and creation operators for *bosons*, such as light quanta, with a given spin and momentum. There the eigenvalue of N is interpreted as the number of bosons of that particular kind. This eigenvalue is usually 0 or 1, so that although it is possible, for instance in a laser beam or at very low temperatures, for the higher integral eigenvalues to be realized, in an electrolyte there is no important difference between ions that are fermions and those that are bosons.

7.4 Quantized Fields and Potentials

In this Section we shall formulate the quantum theory of the electromagnetic field from the unusual point of view of its application to electrolytes and the extracellular field in the brain. For the convenience of the reader, we begin with with a short account of the theory in a more general context that is very similar to Maxwell's classical theory, except that the classical field variables are replaced by matrices. At the microscopic level, the fundamental field variables are the electric intensity ($\mathbf{E}$) and the magnetic induction ($\mathbf{B}$). In a material medium such as an electrolyte, the microscopic charge density (ϵ_M) and the electric current density ($\mathbf{j}_M$) include contributions from atoms and molecules carrying no resultant charge, as well as from the ions.

If we denote the time derivatives of the field variables in the Heisenberg representation by $\dot{\mathbf{E}}$ and $\dot{\mathbf{B}}$ respectively, Maxwell's equations have the form:

$$\nabla \cdot \mathbf{E} = 4\pi\epsilon_M, \qquad \nabla \cdot \mathbf{B} = 0,$$

$$c\nabla \times \mathbf{E} = -\dot{\mathbf{B}}, \qquad c\nabla \times \mathbf{B} = \dot{\mathbf{E}} + 4\pi\mathbf{j}_M, \tag{7.4.1}$$

in electrostatic units, where $c = 2.9979246 \times 10^{10}$ cm./sec. is the velocity of light in empty space. For comparison with the macroscopic theory, however, it is necessary to separate the ionic contributions (ϵ and $\mathbf{j}$) to the charge density and current, and also to introduce the electric displacement ($\mathbf{D}$) by writing

$$\epsilon_M = \epsilon + \epsilon_P, \qquad \mathbf{j}_M = \mathbf{j} + \mathbf{j}_P,$$

$$\nabla \cdot \mathbf{D} = \epsilon, \qquad c\nabla \times \mathbf{B} = \dot{\mathbf{D}} + 4\pi\mathbf{j}. \tag{7.4.2}$$

Here, in the absence of detailed information concerning atomic and molecular structure, ϵ_P and $\mathbf{j}_P$ can be regarded as the contributions to the charge and current densities from the polarization of the medium.

For any field variable F in the Heisenberg representation, it is still true that

$$i\hbar\dot{F} = FH - HF, \qquad -i\hbar\nabla F = F\mathbf{P} - \mathbf{P}F, \tag{7.4.3}$$

but $\dot{F}$ and ∇F may be interpreted as derivatives of F with respect to time and position, in the usual way. The corresponding variable in the Schrödinger representation is

$$F_S = UF\overline{U}, \tag{7.4.4}$$

where $U = U(t, \mathbf{x}, \mathbf{0}, \mathbf{0})$ is the unitary matrix introduced in Section 7.2, and the expectation value of the field variable F at time t is

$$< F >= \mathrm{tr}(F_S P) = \mathrm{tr}(UF\overline{U}P), \tag{7.4.5}$$

where P is the statistical matrix at time t. When $t = 0$ and $\mathbf{x} = 0$, $U = 1$ (the unit matrix), and it is evident from (7.4.4) that F

reduces to F_S. In the Schrödinger representation, the field variables are independent of time and position, so that the solution of the matrix version of Maxwell's equations with prescribed initial conditions can be effected in principle by the determination of the unitary matrix U.

In the classical solution of Maxwell's equations, it is usual to introduce the potentials φ and $\mathbf{A}$, satisfying

$$\mathbf{B} = \nabla \times \mathbf{A}, \qquad \mathbf{E} + \dot{\mathbf{A}}/c = -\nabla\varphi, \qquad \nabla \cdot \mathbf{A} = 0, \tag{7.4.6}$$

The first two of these equations are general solutions of the second and third equations of (7.4.1), while the third signifies the choice of the Coulomb gauge, which is most convenient in a non-relativistic context. By substitution in the first and fourth equations of (7.4.1), it is easy to verify that the potentials are solutions of the equations

$$\nabla^2\varphi = -4\pi\epsilon_M, \qquad \Box\mathbf{A} = 4\pi\mathbf{j}_M/c, \tag{7.4.7}$$

in which $\Box = (\partial/\partial t)^2/c^2 - \nabla^2$ is the D'Alembertian differential operator. In empty space where $\epsilon_M = \mathbf{j}_M = 0$ and $\varphi = 0$, the solutions for $\mathbf{A}$ represent transverse waves travelling with the velocity of light. But here we are more interested in the application to the interior of an electrolyte, where there is a charge density ϵ_M that in general includes contributions from polarized atoms and molecules as well as ions.

Although all the variables are quantized microscopic quantities, since the equations are linear they are also satisfied by the set of macroscopic variables $< \mathbf{E} >$, $< \mathbf{B} >$, $< \mathbf{D} >$, $< \varphi >$, $< \mathbf{A} >$, $< \epsilon >$ and $< \mathbf{j} >$. In a classical theory such as that presented in Chapter 4, the brackets $< \cdot >$denoting expectation values are omitted. It is a result of statistical mechanics that

$$< \mathbf{D} >= \kappa < \mathbf{E} >, \tag{7.4.8}$$

where κ is the dielectric constant of the medium, and the generalized form of Ohm's law in (4.3.13) has been given a quantal derivation in terms of the statistical matrix by Kubo and his associates[43]. Thus, all the essential results obtained in Chapter 4 retain their validity in quantum mechanics. In particular, small fluctuations in the potential can be resolved into components with a definite frequency.

According to (7.4.4), in the quantized theory, the solution of the equations (7.4.7) for the the electromagnetic potentials may be written formally as

$$\varphi = \overline{U}\varphi_S U, \qquad \mathbf{A} = \overline{U}\mathbf{A}_S U, \tag{7.4.9}$$

where φ_S and $\mathbf{A}_S$ are the potentials for $t = \mathbf{x} = 0$. It is clear from (7.2.16), however, that to make use of this result it is necessary to have matrix representations of the energy E . For this purpose, we again consider the electrolytic system S occupying the rectangular region R, We may regard the electromagnetic field and the charged matter as two systems S′ and S″ in interaction with one another. The energy of the charged matter is simply its kinetic energy of motion. As in Maxwell's theory, the energy density of the electromagnetic field is $(\mathbf{E}^2+\mathbf{B}^2)/(8\pi)$, but since

$$\mathbf{E}^2 = \dot{\mathbf{A}}^2/c^2 + \nabla\cdot(2\varphi\dot{\mathbf{A}}/c + \varphi\nabla\varphi) + 4\pi\varphi\epsilon_M,$$

the energy is given by

$$H = H' + V,$$

$$H' = \frac{1}{8\pi}\int\{\dot{\mathbf{A}}^2/c^2 + (\nabla\times\mathbf{A})^2\}d^3x, \quad V = \tfrac{1}{2}\int\varphi\epsilon_M d^3x, \tag{7.4.10}$$

where the integrations extend over the entire region R. The second term, V, is is clearly the energy of interaction of the charge with the electric field that it generates; the factor $\frac{1}{2}$ is needed to avoid counting the energy of interaction of the charges twice. Since c is very large, it can be seen from (7.4.7) that V is the main contribution to the energy of the field. By substituting the expression for ϵ_M from the first equation of (7.4.7) and using Gauss's theorem, the latter can also be written in the form

$$V = \frac{1}{8\pi}\int(\nabla\varphi)^2 d^3x. \tag{7.4.11}$$

In the application to the cortex, a similar transformation can be made of the energy of interaction V^{c} of the ions of the electrolytic fluid with the electric field generated by charge associated with the cell; this is

$$V^{\mathrm{c}} = \int\epsilon_M\varphi^{\mathrm{c}}d^3x = \frac{1}{4\pi}\int\nabla\varphi\cdot\nabla\varphi^{\mathrm{c}}d^3x = \int\varphi\epsilon_M^{\mathrm{c}}d^3x, \tag{7.4.12}$$

where φ^{c} is the potential generated by the charge density ϵ_M^{c} of the cell. From the second of these expressions it is easy to infer where in the brain the interaction of the extracellular field with a cell will be of most significance. We have seen that, as a consequence of the metabolic activity of the cells, a potential difference of up to 100 mV is developed across the cellular membrane; and in the channels through the membrane, only $\sim$ 50 Å in length, the expectation value of the potential gradient is therefore not only large but very much greater than anywhere else in the electrolytic fluid. The same potential difference polarizes the membrane of the cell. Thus, in and only in the channels of the membrane, values of both $\nabla\varphi$ and $\nabla\varphi^{\mathrm{c}}$, which are not only large but normal to the surface of the membrane, predominate. This indicates the importance of electric phenomena in the channels for the vital functions of the cells.

The radiation field

Although the energy of the radiation field generated by the ionic currents denoted by H' in (7.4.10) is very small in an electrolyte compared with that of the electric field responsible for graded and action potentials, it is not without significance, especially for the external interactions of the ions such as those which permit the monitoring of superficial activity in the brain by magnetoencephalography. It is this radiative component of the electromagnetic field that is given most prominence in standard works of quantum electrodynamics; for this reason we shall not discuss it in depth here.

The energy of the field in the interaction representation can be evaluated explicitly in terms of the vectorial Fourier coefficients $\mathbf{c}_k$ of the transverse component of the vector potential $\mathbf{A}$ and their time derivatives $\dot{\mathbf{c}}_k$, thus:

$$H' = \sum_{\mathbf{k}} \tfrac{1}{2}(\dot{\mathbf{c}}_k^2 + \omega_k^2 \mathbf{c}_k^2), \tag{7.4.13}$$

and the expression under the summation is the same as the energy of a harmonic oscillator with unit mass and frequency ω_k. The quantum mechanics of the oscillators is the same as that developed in the last Section, and shows that the energy associated with each wave vector $\mathbf{k}$

is of the form $N_k \hbar\omega_k$, where N_k is interpreted as the number of particles with energy $\hbar\omega_k$. These particles are the photons which, coming from external sources, are capable of activating neurons in the retina, and escaping from the electrolytic layer at the surface of the brain, provide an indication of the ionic currents below the scalp.

Particle fields and densities

In quantum mechanics, it is still possible to express the charge density ϵ_M that appears in (7.4.10) and (7.4.12) in terms of the number densities n_a of the particles carrying a charge:

$$\epsilon_M = \sum_a e_a n_a; \tag{7.4.14}$$

however, the n_a are no longer simply functions, but matrices n_a that depend on the time t and the position $\mathbf{x}$ in the Heisenberg representation. The corresponding classical quantities introduced for the ions in Section 4.3 may be interpreted as expectation values $< n_a(t, \mathbf{x}) >$, computed as in (7.4.5), with the help of the statistical matrix for the entire electrolyte.

To obtain explicit expressions for the number densities, it is necessary to introduce a matrix field variable ψ_a for each particle, including water molecules, carrying a charge. Each field ψ_a can be expressed in terms of a set of complex orthonormal functions $\chi_{ak}(x)$ of position within any region of interest (R) within the electrolyte, thus:

$$\psi_a = \sum_k c_{ak}\chi_{ak}(x), \qquad \int_{\mathrm{R}} \chi^*_{ak}(x)\chi_{al}(x)d^3x = \delta_{kl}, \tag{7.4.15}$$

where the three-dimensional integration is over the interior of R and, as usual, δ_{kl} has the value 1 if $k = l$, but 0 otherwise. For a rectangular region of volume V_{R}, $\chi_{ak}(x) = V_{\mathrm{R}}{}^{-\frac{1}{2}} \exp(i\mathbf{k}\cdot\mathbf{x})$, and the c_{ak} are Fourier coefficients. But for any region, since ψ_a is a matrix, each c_{ak} is also a matrix depending in general on the time. In fact c_{ak} is an annihilation matrix, with properties similar to c in(7.3.9) when the particles of the a-th type are fermions, or c_0 in (7.3.17) when they are bosons. In any event the matrix

$$\nu_{ak} = c^*_{ak}c_{ak} \tag{7.4.16}$$

represents the number of particles of the a-th type in the k-th mode within the region, and has eigenvalues 0 and 1 for the particles that are fermions, and also for bosons if the very small probability of an integral value greater than 1 is neglected. We may therefore safely assume that $\nu_{ak}^2 = \nu_{ak}$, so that ν_{ak} represents a bit of information as defined in the last Section.

If ψ_a^* is the hermitean conjugate of ψ_a, then $\psi_a^* = \sum_k c_{ak}^* \chi_{ak}^*(x)$ and the number densities n_a and the charge density ϵ_M in (7.4.7) and (7.4.12) are given by

$$n_a = \psi_a^* \psi_a = \sum_{k,l} c_{ak}^* c_{al} \chi_{ak}^*(x) \chi_{al}(x),$$

$$\epsilon_M = \sum_a e_a \sum_{\mathbf{k}} c_{ak}^* c_{al} \chi_{ak}^*(x) \chi_{al}(x), \qquad (7.4.17)$$

With this expression for the charge density, (7.4.7) can be solved explicitly to obtain the potential φ as a function $\varphi(x)$ of position, in the form

$$\varphi = \sum_a e_a \sum_{k,l} c_{ak}^* c_{al} f_{kl}(x), \qquad \nabla^2 f_{kl}(x) = -4\pi \chi_{ak}^*(x) \chi_{al}(x), \quad (7.4.18)$$

within R. If R is a rectangular region,

$$f_{kk}(x) = -(2\pi/V_{\mathrm{R}})(\mathbf{k} \cdot \mathbf{x})^2/\mathbf{k}^2,$$

$$f_{kl}(x) = (4\pi/V_{\mathrm{R}}) \exp[-i(\mathbf{k} - \mathbf{l}) \cdot \mathbf{x}]/(\mathbf{k} - \mathbf{l})^2 \ \ (\mathbf{k} \neq \mathbf{l}). \qquad (7.4.19)$$

The quantized potential is what might be detected in an electrolyte by some microscopic measurement at the point $\mathbf{x}$ at time t, and includes contributions from the charge of polarized water molecules. It is necessary to take the expectation value of φ to obtain the macroscopic potential $< \varphi >$, and the contributions from the polarization charge serve to reduce the effective ionic charge by the factor $1/\kappa$, according to (7.4.8).

The field as a quantal 'tape'

Since $f^*_{kl} = f_{lk}$, the infinite matrix f with elements f_{kl} is hermitean and can therefore be reduced to diagonal form by a unitary transformation, thus:

$$f_{kl} = \sum_m u_{km} f_m u^*_{ml}, \qquad \sum_m u_{km} u^*_{ml} = \delta_{kl}, \tag{7.4.20}$$

where the f_m are the eigenvalues of f; but since f depends on position and time, so do its eigenvalues f_m in general. It follows from (7.4.18) and (7.4.20) that

$$\varphi = \sum_{a,m} e_a f_m d^*_{am} d_{am}, \qquad d_{am} = \sum_k c_{ak} u^*_{km}. \tag{7.4.21}$$

Moreover, because of the unitary condition satisfied by u_{km}, as shown in (7.4.20), the d_{am} satisfy the same relations as the c_{ak} in (7.4.16), and it follows from $\nu^2_{ak} = \nu_{ak}$, under the same conditions, that

$$n^2_{am} = n_{am}, \qquad n_{am} = d^*_{am} d_{am}. \tag{7.4.22}$$

Finally, we note that the expression for the potential in (7.4.21) may be written

$$\varphi = \sum_{a,m} f_m n_{am} = \sum_B f_B n_B, \tag{7.4.23}$$

where the subscript B stands for a and m.

The interaction energy V^c of the extracellular field with the charge of the cell is defined in (7.4.12) and is easily evaluated with the help of (7.4.23), yielding

$$V^c = \sum_B \int f_B n_B \epsilon^c_M d^3x, . \tag{7.4.24}$$

where the integration is now over the cell.

As they are idempotent matrices of the same type as introduced in (7.3.3), *we identify the n_B as bits of the 'tape' of a quantal Turing machine.* In principle, they may depend on position and time. In the absence of variable external interactions, it is possible to find not only *static* representations in which they are diagonal, and therefore independent of time, but *dynamic* representations, where they depend on time in any way consistent with the macroscopic equations; they may, in fact, be periodic functions of the time. In the following Section we shall make use of what is known as the *interaction representation*, in which a static or dynamic representation is adopted for the bits of the electrolytic fluid, but the statistical matrix of the 'tape' is constantly changing as a result of its interactions with the cellular environment. We shall also examine the process by which the 'machine', consisting of the cells of the cortex, is able to scan and modify the tape; and, since the modification of the tape requires interaction with the machine, the state of the machine will naturally be modified in the same process.

7.5 Measurement and Observation

The Interaction Representation

In the following paragraphs we analyse the requirements for the detection of a microscopic system in detail, and so obtain a better insight into the mechanism by which, in the process of measurement, an indeterminate observable acquires a definite value.

When two or more systems interact there is, in general, an exchange of both energy and information; and while the total energy is unchanged, there is a loss of information concerning each of the systems. This applies in particular to the interaction between a microscopic system and a macroscopic detector, to be studied below with the help of a technique based on the use of the *interaction representation*.

Let us consider a composite system S consisting of two subsystems S$'$ and S$''$, and suppose that the statistical matrix of the composite system at some initial time $t = 0$ is P_0. As shown in (7.2.18), the statistical matrices of the subsystems at the initial time are $P_0' = \mathrm{tr}''(P_0)$ and $P_0'' = \mathrm{tr}'(P_0)$, but P_0 can only be expressed as the direct product of P_0' and P_0'' when the subsystems have not been in interaction up to that time. It follows that the information to be gained from the composite system is the same as the joint information to be gained from the two subsystems only if they have not interacted previously.

If A is the action, the statistical matrix P of the composite system, and the quantal information I to be gained, in any observational frame at time t are given in terms of P_0 and I_0 by

$$P = UP_0\overline{U}, \qquad I = UI_0\overline{U}, \qquad U = \exp(-iA/\hbar), \qquad (7.5.1)$$

in the Schrödinger representation, according to (7.2.9), (7.3.1) and (7.2.16).

We choose an observational frame of reference so that the centre of mass of the composite system is at rest ($\mathbf{v} = 0$) and is appropriately oriented ($\mathbf{u} = 0$) at the origin of coordinates ($\mathbf{x} = 0$). Then, as in (7.2.21), the action reduces to the energy H and

$$U = \exp(-iHt/\hbar), \qquad H = H^{(1)} + H^{(2)} + V. \qquad (7.5.2)$$

Here H, $H^{(1)}$ and $H^{(2)}$ are the energies of the composite system and the two subsystems, respectively, and V is the interaction energy; also, $\overline{U}$ is the hermitean conjugate of U, which satisfies $U\overline{U} = 1$. It is obvious that the unitary matrix U satisfies

$$i\hbar\frac{\partial U}{\partial t} = (H^{(1)} + H^{(2)} + V)U, \qquad (7.5.3)$$

and if we write

$$U = \exp[-i(H^{(1)} + H^{(2)})t/\hbar]T = U_0T, \qquad (7.5.4)$$

it follows from (7.5.3) that $T(t)$ satisfies an integral equation

$$T(t) = 1 - i\int_0^t \tilde{V}(\tau)T(\tau)d\tau/\hbar, \qquad \tilde{V} = \overline{U}_0VU_0 \qquad (7.5.5)$$

which can be solved, for instance, by iteration. The expression given in (7.2.9) for the statistical matrix is then expressible in the form

$$P = U_0\tilde{P}\overline{U}_0, \qquad \tilde{P} = TP_0\overline{T}, \qquad (7.5.6)$$

where $\tilde{P}$ is the statistical matrix in the interaction representation.

The expectation value $< O >$ of an observable O at time t is $\mathrm{tr}(PO)$, where P obviously depends on the time in the Schrödinger representation, so that although O is independent of the time, its expectation value $< O >$ varies with time, as it should. However, it follows from (7.2.7) that

$$< O > = \mathrm{tr}(PO) = \mathrm{tr}(\tilde{P}\tilde{O}), \qquad \tilde{O} = U_0O\overline{U}_0, \qquad (7.5.7)$$

where $\widetilde{O}$ is the observable in the interaction representation.

It is evident that, in principle, the last three results provide a method for the calculation of the expectation value of any observable of the composite system as a function of time. But since the matrix U_0 in (7.5.4) is the direct product $U_0' \otimes U_0''$, where $U_0' = \exp(-iH't/\hbar)$ and $U_0'' = \exp(-iH''t/\hbar)$ are unitary matrices of the subsystems, we shall need an explicit evaluation of matrices of this type, which is developed below.

Measurement and Observation

We are now in a position to make a study at the most fundamental level of the interaction between the collection of cells forming the brain and the electrolytic fluid that envelops it, interpreted as the interaction between a quantal Turing machine and its 'tape'. In the brain, the 'bits' of the quantal tape are represented by the matrices n_B in (7.4.23) and (7.4.24), and the interaction is with the charge associated with the cells. But it is useful to recognize that this is only a particular example of a natural process that occurs whenever a microscopic system interacts with a macroscopic system in a sufficiently metastable state. We shall therefore consider such a process in a perfectly general context.

The theory of the interaction between two systems is somewhat simpler if they have not experienced any interaction at the initial time $t = 0$. Then the statistical matrix P_0 of the composite system S at that time can be expressed as a direct product $P_0' \otimes P_0''$ of the density matrices of the subsystems S$'$ and S$''$, so that according to (7.5.6), the statistical matrix of S in the interaction representation can be written

$$\widetilde{P} = T(P_0' \otimes P_0'')\overline{T}, \tag{7.5.8}$$

where T is unitary and depends on the time.

We shall make use of this formula to study the interaction between a microscopic system S$'$ and a measuring device D, that in the most general application can be thought of as a set of independently functioning detectors. Because of their independence, S$'$ cannot interact with more than one these detectors simultaneously, and it will be sufficient for our purpose to consider the possible interaction between the microscopic system and just one of them, which we identify with system S″. We are interested in the final form of the statistical matrix $\widetilde{P}$ and wish to show that, under certain conditions, and for all practical purposes, *it consists of two parts, one corresponding to the possibility that the detector* S″ *functioned, and the other to the possibility that it did not.* Although this desired result may seem unremarkable, it has provided one of the most difficult problems of quantum mechanics! The authors[39] have emphasised that it is necessary to assume

(1) that the detector is macroscopic, consisting of an enormous number of microscopic subsystems, and also

(2) that the detector is efficient, implying that it is in a metastable state.

To appreciate the nature of the problem, we note that the T-matrix in (7.5.8) satisfies the integral equation (7.5.5) and can certainly be expressed in the form

$$T = \sum_{r+} g_{r+} \otimes T_{r+} + \sum_{r-} g_{r-} \otimes 1, \tag{7.5.9}$$

where the g_{r+} and g_{r-} are a set of idempotents, in the interaction representation, of a selected observable O' of S′ that is measured by the detector. It is easy to verify from this expression that T is unitary ($T\overline{T} = 1$), provided that all the T_{r+} are unitary. Usually the observable O' depends on the position of S′ and determines whether the interaction energy $\widetilde{V}$ is sufficient to activate the detector. The above expression for T supposes that the g_{r+} correspond to the possibility that the detector is activated, and the g_{r-} to the possibility that it is not. From the substitution of (7.5.9) into (7.5.8), we find that

$$\widetilde{P} = P_{++} + P_{+-} + P_{-+} + P_{--},$$

$$P_{++} = \sum_{r+,s+} g_{r_+} P_0' g_{s+} \otimes T_{r+} P_0'' \overline{T}_{s+}, \qquad P_{+-} = \sum_{r+,s-} g_{r+} P_0' g_{s-} \otimes T_{r+} P_0''$$

$$P_{-+} = \sum_{r^-,s^+} g_{r-} P_0' g_{s+} \otimes P_0'' \overline{T}_{s+}, \qquad P_{--} = \sum_{r-,s-} g_{r-} P_0' g_{s-} \otimes P_0''. \tag{7.5.10}$$

It thus appears that the statistical matrix of the composite system is a sum of *four* terms. The first and the last correspond to the possibilities that the microsystem is detected and that it is not detected. But P_{+-} and P_{-+}, which are hermitean conjugates of one another, correspond to the possibility that the microsystem is neither detected nor undetected, and the whole system is in an indeterminate state rather similar to Schrödinger's cat. If the two conditions listed as (1) and (2) above are satisfied, these indecisive terms should surely be zero, or sufficiently near to zero for all practical purposes; this is what remains to be shown.

The statistical matrices of the separate subsystems S′ and S″ are $\widetilde{P}'$ and $\widetilde{P}''$, respectively, given by

$$\widetilde{P}' = P'_{++} + P'_{+-} + P'_{-+} + P'_{--}, \qquad P'_{++} = \sum_{r+,s+} \mathrm{tr}''(T_{r+}P''_0\overline{T}_{s+})g_{r+}P'_0g_{s+},$$

$$P'_{+-} = \sum_{r+,s-} \mathrm{tr}''(T_{r+}P''_0)g_{r+}P'_0g_{s-}, \qquad P'_{--} = \sum_{r-,s-} g_{r-}P'_0g_{s-} \qquad (7.5.11)$$

and

$$\widetilde{P}'' = P''_+ + P''_-, \qquad P''_+ = \sum_{r+} p'_{r+}(T_{r+}P''_0\overline{T}_{r+}), \qquad p'_{r+} = \mathrm{tr}'(g_{r+}P'_0),$$

$$P''_- = (1 - p'_+)P''_0, \qquad p'_+ = \sum_{r+} p'_{r+}. \qquad (7.5.12)$$

Here p'_+ is identified as the total probability that measurement of the observable O' at time t should yield the value o'_+, with contributions given by

$$p'_+ = \sum_v p'_{r,v}p^*_v, \qquad p'_{+,v} = \mathrm{tr}'(\sum_{r+} g_{r+}g^*_v) \qquad (7.5.13)$$

where p'_+ is the probability that the selected observable O' of S′ has the value o'_+ and, as in (7.2.8), $p'_{+,v}$ is the probability for a transition between states represented by the idempotent g^*_v, and any of the g_{r+}.

Of course $1 - p'_+$ is then the total probability that the measurement yields some other value, or that the microsystem is not detected. These results are entirely consistent with Born's statistical interpretation of quantum mechanics. The fact that the statistical matrix (7.5.12) is expressed as a sum of two terms (non-trivially, when the T_{r+} are different from 1) implies not the existence of more than one world, but that following the interaction, additional information may be gained from examination of the component S″ of the measuring system.

However, the nature of the information is encoded in the statistical matrix $\widetilde{P}'$ of the system S′, and it should be expected that, with an efficient measuring device, this also reduces effectively for large t to the sum $P'_{++} + P'_{--}$ of two terms, since the component P'_{+-} of $\widetilde{P}'$ is a measure of the residual indeterminacy of the measurement of O'. From (7.5.11) it is evident that this component is given by

$$P'_{+-} = \sum_{r+,s-} C_{r+}(g_{r+}P'_0 g_{s-}), \qquad C_{r+} = \mathrm{tr}''(T_{r+}P''_0). \qquad (7.5.14)$$

where the coefficients C_{r+} are determined by the interaction of the microscopic system with the measuring device. We shall now carry out the evaluation of these coefficients, with the object of showing that, under the specified conditions, they are completely negligible.

The Conditions for Observation

The results obtained so far would remain correct if S″ were itself a microsystem, or for some other reason S′ escaped detection. Then it would be quite possible for the interaction of these two systems to remain indeterminate. The conditions for observation, in more detail, are as follows.

Some macroscopic feature of the detector must change rapidly and significantly as a result of the interaction. It follows not only that the detector S″ should be a macroscopic object, but that the interaction with the microscopic system S′ should result in an appreciable change in the expectation value of an observable O'' of the component S″ of the measuring device, corresponding to an eigenvalue of O'. The interaction must therefore affect very many (R) of the disjoint microscopic subsystems from which S″ is made. If $O'' = -\log P''$, where P'' is the statistical matrix of S″, the expectation value is the information I'' associated with S″, or the entropy in suitable units. A significant and rapid change in the entropy can result if S″ is in a thermodynamically unstable or metastable state. Subject to these requirements, we shall show that, when the observable O' is measured, the statistical matrix $\widetilde{P}'$ appearing in (7.5.11) reduces effectively to the form $P_{++} + P_{--}$ after the interaction with the detector has occurred and the coefficients C_{r+} in (7.5.14) are effectively zero.

To formulate the required conditions, the statistical matrix P_0'' of S″ at the initial time is first expressed in terms of the idempotents g^*_{m,s_m} $(m = 1, ...R)$ of its microscopic subsystems, thus:

$$P_0'' = \sum_{s_1} p^*_{s_1} g^*_{1,s_1} \otimes P_{s_1}, \qquad P_{s_1...s_{m-1}} = \sum_{s_m} p^*_{s_1...s_m} g^*_{m,s_m} \otimes P_{s_1...s_m}. \tag{7.5.15}$$

Here the coefficient $p^*_{s_1...s_m}$ is a conditional probability, and $P_{s_1...s_m}$ is the reduced density matrix for the part of the detector excluding the first m of its microscopic subsystems. As foreshadowed in Section 7.2, the subscript $s+$ that labels the states of the detector is being treated as an R-component vector $(s_1, ...s_r)$. In the absence of interaction with S′, the statistical matrix P'' of S″ at time t, and also any selected observable O'' of S″, can be expressed in the same way. However, at time t the statistical matrix of S″ in the interaction representation is given by (7.5.12), in which the unitary matrix T_{r+} can be written

$$T_{r+} = \sum_{r_1} t_{r_1} g_{1,r_1} \otimes T_{r_1}, \qquad T_{r_1...r_{m-1}} = \sum_{r_m} t_{r_1...r_m} g_{m,r_m} \otimes T_{r_1...r_m}, \tag{7.5.16}$$

where the coefficient $t_{r_1...r_m}$ is a complex number of modulus 1, and $T_{r_1...r_m}$ is unitary. All of these vary with the time.

Assuming that the detector functions, the change in entropy or information can be determined from the components $T_{r+}P_0''\overline{T}_{r+}$ of the statistical matrix, which may be developed by successive substitutions from (7.5.15) and (7.5.16). After the first substitution, for example,

$$T_{r+}P_0''\overline{T}_{r+} = \sum_{s_1} p^*_{s_1} g_{1,r_1} g^*_{1,s_1} g_{1,r_1} \otimes T_{r_1} P_{s_1} \overline{T}_{r_1}, \tag{7.5.17}$$

Subsequent substitutions make use of the results obtained by setting $m = 2, 3, ...$ in (7.5.15) and (7.5.16). The trace of any function of the matrix in (7.5.17) and similar matrices obtained on further substitution can be evaluated in terms of the traces

$$c_{r_m s_m} = \mathrm{tr}(g_{m,r_m} g^*_{m,s_m}), \tag{7.5.18}$$

and these are the only time-dependent factors. Thus a macroscopically significant change in the entropy requires a significant change in a large number of these transition probabilities. In fact, at time $t = 0$, $T_{r+} = 1$, and $g_{m,r_m} = g^*_{m,r_m}$, so that the $c_{r_m s_m}$ all reduce to 1; but for $t > 0$, when the stated conditions are met, very many of them must rapidly deviate from their initial values. A particular example of this, in which the detector is modelled by a set of coupled oscillators in a metastable state, is given in an earlier publication[360].

It is now easy to obtain an explicit expression for the indeterminacy coefficients C_{r+}, as defined in (7.5.14), by a similar method. Again with the help of (7.5.15) and (7.5.16), we have

$$C_{r+} = \prod_{m=1}^{R} \sum_{r_m} t_{r_1 \ldots r_m} \sum_{s_m} p^*_{s_1 \ldots s_m} c_{r_m s_m}. \tag{7.5.19}$$

The transition probabilities $c_{r_m s_m}$ are always non-negative real numbers not greater than 1, and for $t >> 0$, under the conditions stated, many of them will have values significantly less than 1 (typically $\frac{1}{2}$). This is therefore true of the statistical averages $\sum_{s_m} p^*_{s_1 \ldots s_m} c_{r_m s_m}$, which may also be interpreted as probabilities. The coefficients $t_{r_1 \ldots r_m}$ under the summation in (7.5.19) are of modulus 1, and it follows that their average value must have a modulus not exceeding 1. Thus C_{r+} is a product of R factors many of which have a modulus appreciably less than 1, and if R is sufficiently large, this product will be immeasurably small in absolute magnitude. Thus, the effect of the measurement is to reduce the indeterminacy amplitudes C_{r+} of the observable O' to a completely negligible level.

In summary, one of the essential features of the detector is its macroscopic character, required to ensure that the amplitudes C_{r+} are completely negligible. The metastability of the functional components of the detector is also required to ensure a sufficiently rapid and readily observable change in entropy following the detection of the microscopic system.

The statistical matrix $\tilde{P}'$ of S′ in (7.5.11) is thus reduced effectively to the form

$$\tilde{P}' \simeq P'_{++} + P'_{--}. \tag{7.5.20}$$

and as $\mathrm{tr}'(P'_{++}) = p'_+$, the classical information to be gained concerning S′ from the operation of the detector is

$$< I' >= - < \log \tilde{P}' >= -p'_+ \log p'_+ - (1 - p'_+) \log(1 - p'_+). \tag{7.5.21}$$

This has a maximum value of log2, or one bit, when $p'_+ = \frac{1}{2}$ and nothing is known initially concerning the microscopic observable O' responsible for the functioning of the detector. This information is very small and is important only because of its exact correspondence with the macroscopic information to be gained from the detector. However, the information I' in (7.5.21) could only be zero if the value of O' were already known, and indeterministic quantum mechanics does not allow the prediction of the result of the measurement, or the content of the information actually gained by the measurement. Nor does it allow the prediction of the result of the observation in the animal cortex, but the process by which the information is gained by an observer is precisely similar to the process by which information is gained concerning any other macrosopic event.

After the event of the functioning, or failure to function, of the detector, a new statistical matrix $\widetilde{P}'_i$ (where $i = +$ or $i = -$) for the microsystem can be constructed by a conscious observer, incorporating the information I' gained from the measurement. This is the construction we called 'revision of the statistical matrix' in Section 7.3, instead of using the ubiquitous but misleading description 'collapse of the wave packet'. The relevance of these results to a theory of consciousness will be discussed in the final Chapter.

The above theory of measurement is very general, and it remains to consider the application to the acquisition of information about the external world by the animal brain. An account of the internal processing of this information was given in Section 6.5, but was also very general and did not take into consideration the nature of the information conveyed by the senses. Auditory and tactile information has a significant role, but visual information is most important in conveying perceptions of space and time, and depends on the sensitivity of the eye to light, which is made up of photons emitted as a consequence of quantal events at very many points of space-time. Although the eye is sensitive to very small numbers of photons[26,27], it is their statistical effect that is primarily responsible for our perceptions of the external world.

The information transmitted from a distant event by a photon is encoded mainly in its momentum, though the spin (polarization) may also be significant for some animals such as bees. The direction of the momentum is interpreted as the direction of the source from which the photon was emitted, and its magnitude as the colour of the source. The direction is adequately represented by a pair of angular variables θ and ϕ, which, according to (7.3.3), form a single bit of quantal information. The angles depend on the orientation of the observer, who is able to explore the field of vision by movements of the eye and head. Bits of visual information acquired in this way are of a few types distinguishable by colour, and are processed internally to construct a two-dimensional image of the environment. With the help of binocular vision, the information can be processed further to gain some idea of distance, and with the help of hippocampal circuits[197] it can be recorded sequentially in memory, as described in Section 3.3. The effect of all these processes is to build a self-centred perspective of the external world in space and time from quantal bits of information.

Perhaps the most fundamental of the internal processes described is the assembly of two-dimensional images from quantal bits, and we can conjecture how this is done. We have pointed out earlier that the effect of the transmission of visual information can often be detected as potentials in the extracellular fluid of the brain. Bits of information can be combined in different ways, but the most important combination is the *join*. The join of two different bits of information, $n^{(1)}$ and $n^{(2)}$, in a multi-dimensional representation is the *piece* of information

$$p = (n^{(1)} + n^{(2)} - n^{(1)}n^{(2)} - n^{(2)}n^{(1)})/[1 - \mathrm{tr}(n^{(1)}n'')] \qquad (7.5.22)$$

which satisfies $n^{(1)}p = n^{(1)}$ and $n^{(2)}p = n^{(2)}$. If the bits represent information concerning the directions of two sources of light, the piece represents information concerning the line joining them. In these circumstances the piece is an integral component of the extracellular potential, and it is therefore an observable that can be detected by neurons by parallel processing. Other observables, corresponding to areas or more complex geometrical patterns may be detected in a similar way. Thus, through its capacity for the quantum parallel processing of potentials in the extracellular fluid, it is possible for the brain to acquire intuitive perceptions of space and time.

Summary

In the context of indeterministic quantum mechanics, a new meaning must be given to the concept of an *observable* quantity. This was defined in (7.2.1) as a matrix constructed from all possible values, called *eigenvalues*, that could result from the measurement of the observable. The measurement of any observable of a microscopic system precludes the possibility of measuring some related *complementary* observables; therefore, the maximum information that can be gained from a measurement is the value of each of a set of observables, whose nature depends on the measuring device. The exact values of all of a complete set of observables cannot be known without or in advance of measurement, but quantum mechanics permits the determination of the probabilities that observables have any specified values. For *selected* observables these probabilities can be used to construct a *statistical matrix*, defined in (7.2.5), which encodes all the information that can be obtained concerning a microscopic system.

The *fundamental* observables of any system are its energy, momentum, angular momentum, central vector and mass, the last two of which determine the position in space of the system. As shown by (7.2.9) and (7.2.16), the fundamental observables determine the way the statistical matrix depends on the time, and the position, orientation and velocity of the measuring device.

As in classical physics, the concept of *information to be gained* can be given the quantitative meaning formulated in (7.3.1). No information can be gained from a system in a pure state; therefore the latter can be only the reconstruction by a conscious observer of the *former* state of a system in the light of information actually gained. But indeterministic quantum mechanics imposes important restrictions on information to be gained concerning a microscopic system, depending on the measuring device employed. Information may also be *created* in the process of measurement. The information to be gained is localized in the measuring device, and the transfer of information does not require action at a distance.

In Section 7.4 an account is given of the quantization of the potentials of the electromagnetic field and particle fields, and of its application to the electrolytic fluid of the brain. It is pointed out that the classical electromagnetic fields and potentials can be interpreted as expectation values of the corresponding quantal fields and potentials, so that the essential results of Chapter 4 retain their validity in the quantum theory. Because of the large potential gradient in the channels of the cell membrane, it is found that these channels are the focus of the interaction of the extracellular fluid with the cell. The principal results, formulated in (7.4.23) and (7.4.24), are the decomposition into wave-like components of the electric potential, and the energy of their interaction with the charge associated with a cell. In quantum theory, the components of the extracellular potential all have quantized (discrete) amplitudes subject to the same indeterminacy as other quantum mechanical observables. They are described formally as 'bits' of a quantal 'tape' that can be both scanned and modified by the cells of the cortex.

The interaction of a quantal 'bit' with a cell is treated as a particular example of the interaction of a microscopic system with a measuring device. In this Section the interaction of any two systems is studied in what is known as the *interaction representation*, and the results are applied to the interaction of the microscopic system with a detector that is part of the measuring device. The result of (7.5.11) shows that after some time the statistical matrix of the microsystem is always a sum of four terms: one corresponding to the possibility that the microsystem interacted with the detector; one to the possibility that it did not; and two to the possibility that the result of the interaction remained indeterminate, as in Schrödinger's cat paradox.

Two conditions are proposed for the reduction of the indeterminacy to completely unobservable proportions: (1) that the detector should be a macroscopic object, so that a very large number of microscopic particles are affected by the interaction; and (2) that the detector should be in a metastable state, so that a microscopic interaction results in a large change of the entropy of the detector. By making use of these conditions, it is shown, in (7.5.20), that the statistical matrix is effectively reduced to two terms.

The information to be gained concerning the microsystem from the detector in the final state of the combined system is given by (7.5.21); but this can also be described as information created by the system, since it was not available in the initial state.

Chapter 8

Aspects of Consciousness

8.1 Awareness and Volition

Throughout this volume, we have identified consciousness pragmatically as a combination of *awareness*, implying the attention given to sensory impressions and other elements of short-term memory; and *volition*, implying the the decision making that guides the direction given to a train of thought, or the performance of a sequence of voluntary motor actions. The importance of the formation of sequential memory and constant access to this memory has been emphasised, and we have developed a quantitative description of all cortical processing in terms of information, insisting on a fundamental role for quantal indeterminism.

But the *instant of perception* is a fundamental element of awareness, just as the *instant of choice* is a fundamental element of volition. Our initial aim is to provide a detailed description of such events in physical and biological terms, in order to provide a scientific basis for understanding of events that some scientists of great distinction have invested with mysterious if not magical qualities. The sense of mystery is most vividly conveyed in a variety of paradoxes that are of a physical, rather than a logical or mathematical character. Some simple examples have already been introduced in Sections 1.3 and 7.3, and given an interpretation consistent with common sense; but there is one other that may seem to have special relevance to our theme.

This is a paradox that has features different from those so far considered, and that seems at first encounter even more puzzling. In the version due to de Broglie[361], a box containing a single elementary particle is sealed in Paris. The box is separated into two halves by inserting an impermeable partition, and one half is sent to Tokyo, while the other half remains in Paris. It was natural for de Broglie to represent the particle as a wave function and reason that, even after separation part of the wave function would be in each half of the box. But if the half of the box in Paris is opened and examined, then it either will or will not be perceived to contain the particle. The examination requires conscious intervention, of course, but at that instant it also becomes certain that the other half of the box in Tokyo either does or does not contain the particle. Because of this, some authors have concluded that action at a distance is a necessary consequence of quantum mechanics. But in fact the experiment could be done with a tennis ball, instead of an elementary particle, with a similar result, and although the detection of the particle has to be modelled by quantal methods such as those of Section 6.5, in terms of information theory there is little difference, because the presence of the particle in one half of the box is a *selected* observable from the time the box is divided. This is the type of situation in which the results of classical and quantal information theory have been shown to be identical. No one would suggest that action at a distance is implied by the discovery of a tennis ball in one place instead of another.

It may still be asked why the theory of the previous Section should be considered to apply to the process of dividing the box, and not just to the actual process of detection of the particle. This is a pertinent question, since the separation of the two halves does not appear to require any substance that is in a metastable state. However, the important circumstance, which can be verified by an explicit calculation using (4.2.15), is that there is a change in the entropy of the system of particle and box which occurs at the time when the partition of the box is effected. The change in entropy, or information to be gained, is significantly large if the box is of macroscopic dimensions; if it is not, de Broglie's paradox is in principle similar to the EPR paradox that was discussed in Section 7.3. The change in entropy must be supposed to initiate the process described in Section 6.5, while the time at which the observational process is completed is not important, except insofar as it involves a conscious observer.

This paradox shows how the formulation of a problem in terms of a single wave function or state vector can be misleading, and illustrates the circumstances in which the use of the statistical matrix and quantal information theory is most advantageous. In general, a macroscopic object such as a box must be represented by a statistical matrix. But, as we have seen in the previous Section, there is an important role for consciousness in the revision of the statistical matrix in the light of information gained, and this must be taken into account to reach a complete understanding of any observational process.

The revision of the statistical matrix is a process governed by the laws of quantum mechanics, and to obtain further insight into the nature of consciousness, we must consider the structure of the statistical matrix of the cortex, which exhibits in minute detail the interdependence of the observer and observed. The quantum mechanical relations satisfied by this matrix determine certain probabilities that represent the limits of definite knowledge; and they provide the only quantitative information we now possess relating mental processes to observable phenomena. In Section 7.3 we have seen how the commutation relations imply indeterminacy in the values of complementary observables of a physical system, detected by the external process of measurement. But since the observing nervous system is an essential part of the total system, similar relations must also hold for its internal processes. It is the implications of this fact that, with the help of the principles developed in the preceding Sections, we now wish to explore.

Let us consider the state of the human cortex produced by a single aspect of an observation, say the noting of a particular pointer position on a dial in an experiment to detect the presence of a particle in some well defined region of space. This state is represented by the statistical matrix of the cortex, obtained by reduction of the statistical matrix for the combined system of the observer and observed. Disregarding the details of neural transmission and processing for the moment, a reduced statistical matrix for the cortex represents a unique electrical field configuration determined by the potentials in and around the neurons at the instant of recognition. These potentials depend, of course, not only on recognition of the pointer position, but also on a variety of other sensory inputs received at the same time, as well as a series of internal transmissions and feedback effects occurring prior to recognition. Further, this field must change smoothly in time to other slightly different configurations to permit the recognition of subsequent pointer positions. It is on the informational properties of such complex cortical fields and the dynamics of their changes that we concentrate attention in the following Sections.

Awareness we take to consist entirely of the information conveyed by dynamical patterns of images and symbols, interpreted in various specialized regions of the cortex that activate short-term memory. Actually, the term 'transient memory' is more appropriate to emphasize the fact that memories vary continuously in duration, depending on how many times the patterns of pulses of which they consist are renewed; that is, how many times the inevitable exponential decay of the potential in the neurons affected will be arrested prior to entering refractory states, by repetition or periodic extracellular potential waves. If unrenewed any transient pattern will quickly fade from awareness; but repeated renewal will first create a 'mid-term' memory by long-term potentiation of these neurons, and eventually, if continued, cause organic changes at their operational synapses resulting in a long-term memory.

Recent results in neuroscience and cognitive science research suggest that the thalamic and hippocampal systems function as both the distribution center for incoming pulse patterns, and as the arena for the returned interpreted patterns. However, it is the latter only of which we are aware, a complex flux consisting of images and symbols from both external and internal sources input to this arena after their interpretation. Thus, it will be necessary to model the functioning of these midbrain systems to simulate conscious processes: necessary but not sufficient, for the volitional action of the will, of which we are unaware, is also required to fix attention on successive elements of the interpreted flux.

Further, awareness of sensory input from the environment and body is always very limited, and progressively suppressed when attention is increasingly concentrated on a single subject. It is known to vanish almost entirely, for example, in hypnotic states produced by prolonged visual fixation on some single object. Conversely, when attention is released during sleep, foreground and background states of awareness merge, an undifferentiated mental state develops, and unconsciousness results. These are empirical facts that establish, not only that a differentiated state of foreground and background activity is required to support awareness, but that in such a state the fixation of attention required to gain definite information necessarily causes the remaining informational content of the brain to become less definite, just as fixing the value of one conjugate variable by a measurement causes the value of the other to become uncertain.

To observe a pointer reading, for example, it is evident that the observer's attention must temporarily be fixed on the pointer position and its value; that is, for this brief interval the associated mental processes must occupy the foreground of that particular brain state, while all other sensory inputs and internal activities are relegated to the background. But it is equally evident that an act of will is required to fix the attention in this way; and that such voluntary actions are manifestations of the volitional aspect of consciousness, to be discussed in more detail below. However, since the example makes it clear that both awareness and volition play important parts in the process of observation, it will be useful to emphasize in advance that this process can be treated as a specialized application of the theory of measurement.

We have pointed out previously that there is a parallel between the observation of an event by a conscious observer and the detection of a microscopic event by a macroscopic measuring device. As a specific example of the latter, consider the observation of water droplets formed around ions produced by a charged particle in its passage through a cloud chamber. All events of this kind involve the amplification of an extremely small perturbation through its effect on macroscopic matter in a metastable state. Many water droplets produced by the passage of particles through a supersaturated vapour high in the atmosphere will probably never be detected, just as many of the sensory stimuli registered by the nervous system may have no effect on the consciousness of the observer. On the other hand, if sensors are activated by the passage of a charged particle, analogous to the activation of transient memory in the cortex, an observation is made by providing a temporary or permanent record. It follows that the general theory of the detection of events contained in the previous pages may be applied to the modelling of the mechanism of awareness, if not that of the formation of and retrieval from memory.

An important aspect of this theory, peculiar to indeterministic quantum mechanics, is the distinction between information to be gained and information actually gained from the same event. The former is calculable and determinate; but the latter is in general unpredictable, indeterminate before the process of detection and certain afterwards. *We identify awareness with information actually gained*, which because of the technical definition of information in this context, gives precise meaning to what has hitherto been an intuitive concept.

The information gained by awareness of a particular sequence of sensory stimuli is not subjective, but objective in the sense that it corresponds to macrosopic physical processes in the brain. The immediate effect of the gain of information is a sequence of neural events, such as those described above, leading perhaps to long term potentiation, and possibly to progressive enhancement of specific synaptic connections within the cortex. The result of such activity, much of which may be unconscious, is to leave the brain in a physical state with a significantly lower entropy than previously; and this change can be detected in principle by an external observer in various ways: by electroencephalography and magnetoencephlography, by its effect on behaviour, and finally by various invasive techniques. Like all information gained in this way, its content may ultimately be lost by decay, but for a time it is measurable and even attains a stable value.

For these reasons, in more explicit terms we identify awareness with the information gained from a continuously changing sequence of states determined by neural potentials, each associated with the attention fixed on a specific element of a transient memory pattern. On the other hand, we shall identify *volition* with information created, in this context by the resolution of quantum indeterminacy required to fix attention by the action of the will. In the imagery of computer science, this action may be pictured as consisting of commands generated by a separate internal source, a 'master program' running continuously in the conscious state and calling behavioural 'subroutines', learned from experiences, as they are needed. Some simple subroutines of this type, and a typical segment of the master program, were modelled in Section 6.4.

It should be noted that in a completely deterministic theory volition would be of no significance, since the history of the universe would be determined from the very beginning. But quantum mechanics is a indeterministic science that, though useful for the calculation of probabilities for both microscopic and macroscopic events in the future, simply sets the limits of definite knowledge and does not allow the possibility of making more accurate predictions. This is the conclusion of the Copenhagen interpretation, which is entirely consistent with experience, and has important implications for information theory. In particular, it makes an important distinction between information to be gained by observation, which is an objective concept, and information actually gained or created internally by the observer.

There is also a less sharp distinction between microscopic phenomena, that are subject to the laws of quantum mechanics and therefore unpredictable, and macrosopic phenomena which can be modelled quite accurately by classical theories, such as those treated in Chapter 4. Classical mechanics allows the determination of changes in time of the information to be gained by a macroscopic system, including exchanges of information with other systems and losses of information to its environment. But in practice the predictions are verified only over a characteristic time scale, which is long for the orbital motion of satellites and planets, and short for chaotic phenomena like turbulence for which only statistical predictions are possible. Macroscopic observables are best defined as expectation values; the variances that measure the expected departure from the expectation values may be quite small but tend to increase with time. Because of its deterministic character, classical theory can provide no more than a statistical account of the information derived from microscopic events. On the other hand, the variances of measured values of microscopic observables are determined largely by the experimental conditions from which the information is gained.

After it reaches a macroscopic level, the conversion of information from one form to another has little to do with quantum mechanics until it is acquired by the conscious observer, in a process variously described in the literature as the 'collapse of the wave function' or the 'reduction of the wave packet'; but, as we have suggested, more aptly as the 'revision of the statistical matrix'. It is this type of event that is an important feature of quantum mechanical information theory. In principle the determination of the information to be gained by cortical activity is allowed, but this is not the same as the information created. We have identified awareness with the information gained, and *volition is now identified with the information created internally by the brain.* Since information can be quantified, these are both quantitative as well as intuitive concepts.

The effects of volition can be monitored in the way described in Section 7.1, and can be conceived as contributing to the operation of the 'master program' created largely by experience, as noted above and described in Sections 6.4 and 6.5. *The actual mechanism of volition is the converse of that responsible for awareness*; the former is the result of the amplification of selected microscopic components of the intracellular potential in outward transmission through the neural membrane, just as awareness is the result of the amplification of selected microscopic components of the extracellular potential in inward transmission through the neural membrane, as described in Section 4.5. Since the selection is related to the frequency, however, perception and decision, the elements of awareness and volition respectively, are not mutually exclusive, and both are normally operative in the same event.

We have suggested an analogy in quantal theory between such effects and the formation of water droplets along the track of a charged particle in a cloud chamber. There are, however, important differences between the action of an observational device such as a cloud chamber and the action of the animal cortex. While the information created by the former has a random character, that created by the latter is well correlated, since it is derived from of a sequence of internal states that involve continuous retrieval from memory and constitute part of a train of thought or an unfolding pattern of motor activity. As described in Section 3.2, studies of the time correlations of such states have established that, though the information created to form an isolated state may be random, the information produced by sequences of this type cannot be described as 'noise'. Consequently, it is possible to model volitional effects, like those which have been shown to lead to motor activity, as demonstrated in Section 6.5.

Because of its relation to information, *entropy* is another useful variable for modelling volitional effects within the cortex. One of the remarkable characteristics of life is its ability to adapt to its environment by the local and temporary reduction of entropy; in the higher animals the fixation of attention, and the initiation of motor activity, both of which decrease informational entropy by organization, must be regarded as an inevitable life process. According to the second law of thermodynamics, the total entropy of a system cannot decrease if there is no resultant transfer of entropy across its surface; and all irreversible processes, such as viscosity, thermal conduction, diffusion and chemical reactions, are accompanied by a spontaneous increase in the total entropy. But this law has only a statistical validity; within short periods of time, especially in the presence of non-linear processes, local fluctuations resulting in a decrease of entropy may occur.

This is particularly so in the animal cortex with its metastability, non-linear ionic currents and corresponding fluctuations in potential. The low entropy of the individual cells is maintained by the metabolic processes responsible for the exchange of sodium, potassium and calcium across the membrane surfaces, and the low entropy of the extracellular fluid by related exchanges across the same surfaces. These processes require a steady supply of energy from the blood, and though some of the activity of the cortex is reversible, as a whole it is irreversible. A substantial amount of entropy must be exported to the blood by localized fluctuations, and this too proves useful for modelling purposes. All of these well known biological processes have a transparent interpretation in terms of information theory.

8.2 Computing the Uncomputable

In Section 1.5 we have highlighted the properties of the classical Turing machine, the prototype of all automatic computers. Turing's formulation of these properties[103] was an incidental, though indispensable, step towards furnishing a canonical definition of what is 'computable' by procedures that can be implemented by a machine. He was able to show that there must be some functions that are uncomputable by finite deterministic procedures and to provide an example of what is definable but not computable. We shall not reproduce the proofs here, but shall discuss the principles involved, which are similar to those used by Gödel[104] in his well known mathematical proof that that there must be some propositions that are true but unprovable by the use of any finite set of axioms. Both proofs clearly owe something to Cantor's much simpler demonstration that the set of real numbers is uncountable. A countable set can be listed, at least in imagination, and given any list of real numbers in decimal form, a real number that is not on the list can then be formed whose n-th digit is different from that of the n-th real number on the list. It is also possible to find true propositions that are not on any list.

Though they are logically impeccable, Turing's theorem about what is computable, and Gödel's about what is provable, are reminiscent of the classical logical paradoxes. Berry's paradox, about "the least integer not nameable in less than 18 syllables", is an example of the difficulties that arise when descriptions or propositions are applied to themselves; Russell's paradox, which amounted to the assertion "This statement is false", was a sophisticated version of Epidemes the Cretan's "All Cretans are liars". The assertions "This theorem is unprovable" and "This function is uncomputable" are very similar, and while they are gross oversimplifications of Gödel's and Turing's propositions, they may serve to convey the sense of mystery that many people experience when confronted with them[12].

But there is nothing in Gödel's and Turing's work, still less in the logical or linguistic paradoxes, to suggest that they have a bearing on consciousness, or that there is any fundamental impediment to the understanding of consciousness by the conscious mind. Turing's uncomputable function has no obvious relation to quantities that are uncomputable in the context of quantum mechanics.

According to the most widely accepted Copenhagen interpretation of quantum mechanics there are always observable quantities associated with a physical system that are uncomputable because their values are indeterminate unless or until they are measured. In Section 7.1 we have described the deterministic alternatives to Born's statistical interpretation of quantum mechanics[22], such as Bohm's 'hidden variables'[16] and Everett III's 'many worlds'[20]; and have suggested that they may be safely disregarded so long as it is impossible to compute, except in terms of probability, the outcome of many events, notably those resulting from the intervention of consciousness.

In recent years there has been a widening interest in the possibility of quantum computing, suggested by Benioff[109] and explored in some detail by Deutsch[111]. The interest in these ideas has been heightened by the realization[112,113] that quantum processors might be very much more efficient in certain types of computation than their classical counterparts because of their inherent parallelism. In principle, an unlimited amount of information can be obtained from a single measurement by such a processor. However, there are difficulties in both the selection and detection of the information in quantum computation[362], some of them well-recognized but others still to be generally appreciated.

The bits of the 'tape' of the quantal Turing machine have usually been conceived as quantum-mechanical spin components. An interesting example has been described by DiVincenzo[363], consisting of a 'quantal gear-box', with two intermeshing gear wheels. The wheels are conceived as macroscopic objects, but the cogs of both wheels are supposed to carry protons, with spins that interact in pairs as the wheels rotate. If the spins initially have selected values, and interact only with one another, the statistical matrix of the entire set of spins evolves unitarily with time in the manner shown in (7.2.9). This unitary behaviour is entirely computable and predictable as long as it continues; but as DiVincenzo points out, unitarity is possible only if the protons do not interact with the wheels and there are no external interactions of any kind. Unfortunately, there is no way of obtaining the result of the computation except by allowing external interactions, so that, even in principle, the utility of the quantal gearbox as a processor of information still has to be demonstrated. The spins of the protons are quantal bits in the sense that they can be represented in terms of matrices like (7.3.3), and together form a system that may be described as a quantal tape; but if the wheels do not interact with the spins, they cannot constitute a Turing machine. To obtain a better idea of what *is* possible, we next examine the relationship of action to information in the context of quantum mechanics.

Quantal Action and Information

In Section 4.1 we have seen that the fundamental quantities of classical physics are action and information. They depend only on the observer, and all other physical quantities can be derived from them. The same is true in quantum physics, where, however, action and information are observables represented by hermitean matrices instead of real numbers. The classical quantities are identified with expectation values of the quantal observables defined in (7.2.15) and (7.3.1).

The matrix I representing the selected information to be obtained from a system is simply related to the statistical matrix P of the system. As probabilities of independent events are multiplicative, but information concerning those events is additive, the relation is

$$I = -\log P. \tag{8.2.1}$$

On the other hand, the matrix A representing the action associated with the system determines the way the statistical matrix, and therefore the information, depends on the time, position, orientation and velocity of the observer. If the system is isolated, there is no change in the information to be gained, but information is usually lost as a result of external interactions; and over a period of time such interactions contribute to the action. According to (7.5.1), the information (I) to be gained by the observer at time t is connected with that to be gained by another observer at time $t = 0$, (I_0), by the relation

$$I = \exp(-iA/\hbar)I_0 \exp(iA/\hbar), \tag{8.2.2}$$

where $\hbar$ is the quantal unit of action.

It is convenient to use the interaction representation where, if the external interactions of the system are neglected, the action is reduced to zero, so that P and I are both unchanged. More generally, the action A is obtained by the integration of interactions over the time t. For a microscopic system the action can be treated as a perturbation, at least until non-linear effects come into play, so that the above relation can be replaced by

$$AI - IA = i\hbar(I - I_0). \tag{8.2.3}$$

But if the observables A and I satisfy this relation it follows from (7.3.7) that their uncertainties ΔA and ΔI satisfy

$$\Delta A \Delta I \geq \tfrac{1}{2}\hbar \, |< I - I_0 >| \, . \tag{8.2.4}$$

Implications for Quantum Computing

This new uncertainty relation evidently governs the processing of information by any quantal machine. Its application to mental processing will be discussed in the next Section, but here we note its more general implications. It sets a limit to the information that can be gained from a quantal system, and in doing so complements the theory of Section 7.5, which reveals the conditions under which this information may be gained. The scanning of a single bit by a quantal computer must result in a change in the information to be obtained from the bit, so that the right side of the above equation has a definite value different from zero, and the left side cannot be smaller. If the uncertainty in the value of I (or I_0) is to be very small, the uncertainty in the action must be correspondingly large, and very large fluctuations in A must be possible. This means that weak interactions are unlikely to be useful for quantum computation. Information concerning microscopic events is very hard to obtain from weakly interacting particles like neutrinos, and even more so from gravity! The magnetic interactions required to determine the value of a spin component of a particle are favoured only if they are strong enough, or are allowed to act over a sufficiently long period of time.

But a system consisting of the spins of a set of particles is only one example of what might be the tape of a quantal Turing machine. Any quantal system with many independent degrees of freedom would do as well, if it has an observable that can be expressed in terms of a finite number of quantal bits. However, the precise specification of a machine that solves the practical problem of 'scanning' an extended sequence of quantal bits of this kind is a difficult task that can be accomplished only in the light of the theory of the measurement of quantal observables[39].

In the literature there are widely different proposals concerning the nature of the quantal processes important for the appearance of consciousness. In the previous Chapter we have developed a model of submicroscopic cortical processes that necessarily treats the bits of the quantal tape not as spins, but as components of the electric field in the electrolytic fluid with definite frequencies. Like the spins of elementary particles these are observables which normally have two components that can serve as bits of a quantal computer; and the amount of information to be obtained from the parallel scanning of such bits is indeed unlimited. This enables us to create a realistic model of the process in which such observables are selected and detected by the nervous system, a process which, insofar as the analogy applies to the phenomenon of consciousness, may be described aptly as 'computation of the uncomputable'.

8.3 A Theory of Consciousness

As emphasised in the Introduction, we regard consciousness as dependent on the information content of a continuously changing sequence of states, determined by neural potentials associated with the attention given to external objects of perception or those spontaneously generated within the brain. Ultimately, this is the result of the resolution of quantum indeterminacy in the mind of the observer. Consequently, we treat the processes of observation and decision-making as special applications of the quantal theory of measurement.

Perception and awareness are the momentary and continuing aspects of the process by which information is gained, while decision and volition are the momentary and continuing aspects of the process by which information is created. They are not essentially different processes; one is the converse of the other, and both depend for their operation on the formation of and retrieval from memory. In its information processing capacity the brain performs all the functions required of a quantal Turing machine. Analogously, awareness is equivalent to information acquired from the 'tape', while volition is equivalent to the creation of new information on the tape. A perception is a component of awareness, and a decision is a component of volition, evolved in the 'scanning' of the tape, and both require the quantum parallelism that distinguishes the quantum computer from its classical counterpart. Memory is defined by the internal state of the 'machine'.

We have already pointed out that the implied definition of consciousness, though more precise, is consistent with that sanctioned by common usage, which has also guided the experimental investigation of conscious phenomena. According to well known dictionaries, 'conscious' implies 'awareness of something when one allows it to enter his mind and usually fixes his attention upon it' and 'consciousness' is a 'concomitant of all thought, feeling and volition'.

However, in substance the theory requires:

(1) not only the applicability of quantum theory, but the inapplicability of classical theory to the distinctive neural processes of consciousness;

(2) the identification of the 'tape' of the quantal processor as the electrical potential in the extracellular fluid of the cortex;

(3) the identification of the 'machine' as the set of cells that interact with the extracellular fluid;

(4) a quantitative account of the processes by which information is acquired from the tape by the machine, and by which the information to be gained from the tape is modified;

(5) a macroscopic model for the formation of memory, and the retrieval of information from memory

Our proposal to satisfy the first of these requirements is very similar in essential respects to others in the literature, and will be treated first in the following discussion. This is followed by proposals to meet the requirements (2) through (4), taken from recent papers by the authors[364,365]. Progress made towards meeting the last requirement has been described in earlier Chapters, but will be summarized briefly to complete this Section.

The Relevance of Quantum Mechanics

Quantum mechanics is generally accepted as a modern formulation of the relevant laws of physics, and there is no scientific evidence that biological systems are exempt from these laws. In principle, therefore, there is little doubt that experimental observations can be interpreted in terms of quantum theory, but there is room for clarification of its importance for consciousness and the manner in which it is to be applied.

Earlier in this book we have have pointed to abundant evidence that quantum mechanics does have a decisive role, including the unpredictability of conscious action, the way in which it differs from purely mechanical action, and above all the concurrence of experiments and theory in demonstrating the escalation of events from the ionic and microscopic levels in the cortex. For these reasons we are in basic agreement with a number of recent discussions in the literature which have advanced the hypothesis that quantum mechanics is somehow involved in the operation of consciousness. Since the suggestions of how this may occur vary widely[12–15,39], however, there is an obvious need for a clearer understanding of the phenomenon. The definition of consciousness that we have given is designed to achieve this, and offers the possibility of gaining further insight and resolving such differences by modelling the computational processes of the cortex as those of a *quantal Turing machine.*

The Biological Quantal 'Tape'

The considerations of the last Chapter and the previous Section lead naturally to the identification of the 'tape' of the biological Turing machine with periodic fluctuations in potential in the electrolytic fluid. Normally the crucial indeterministic events underlying patterns of conscious activity escape notice; only their macroscopic consequences are accessible to experimental observation. But, as described in Sections 3.2 and 7.1, certain patterns clearly associated with conscious activity, such as the of evoked potentials where a human subject responds to a sensory stimulus with a prearranged motor action, reach a level where they can be studied experimentally[191].

The quantized potential in an electrolyte at ordinary temperatures can be resolved into components, each of which satisfies the definition of a bit; collectively, therefore, these components form a quantal 'tape' in the sense of the definition. An observable bit can be represented as a matrix with two eigenvalues, which can be taken to be 0 and 1, but can not be assumed to have definite values unless and until the bit is observed. In its most general form, as shown in (7.3.3), a bit is determined by a pair of angular variables θ and ϕ, of the kind that determine the co-latitude and longitude on a sphere. The poles correspond to the states of absolute certainty, where the result of a measurement must yield values 0 and 1 respectively; however, normally the angular coordinates are not only indeterminate but vary with time at a rate determined by the energy, which is also indeterminate.

In an electrolytic environment, and most probably as a consequence of the advantages derived from the exchange of information, the cells of the cortex seem to have evolved the basic requirements of a quantum computer, using the potential in the extracellular layers as a 'tape'. In Section 7.4 it was pointed out that in quantum as in classical theory, the potential is related to the charge density by Coulomb's law. But the charge cannot have arbitrary values, as it could in Maxwell's theory, since it is associated with ions, each of which has its characteristic charge. Ions of a particular type can be represented by a field very much like a radiation field, except that whereas photons propagate with the velocity of light and have no rest mass or charge, the ions have a characteristic mass and charge. In a quantized theory, the field variables are matrices, and as the charge density is constructed from these matrices, it is likewise a matrix, though it depends on position and time. *The quantized potential in an electrolyte is therefore a linear superposition of commuting observables which can be regarded as the 'bits' of a quantum 'tape';* and, in principle, an unlimited amount of information can be gained from the scanning of such a 'tape'.

The Nature of the 'Machine'

Various quantal mechanisms have been suggested in the past that could have significant consequences for the action of the brain, but few of these proposals would be effective in information processing. The quantal Turing machine, on the other hand, is at present the most general known type of information processor, and what is clearly needed is an unambiguous identification of those parts of the cortex that could serve as a quantal 'tape' and those that could perform the functions of the machine. In such terms, the choice is very limited, but nevertheless suitable identifications of both tape and machine have emerged from the considerations of the last Chapter. The result is a model of what we believe to be a 'source of consciousness', wherein the electrolytic fluid in which the cells of the cortex functions are bathed serves as the quantal 'tape', and the network of cells as the quantal 'machine' In modelling the computationally conscious action of the cortex, it is supposed that the scanning is effected by those interactions between individual cells and 'bits' of the tape that have lasting macroscopically observable consequences.

A simple computer program can be constructed [see Appendix 8.3] to simulate the interaction in real time of the 'machine' with the 'tape'. A set of bits is supposed to be in interaction with channels of different cells of the machine. The state of each bit is sufficiently specified by a selected phase angle of the type denoted by θ in (7.3.3); normally this is assumed to increase linearly with time, so that though the eigenvalues of the bit are 0 and 1, the probability $\frac{1}{2}(1 + \cos\theta)$ that the bit has the eigenvalue 1 fluctuates with a characteristic frequency between 0 and 1. At regular intervals the bits are scanned, and if the value 1 is found, the value of θ is revised to the next multiple of 2π above. The phase angles of bits of the tape associated with neighbouring neurons are assumed to be affected by the interaction, in such a way that the firing of one neuron would tend to inhibit its neighbours. Nevertheless this correlation is sufficient to ensure that a potential wave develops and that ultimately the firing of large numbers of neurons sensitive to the frequency is synchronized by the wave. The program models the stochastic process by which the tape is scanned, but not in quantum mechanical detail.

In artificial quantal computers, the scanning of the tape is likely to prove a difficult process, which must be performed with equipment similar to that required for the measurement of any other submicroscopic quantity. But to compensate for the difficulty, a suitable machine would have the ability to scan an unlimited number of bits in the same operation through inherent quantum parallelism which, as in the last Section, is an important motive for the development of quantum computing[112,113].

Scanning the 'Tape'

The ways in which such information can be created on and retrieved from the 'tape' can be regarded as problems of the indeterministic quantum theory of measurement; and the fact that this theory does not permit complete determination of the future constitutes its special strength in the present context, since it is exactly this indeterminacy which permits the continuous creation of new information outside the bounds of strict determinism. Thus, like Brillouin[220], we adopt a generalization of Shannon's theory[46], in which the information concerning any system, though never complete, is encoded in a set of probabilities that in our application form the statistical matrix of a quantal Turing machine.

But if the potential in the extracellular fluid of the brain is the 'tape' of a quantal computer, the interconnected collection of cells forming the brain must constitute the 'machine' itself. The contact between a neural cell and the extracellular fluid is made in the channels known to permeate the cellular membrane. These channels are no more than 10 Å in diameter, which is both necessary and sufficient to prevent the normal diffusion of hydrated ions across the membrane.

This does not mean that the brain, considered as a 'machine', is controlled by its extracellular fluid 'tape', only that the resulting interactions constitute an important additional source of information which must be included in the study of consciousness. As shown by (7.4.12), the interaction energy of a cell and the extracellular fluid is localized almost exclusively in channels of the neural membrane where the gradients of the electrolytic and cellular components of the potential are parallel and both extremely large. It has also been confirmed experimentally that the macroscopic effect of the interaction is small everywhere except in and around these channels.The 'bits' of the quantal tape correspond to components of the potential with a sharply defined frequency; and since these are typically a few nV in amplitude, a quantal treatment of the interaction of a bit with a neural cell is most appropriate in the initial stages of the acquisition or creation of such information by the brain. But because of the rapid amplification of the potentials in transmission across the membrane, a classical treatment such as that given in Section 4.4 is also valid.

In (8.2.4) we have reached the general conclusion that the observables A and I, representing action and information in the scanning of the tape by a quantal Turing machine, have variances, or uncertainties, ΔA and ΔI which satisfy

$$\Delta A \Delta I \geq \tfrac{1}{2}\, \hbar \, |< I - I_0 >| \, .$$

This uncertainty relation evidently governs information processing by the brain on its lowest neural level. It means that there is a fundamental unpredictability affecting any process in which information is gained or created, and that large dynamical fluctuations are required for the ordering of certain 'bits' of information in the 'stream of consciousness'. It also has consequences for the cell: since this is the macroscopic detector of the bits, a large change, proportional to the change in information, occurs in its entropy.

Macroscopic Processes

In previous publications the authors have developed quantitative descriptions of various aspects of cortical processing consistent with physical and chemical law and neurobiological fact[39,45,209,364]. In particular, by applying the methods of mathematical physics, field-coupled motions of bioactive ions in and near synaptic junctions have been modelled in such a way that quantum effects are incorporated and the Hodgkin-Huxley equations are reproduced in the classical limit[239].

These results, together with the successful simulation[9,311] of certain types of conscious processes with programs running on digital computers, are what suggested[365] that it might prove possible to model such processes, at least those of a computational character, by pursuing an analogy with the Turing machine, suitably generalized to incorporate quantum effects. The specifications of the classical Turing machine have been given in Section 1.5, and the quantal machine is similar in several respects. In particular, the 'scanning' of the tape by the machine changes the internal state of the machine, and may also modify individual bits of the tape, in a way that depends on its existing state. There are, however, some important differences: until scanned, the bits are indeterminate in value, but to compensate for this, many bits may be scanned simultaneously by 'quantum parallelism'.

At the macroscopic level, the mechanism by which information is passed from one neuron to another is now relatively well understood and need not be repeated here. For present purposes, however, it is necessary to stress that in equilibrium, the electrical potential is determined by the chemical potentials of the ions, and because of their differences in potential across the membrane, there is also a difference in electrical potential which is normally 50 to 100 mV lower within the cell. *The neural cell is therefore in an electrically metastable state*, which is easily disturbed by the cumulative effect of small external activations. When a certain threshold is reached, the cell experiences a graded or action potential characterized by a flux of ions through the channels of the membrane in its transition to a more stable state.

One especially important form of activation occurs at synapses, where one neuron is separated from another neuron only by the thin layer of extracellular fluid that fills the synaptic cleft; but transmission there is facilitated by a variety of neurotransmitter substances and associated receptors in the cell membrane. Activation of this type involves macroscopic processes subject to deterministic laws that can be successfully simulated by mathematical modelling[9,89,311] and replicated by *in vitro* experiments, such as the well known voltage clamp experiments of Hodgkin and Huxley[229].

However, the processes involved in the potentiation of neurons and the initiation of graded and action potentials in living creatures are much less predictable. It has become clear in recent years[152] that synaptic transmission is often modulated by rhythmic potentials in the extracellular fluid, so that many graded and action potentials are synchronized with these rhythms. Electrical activity patterns obtained from full scalp EEG recordings have been shown to be unambiguously related to certain types of conscious as well as unconscious activity[191,192]. For example, the sinusoidal α-rhythm found in tranquil states of mind is rapidly transformed to highly irregular fluctuations when attention is attracted to sensory stimuli, and recognizable patterns of activity extending over the whole cortical surface follow decisions to respond with motor actions.

Recently it has been shown that even such highly irregular fluctuations as often accompany conscious activity cannot be regarded merely as noise; there are underlying periodicities and other features of 'chaos' which are now recognized to have an important informational content[199]. Still more recently, interesting studies have been made[82] of a $6-7$ Hz θ-rhythm in the frontal cortex that accompanies mental tasks such as calculation or tracing a maze. In the last few years, in fact, there has been what Mountcastle[199] has described as a 'paradigm change' regarding such field effects.

8.4 Summary and Conclusions

In the previous Section, we have enumerated the basic requirements of a theory of consciousness, and the way in which these requirements have been met in the course of this book. The guiding principle has been that in its conscious functions, as distinct from its biological functions, the brain is a processor of information, though not a classical computing machine. It does, however, compute the uncomputable, in the sense that many of the results of its information processing cannot be predicted in advance; it can therefore be characterized computationally as a quantal Turing machine.

In retrospect, it can be seen that, using only a few firmly established physical laws, we have modelled the consequences of the detection of a 'bit' by the 'quantal computer' from microscopic beginnings to large scale macroscopic effects, and shown these to correspond to known effects of information processing in the cortex. Wherever possible, theory has been supported by calculations that are in good qualitative and quantitative agreement with experiment. We shall conclude by summarizing some of the more striking results.

The focal points of consciousness are within the channels that permeate the membrane of each cell of the cortex and are the avenue for the exchange of information with other cells and with the external environment. The transmission of information by a single channel is specific to ions of a particular type and characterized partly by the frequency of fluctuations of potential, which must match the frequency of similar small fluctuations in the extracellular fluid, but also depend sensitively on the geometry of the channel and on the differences in concentration across the membrane of the various types of ions. There are many channels in the membrane capable of detecting different components of the extracellular potential in parallel, with the consequence that the cell is potentiated and a memory trace may be formed.

The frequencies to which a cell is sensitive vary somewhat from cell to cell, but the lowest are of the order of the frequencies of the θ- and α-rhythms that are commonly seen in electroencephalographic records. Inwardly as well as outwardly directed components of the potential are always present, and fluctuations within individual cells may contribute to potentials with particular frequencies in the extracellular fluid. Together, these effects allow information to be transferred in both directions, providing the basis for a method of communication between cells that underlies and complements synaptic transmission, and helping to explain why many action potentials are synchronous with extracellular activity. .

These results can be obtained from purely macroscopic considerations. But macroscopic theory can not elucidate the quantal initiation of the acquisition and creation of information. Therefore, an analogous quantal treatment of the processes of observation and modification of the 'bits' of the extracellular 'tape' is required. In microscopic theory the fundamental variable is the statistical matrix, which determines the information to be gained from any system.

On account of the electric metastability of the membrane, microscopically small but non-vanishing potentials with the right frequency will be amplified in channels of the membrane, and macroscopically significant changes of the potentials and their gradients will occur. It follows from the theory of irreversible processes that there must also be a macroscopically significant change of entropy. This is necessarily positive and, since entropy is proportional to deficit of information, is equivalent to a loss of information concerning the microscopic state of the cell, which is compensated not only by the minuscule gain of information concerning the value of a bit of the electric tape, but also in much greater measure by the subsequent formation of a record of that information. In potentiated states, this information may take the form of an enduring memory trace, and contribute to the development of graded and action potentials leading to the initiation of some thought process or motor action.

Provided that a macroscopically significant change of entropy occurs as a consequence of the interaction of the cell and the bit, the quantal indeterminacy affecting the value of the bit will be removed; but it is necessary for very many ions or molecules of the cell to be affected by the interaction if it is to result in such a change in the state of the cell. This conclusion is supported by the new uncertainty relation featured in the preceding Sections. Entropy is proportional to the information to be gained, and if the change of entropy due to interaction with the bit is macroscopically significant, and thus much larger than the resulting quantal uncertainty in the entropy of the cell, then the uncertainty (fluctuation) in the interaction must be much larger.

There is one essential difference between the quantal and classical processing of information. In quantum theory the gain of information concerning a microscopic event implies a retrospective revision of the statistical matrix. This revision, often called a 'collapse of the wave packet', follows an observation of the previously unpredictable outcome of the measurement of a microscopic variable. It affects only the matrix of the system before the observation was made, which will probably be entirely changed by the observation. The revised matrix cannot be calculated in advance because in the process new information has been created; but *the expectation value of the amount of information gained or created* is in agreement with Shannon's classical theory. The revision of the matrix in the manner described in the final Section of the preceding Chapter therefore offers a mathematical representation of the effect of cortical processing that in the future may prove useful for analyzing the phenomenon of human consciousness in more detail.

Discussion

It will be recognized that the preceding conclusions, sufficient in themselves to justify comparing the computational aspects of cortical processing with operations of a quantal Turing machine, have wider implications that deserve further attention.

Perhaps most important is the support given to claims that quantum effects influence consciousness, by showing specifically how they may do so for its computational aspect, and by providing realistic numerical estimates of their magnitude. Insofar as the analogy is valid, this both proves the significance and establishes the limitations of quantal effects. The clear implication of their introduction of indeterminacy at the lowest neural level, as well as of their ability to initiate and sustain the macroscopic potentials of information transfer, is that such effects may influence other states of consciousness in a similar way.

If this is true, then the equations of Chapters 4 and 7 which relate information, entropy and ionic variables at the neural level, the new uncertainty principle, and the analytical methods utilized here may offer the possibility of developing a more comprehensive quantitative model. Of special interest is the fact that the uncertainty of the information being processed depends on that of the action, showing the consequences of the Principle of Least Action affecting processes of this kind. This principle is known to govern the dynamical behavior of quantum as well as classical particles and fields[351], thereby providing an accepted formalism for constructing definitive equations of change.

Such a model must, of course, incorporate established neuroscience, cognitive science, psychological and biological research results to date. It should also feature the most promising system for large-scale information processing by the cortex. But since no general consensus has yet been achieved in this regard, probably the best one can do is to select a system with at least limited interdisciplinary acceptance.

The hierarchical system of interacting cell assemblies originally proposed by Hebb[101] recognizes the existence of specialized regions of neural circuitry, like the unit circuits described by Eccles[99], Szentagothai[338] and Ito[60], and the cortical columns for visual processing defined by Hubel and Wiesel[318]. It is also compatible with functional concepts, such as those proposed by Edelman[213] and systems theories like those of Coward[57], as well as with the processing mechanisms offered by advanced neural network models, such as the ART model developed by Grossberg and his associates, described in Chapter 6. For these reasons it seems a reasonable general system on which to base a more comprehensive model; and, as supplemented by the action of the extracellular fluid, is in fact the system assumed to generate the dynamical potential field featured in the present analogy. Like the individual neurons of which it is composed, each cell assembly of the hierarchy possesses a definite firing threshold[366]; it can therefore equilibrate in a metastable state and must be subject to similar quantum effects.

To make further progress the structural and functional properties of the cell assemblies must be defined in more detail. But in this connection it should be noted that the circuitry columns described by Mountcastle[58], which have been identified in a number of other cortical areas, may qualify as higher-order assemblies of the Hebbian type, and Broca's and Wernicke's areas for learning and processing languages, as still higher-order assemblies. Because these are recurring, well-defined and partially mapped regions of the human cortex, they offer a special opportunity for further microanatomical and cognitive research; and, based on this, a means of extending the analytical and predictive capabilities of the model.

By continuing to model and integrate successive aspects of consciousness documented by experiment we believe, like Crick[125], that it may eventually prove possible to support one or another, or some combination, of the speculative theories advanced by such investigators as Penrose[214], Eccles[15], Searle[217], Dennett[215], and Chalmers[367] by providing the mathematical framework such a theory must have to achieve maturity. To do this, of course, the mechanisms of awareness and volition must be analyzed in more detail so that a master program of the type described in the Introduction can be formulated; but it is interesting to observe that with no more of the model completed than the above, support for certain important concepts in philosophical and psychological theories of consciousness is suggested.

For instance, neuroembryonic studies have established that much of human mental development is genetically determined, while psychological studies have proved that much also depends on environmental input. These competing influences have given rise to widely divergent philosophical systems and behavioral theories emphasizing both extremes. But both can be accommodated by recognizing the full significance of Broca's and Wernicke's areas: that the evolving human brain has developed localized networks of genetically determined neural circuitry predisposed to learn and process a certain type of information[368]. Their slow growth was evidently caused by Darwinian selection because of the advantages they offer for survival in a constantly changing physical and social world; and in all likelihood similar networks exist for the learning and processing other sets of vital information, such as self-preservation procedures, acceptable social behaviors, and one's own self-image. Others may still be developing, primarily in the cerebral cortex, as its greatly increased size and complexity in humans implies.

If we identify these genetically determined networks with Hebbian cell assemblies, then it is evident that they could constitute the physical basis of the 'innate ideas' of Plato and Kant. They would, however, be empty until filled by the sensual and mental experiences of each individual, as insisted by Locke and Hume; and whatever basis patterns were first imposed on them, such as the face of a parent for an infant or a native language for a young child, would surely fill their lowest energy levels to complete such ideas, thereby forming relatively stable informational systems determined both genetically and environmentally.

Historical studies such as those resulting in the Jaynesian theory of the bicameral mind[210], psychological studies such as those resulting in the Freudian and Jungian theories, and neurophysiological studies such as those resulting in the discovery of Broca's and Wernicke's areas, all support the existence of specialized genetically determined networks of this type. But it is equally plain that the basis patterns, being dependent on the particular neural structures of individuals and their specific cultures, would vary within them, causing the resulting innate ideas to vary with time, place and person. Additionally, of course, the information they contain would be constrained by the sensory limitations of the peripheral nervous system, which can be expanded by instruments of greater sensitivity, but ultimately must encounter the barrier of quantum indeterminacy - as in a different context logical processes encounter the barrier of Gödels Theorem.

Nevertheless, specialized brain networks, created over millennia by evolutionary processes, must possess invariant properties independent of particular individuals and specific cultures. Their influence may be responsible for the extrasensory otherworldly experiences induced by extreme concentration or sensory deprivation; but because of their relative stability in the stream of sensation and information that flows through conscious awareness, they must in a sense bound the conscious state by presenting the ideas and images they contain at the limits of active thought. Those containing acceptable social behaviors, for example, may supply ready answers that seem to be true beyond their absolute merit; while those containing one's self-image must supply this to the informational feedback loop of the conscious state to enable interaction with the external world by continuous self-referencing.

These are, of course, implications once removed from those that follow directly from the conclusions which may be drawn from the quantal Turing machine analogy. Requiring Hebbian cell assemblies embedded in the extracellular fluid to generate the complex potential fields assumed to constitute states of consciousness, they too must be classified as speculative, though perhaps less so than theories lacking such a sound neurophysiological foundation. They do suggest a way in which actual partitions of the neural substrate could account for some of the elusive qualities of the human mind.

Appendices

A3.4 Modelling the Quantal Potential

The program listed here was used to obtain the principal features of the Figure in Section 3.4, showing a sequence of action potentials in a small model network of neurons.

The control parameters of the model are called GA, AM(L), E(L), T, and CO. Decreasing GA or increasing CO increases the period and raises the maximum potentials. Increasing AM(L) increases the amplitude for the (L−1)–th neuron, leaving the period unchanged. Decreasing E(L) raises the resting potential for the (L−1)–th neuron. Decreasing T decreases both period and amplitude. The interaction strengths U(L) are also among the data read in near the beginning of the program.

The independent variable X is the time; XL, XG, YL and YG are the least and greatest values of X and the potentials. N is the number of differential equations, NC the number of curves, for each of which a set of data must be provided. There are twelve variables of integration, called Y(1), ... Y(12); these represent the real and imaginary parts of c^{i} and c^{e} for the three firing neurons of the network.

```
   ' "qpots" integrates a system of twelve differential equations
   'simultaneously to determine potentials of three neurons
   '(numbered 0,1,2) in the uantum mechanical neural model
   CLS : SCREEN 9 : DIM R(12),Y(12),YA(12),YI(12)
   LINE (0,0)-(639,349),15,B : NC=2 : GA=1 : EA=EXP(-GA)
   FOR L=0 TO 2 : READ U(L),AM(L),E(L),T,CO : GOTO 10
   DATA 0, 10, 100, .2, -.5
   DATA -.04, 3, 100, .02, .08
   DATA -.005, .4, 100, .001, .2
10 EM(L)=E(L)-AM(L)^ 2 : GM(L)=EXP(-CO*GA*EM(L))
   CH=.5*(T+1/T): SH=CH-T : YI(4*L+1)=AM(L)*CH : YI(4*L+2)=0
   YI(4*L+3)=AM(L)*SH : YI(4*L+4)=0 : NEXT L
   XL=0 : X=XL : XG=5 : YL=-120 : YG=20 : N=12 : CK=1
   XS=640/(XG-XL) : YS=350/(YG-YL) : HI=.5/XS
```

```
   LINE(0,YS*YG)-(639,YS*YG) : 'Integration begins
20 H=HI : XT=X : DXT=DX : K=CK*HI : ND=1
30 IF K>.0625 THEN H=H/2 : K=K/2 : ND=2*ND ELSE 40
   IF H>.01*HI THEN 30
40 XT=X : FOR I=1 TO N : YA(I)=YI(I) : R(I)=0 : NEXT I
   FOR J=1 TO 4 : YP=INT(J/2) : YP=YP*H : X=XT+YP
   FOR I=1 TO N : Y(I)=YA(I)+YP*R(I) : NEXT I : YP=J*(5-J)-2
   YP=YP*H : CK=0 : GOSUB 50 : FOR I=1 TO N : CR=ABS(R(I))
   IF CR>CK THEN CK=CR
   YI(I)=YI(I)+YP*R(I)/6 : NEXT I : NEXT J : I=XS*X
   FOR L=0 TO 2 : COLOR 9+L : J=YS*(YG-Z(L)) : PSET(I,J)
   NEXT L : ND=ND-1 : IF ND>0 THEN 40
   IF INKEY$ ="" AND I<640 THEN 20 ELSE COLOR 15 : END
50 FOR L=0 TO NC : EN=Y(4*L+1)^ 2+Y(4*L+2)^ 2
   Z(L)=Y(4*L+3)^ 2+Y(4*L+4)^ 2-EN-EM(L)
   R=GM(L)*(EA-(EA-1)*EN)*EXP(GA*Z(L))
   IF L=0 OR X<.65 THEN E1=0 : E2=0
   IF L>0 THEN E1=Y(4*L-2) : E2=Y(4*L-3) : 'Synaptic input
   IF (L=0 OR X<.65) OR (L=2 AND X<1.3) THEN E1=0 : E2=0
   R(4*L+1)=Y(4*L+4)+Y(4*L+2)*R+U(L)*E1 : 'R(K)=dY(K)/dX
   R(4*L+2)=-Y(4*L+3)-Y(4*L+1)*R-U(L)*E2 : R(4*L+3)=Y(4*L+2)
   R(4*L+4)=-Y(4*L+1) : NEXT L : RETURN
```

A4.4 Solution of the Dispersion Equation

In the following subroutine to solve the equations (4.4.11), we have written

$$P = p, \qquad Q = q, \qquad R = \omega^2, \qquad X = (q/\omega)^2,$$

$$G_I = \gamma_I, \qquad U_I = (p - \gamma_I)C_I, \qquad V_I = (p - \gamma_I)^2,$$

where I $(= b)$ has the values 1 for the K^+ ion, 2 for the Na^+ ion, 3 for the Ca^{++} ion and 4 for the Cl^- ion. The simplest method begins with the choice of a value of the mean resistance p, in the range bounded by the least and greatest of the γ_I. If N is the number of different types of ions, equations (4.4.11) reduce to

$$Q = X\sum_{I=1}^{N} C_I/(X+V_I), \qquad \sum_{I=1}^{N} U_I \prod_{J\neq I}^{N}(X+V_J) = 0.$$

Then, as the U_I and V_I are known, the second of these equations is a cubic to determine X, when $N = 4$, or a quartic when $N = 5$. When X has been found, the other equation determines Q and hence R.

Units of time (1 ds) and ionic resistance (10^{12} s/c^2) are adopted here and in following programs so that the duration of an action potential and the lowest resistance are of order 1. Concentrations are in dmole, so that the highest concentration is also of order 1. Potentials in units of 25 mV, so that if k is Boltzmann's constant and T is the absolute temperature, $\beta = 1/(kT)$ is of order 1.

The first of the programs assumes that $N = 4$.

```
   '"Resc" solves the cubic as required by the "Res" program.
   'Graph shows value of Q corresponding to mean resistance P.
   'Values of P and Q for resonances are printed on screen;
   'these are upper or lower bounds, since negative values of Q
   'correspond to unstable modes.
   'Vertical lines correspond to ionic resistances.
   CLS : SCREEN 9 : DEFDBL A-H,Q-W
   PI=3.141593 : SW=640 : SL=350 : 'screen dimensions
   LINE(0,0)-(SW-1,SL-1),,B : S=SL/2 : LINE(0,S)-(SW,S)
   I$(1)="K " : I$(2)="Na " : I$(3)="Ca " : I$(4)="Cl " 'ion types
   C(1)=1.35 : C(2)=.05 : C(3)=.0002 : C(4)=.52 : 'concentrations
   G(1)=1 : G(2)=8.5 : G(3)=11 : G(4)=14 : 'resistances
   YL=-4 : YG=4 : XS=SW/G(4) : YS=SL/(YG-YL)
   FOR J=1 TO 3 : I=XS*G(J) : LINE(I,0)-(I,SL) : NEXT J
10 GOSUB 20 : I=INT(XS*X) : FOR K=1 TO 3 : COLOR 8+K
   J=INT(YS*(YG-Y(K))) : IF ABS(J-S)<S THEN PSET(I,J)
   NEXT K : X=X+.02 : IF X<G(4) THEN 10 ELSE END
20 FOR I=0 TO 4 : 'Solve dispersion equation.
   C=X-G(I) : V(I)=C*C : U(I)=C(I)*C : NEXT I
   FOR I=1 TO 4 : A(I)=0 : W(I)=0 : NEXT I : W(0)=1
```

```
   FOR J=1 TO 4 : FOR I=J TO 1 STEP -1
   A(I)=A(I)+A(I-1)*V(J)+W(I-1)*U(J)
   W(I)=W(I)+W(I-1)*V(J) : NEXT I : NEXT J : C=A(1)
   FOR I=1 TO 3 : A(I)=A(I+1)/C : NEXT I : GOSUB 60
   FOR K=1 TO 3 : IF Z(K)=10 THEN Y(K)=10 : GOTO 50
   IF Y(K)=10 OR PY(K)=10 THEN 40 ELSE CA=0
   FOR I=1 TO 4 : YA(I)=Z(K)+V(I) : CA=CA+C(I)/YA(I)
   NEXT I : Y(K)=CA*Z(K)
   IF SGN(Y(K)*PY(K))>0 OR ABS(Y(K)-PY(K))>1 THEN 40
   N=N+1 : LOCATE N+1,2 : IF PY(K)<0 THEN 30
   PRINT "p =";PX;"q =";PY(K) : GOTO 40
30 PRINT "*p =";X;"q =";Y(K)
40 PY(K)=Y(K)
50 NEXT K : PX=X : RETURN
60 'Find real roots Z of cubic Z^3+A(1)*Z^2+A(2)*Z+A(3)=0
   Z(2)=10 : Z(3)=10 : C=A(1)/3 : CB=C*C : CA=CB-A(2)/3
   CB=C*(CB-3*CA)-A(3) : CC=4*CA*CA*CA : CD=CB*CB
   IF CD<CC THEN 70 ELSE CB=.5*(CB+SQR(CD-CC))
   CB=SGN(CB)*(ABS(CB))^ (1/3) : Z(1)=CB+CA/CB-C
   RETURN
70 CC=SQR(CC-CD)/CB : CD=2*SQR(CA) : CC=ATN(CC)/3
   FOR I=1 TO 3 : Z(I)=SGN(CB)*CD*COS(CC+2*I*PI/3)
   NEXT I : RETURN
```

The following program may be used to determine the resonances when there are five types of ions, but the graphical display shows that the structure of the roots of the dispersion equation is very much more complex, and instabilities are correspondingly more difficult to avoid.

```
'"Resq" solves the quartic required when there are five ion types.
'Graph shows values of Q(K) corresponding to mean resistance P.
'Vertical lines correspond to ionic resistances.
'Values of p and q corresponding to resonances are printed on screen.
CLS : SCREEN 9 : DEFDBL A-H,Q-W
PI=3.141593 : SW=640 : SL=350 : 'screen dimensions
LINE(0,0)-(SW-1,SL-1),,B : S=SL/2 : LINE(0,S)-(SW,S) : PI=3.141593
```

```
   I$(1)="K " : I$(2)="Na" : I$(3)="Ca" : I$(4)="Mg" : I$(5)="Cl"
   C(1)=1.35 : C(2)=.05 : C(3)=.0002 : C(4)=.001 : C(5)=.52
   G(1)=1 : G(2)=8.5 : G(3)=11 : G(4)=12 : G(5)=14 : 'resistances
   YL=-4 : YG=4 : XS=SW/G(5) : YS=SL/(YG-YL)
   FOR J=1 TO 4 : I=XS*G(J) : LINE(I,0)-(I,SL) : NEXT J
10 GOSUB 20 : I=INT(XS*X) : FOR K=1 TO 4 : COLOR 8+K
   J=INT(YS*(YG-Y(K))) : IF ABS(J-S)<S THEN PSET(I,J)
   NEXT K : X=X+.02 : IF X<G(5) THEN 10 ELSE END
20 FOR I=0 TO 5 : 'Solve dispersion equation.
   C=X-G(I) : V(I)=C*C : U(I)=C(I)*C : NEXT I
   FOR I=1 TO 5 : A(I)=0 : W(I)=0 : NEXT I : W(0)=1
   FOR J=1 TO 5 : FOR I=J TO 1 STEP -1
   A(I)=A(I)+A(I-1)*V(J)+W(I-1)*U(J)
   W(I)=W(I)+W(I-1)*V(J) : NEXT I : NEXT J : C=A(1)
   FOR I=1 TO 4 : A(I)=A(I+1)/C : NEXT I : GOSUB 50
   FOR K=1 TO 4 : CA=0 : FOR I=1 TO 5 : YA(I)=Z(K)+V(I)
   CA=CA+C(I)/YA(I) : NEXT I : Y(K)=CA*Z(K)
   IF SGN(Y(K)*PY(K))>0 OR ABS(Y(K)-PY(K))>1 THEN 40
   N=N+1 : LOCATE N+1,2 : IF PY(K)<0 THEN 30
   PRINT "p =";PX;"q =";PY(K) : GOTO 40
30 PRINT "*p =";X;"q =";Y(K)
40 PY(K)=Y(K) : NEXT K : PX=X : RETURN
50 FOR I=1 TO 4 : ER(I)=A(I)/16^ I : NEXT I
   FR(2)=ER(2)-ER(1)*ER(1)+EI(1)*EI(1)
   FI(2)=EI(2)-2*ER(1)*EI(1)
   FR(3)=ER(3)-ER(1)*(2*FR(2)+ER(2))+EI(1)*(2*FI(2)+EI(2))
   FI(3)=EI(3)-ER(1)*(2*FI(2)+EI(2))-EI(1)*(2*FR(2)+ER(2))
   'FR(I)+i*FI(I) are coefficients in X^4+6*F(2)*X^2+4*F(3)*X+F(4)=0
   GR=FR(3)+ER(1)*FR(2)-EI(1)*FI(2)
   GI=FI(3)+ER(1)*FI(2)+EI(1)*FR(2)
   FR(4)=ER(4)-ER(1)*(3*GR+ER(3))+EI(1)*(3*GI+EI(3))
   FI(4)=EI(4)-ER(1)*(3*GI+EI(3))-EI(1)*(3*GR+ER(3))
   GR=-4*(FR(4)/3+FR(2)*FR(2)-FI(2)*FI(2))
   GI=-4*(FI(4)/3+2*FR(2)*FI(2))
   SR=FR(4)-FR(2)*FR(2)+FI(2)*FI(2) : SI=FI(4)-2*FR(2)*FI(2)
   HR=16*(FR(2)*SR-FI(2)*SI-FR(3)*FR(3)+FI(3)*FI(3))
   HI=16*(FR(2)*SI+FI(2)*SR-2*FR(3)*FI(3))
```

```
   'GR+i*GI and HR+iHI are coefficients in Y^3+3*G*Y+H=0
   TR=4*GR*GR-4*GI*GI : TI=8*GR*GI
   SR=HR*HR-HI*HI+TR*GR-TI*GI : SI=2*HR*HI+TR*GI+TI*GR
   IF SI=0 THEN SM=SQR(ABS(SR))
   IF SI<>0 THEN SM=(SR*SR+SI*SI)^ (1/4)
   IF SR=0 THEN SA=PI/4 ELSE SA=.5*ATN(SI/SR)
   IF SR<0 THEN SA=SA+PI/2
   CR=.5*(-HR+SM*COS(SA)) : CI=.5*(-HI+SM*SIN(SA))
   IF CR=0 THEN CA=SGN(CI)*PI/6 ELSE CA=ATN(CI/CR)/3
   IF CR<0 THEN CA=CA+SGN(CI)*PI/3
   CM=(CR*CR+CI*CI)^ (1/6)
   IF CM=0 THEN YR=0 : YI=0 : GOTO 60
   YR=CM*COS(CA)-(GR*COS(CA)+GI*SIN(CA))/CM
   YI=CM*SIN(CA)-(GI*COS(CA)-GR*SIN(CA))/CM
60 UR=YR-4*FR(2) : UI=YI-4*FI(2)
   IF UR=0 THEN TA=SGN(UI)*PI/4 ELSE TA=.5*ATN(UI/UR)
   IF UR<0 THEN TA=TA+SGN(UI)*PI/2
   TM=(UR*UR+UI*UI)^ (1/4) : FOR I=1 TO 2 : TR=TM*COS(TA)
   TI=TM*SIN(TA) : IF TM=0 THEN UR=0 : UI=0 : GOTO 70
   UR=.5*(YR+2*FR(2))-2*(FR(3)*COS(TA)+FI(3)*SIN(TA))/TM
   UI=.5*(YI+2*FI(2))-2*(FI(3)*COS(TA)-FR(3)*SIN(TA))/TM
70 'Now TR+iTI and UR+iUI are coefficients in X^2+T*X+U=0
   SR=TR*TR-TI*TI-4*UR : SI=2*TR*TI-4*UI
   SM=SQR(SQR(SR*SR+SI*SI)) : TM=-TM
   IF SR=0 THEN SA=SGN(SI)*PI/4 ELSE SA=.5*ATN(SI/SR)
   IF SR<0 THEN SA=SA+SGN(SI)*PI/2
   HR=.5*(-TR+SM*COS(SA)) : XR(2*I-1)=HR : XR(2*I)=-TR-HR
   HI=.5*(-TI+SM*SIN(SA)) : XI(2*I-1)=HI : XI(2*I)=-TI-HI
   NEXT I : FOR I=1 TO 4 : Z(I)=0 : XR(I)=10*(XR(I)-ER(1))
   XI(I)=10*(XI(I)-EI(1)) : IF ABS(XI(I))<.1 THEN Z(I)=16*XR(I)
   NEXT I : RETURN
```

A4.5 Transmission across the Membrane

The computer program listed below is designed to determine simultaneously the natural frequency and the effective resistance for the transmission of potentials across the neural membrane. The units are the same as adopted in the previous Appendix.

```
'"FREQ" determines frequencies for transmission across membrane.
'Ionic resistances in 70 are in 10^12 s/c^2.
'D is the membrane thickness in Angstrom.
'DV is the membrane potential in units of 25 mV
'W is the frequency in cs^-1; E is the effective resistance. Trial
'values of W and E are entered in the program, and nearest correct
'values are found by trial and error. If error fluctuates or stabilizes,
'touch any key to stop program and obtain one of the following options:
'(1) If error is stable, enter 'e' to end and record values of W, C.
'(2) If error fluctuates, enter 'm' to reduce trial difference T by 10.
'(3) Enter any other character to cause program to resume.
'Enter trial values of W, E and T as data on line below:
DATA 8, 1, .01
JM=11 : DIM FR(JM),FI(JM),XR(JM),XI(JM) : D=80 : DV=4
A=10 : GM=DV/D : EX=EXP(.5*DV) : SH=.5*(EX-1/EX)
'Ion types, and external and internal concentrations in dmole follow:
I$(1)="K " : I$(2)="Na" : I$="Ca" : I$="Cl"
CE(1)=.03 : CE(2)=1.5 : CE(3)=.0025 : CE(4)=1.25
CI(1)=1.5 : CI(2)=.125 : CI(3)=.00015 : CI(4)=.68
G(1)=1 : G(2)=8.2 : G(3)=11 : G(4)=13.4 : 'ionic resistances
FOR I=1 TO 4 : CM(I)=.5*(CE(I)+CI(I))
CD(I)=.5*(CI(I)-CE(I))/SH
NEXT I : READ W,E,T : GL=.25
10 FOR M=0 TO 2 : FOR J=0 TO JM
FR=0 : FI=0 : GR=0 : GI=0 : FOR I=1 TO 4
DR=GL*(J*J-E*E)-A : DI=2*GL*E*J-W*G(I)
DT=DR*DR+DI*DI : FR=FR+CM(I)*DR/DT
FI=FI-CM(I)*DI/DT : GR=GR+CD(I)*DR/DT
GI=GI-CD(I)*DI/DT : NEXT I
GT=GR*GR+GI*GI : FR(J)=2*(GR-FR*GR-FI*GI)/GT
FI(J)=2*(FR*GI-GI-FI*GR)/GT
NEXT J : J=JM-1 : XR(J)=2^(-8) : XI(J)=0
20 K=J : J=J-1 : IF J=-1 THEN 30
```

```
   XR(J)=FR(K)*XR(K)-FI(K)*XI(K)+XR(J+2)
   XI(J)=FR(K)*XI(K)+FI(K)*XR(K)+XI(J+2) : GOTO 20
30 XR=XR(0) : XI=XI(0) : XM(M)=XR*XR+XI*XI
   XR=XR(0) : XI=XI(0) : XM(M)=XR*XR+XI*XI
   IF M=0 THEN W=W+T : GOTO 40
   IF M=1 THEN W=W-T : E=E+T
40 NEXT M : E=E-T : PRINT "W =";W;"E =";E;"error =";XM(2)
   W=W+SGN(XM(0)-XM(1))*T : E=E+SGN(XM(0)-XM(2))*T
   IF INKEY$="" THEN 10
   PRINT "Enter 'e' to end, 'c' to continue, 'm' to multiply T by 1: ";
   LINE INPUT A$
   IF A$="e" THEN 50 ELSE IF A$="c" THEN 10
   T=T/10 : FOR I=0 TO 1 : XM(I)=0 : NEXT I : GOTO 10
50 PRINT "Enter new values of W and E below program and save: "
   'W = 0.810802 E = 0.993400 W = 3.60448 E = 2.429712
   'W = 7.163417 E = 3.591775 W = 11.6871 E = 4.679777
   'W = 17.1992 E = 5.735862 W = 23.70627 E = 6.774956
   'W = 31.21077 E = 7.803846 W = E =
   'W = 2.02213 E = 1.396435 W = 5.95593 E = 2.990108 A=1
   'W= 7.67 E = 2.2 A=10
```

A4.6 Computer Modelling of Potentials

In this Appendix we list and give some explanation of the computer programs used to compute the graded and action potentials, from the physically based theory of Section 4.6.

As explained in the text, many of the solutions of the non-linear equations are unstable, and physically meaningful solutions require very accurately determined initial conditions. The problem is much simplified by integrating the non-linear equations exactly for just two of the electrochemical potentials (for the potassium and chloride ions), and using the linearized equations to determine the others initially in the domain where all potentials are small and the linearized equations are valid.

The first step is to find some values of $p^{(k)}$ and $q^{(k)}$ corresponding to resonances; this can be done with the help of the programs listed in

Appendix 4.4. In the program listed below, four ion types are assumed, and the two values used are $p^{(1)} = 10.75$, corresponding to the calcium resonance, and $p^{(2)} = 8.25$, corresponding to the sodium resonance. The corresponding values $q^{(1)}$ and $q^{(2)}$, with other coefficients required, are found from the subroutine beginning at statement 60, and printed out; note that, for stability, $q^{(1)}$ and $q^{(2)}$ must both be positive.

Here is the program:

```
'"RES" is an updated version of "NEX". This run shows that at the
'small calcium concentration (1/4)*.0002 there is already an action
'potential of 100 mV. Changing concentrations requires correspond-
'ing changes of P(K) and Q(K) with stable values near resonances.
'Increasing Q's by .006 gives a graded potential (remove ' in 92).
'Decreasing Q's by .0005 gives repetitive firing (remove ' in 93).
'X=time in ms; "V " is the electric potential, given by -Y(0)-Y(1)
'For K>0, I$(K) is an ion type; the ionic potentials are Y(K).
CLS : DEFINT I,N : SCREEN 9 : SW=640 : SL=350 : 'screen
I$(0)="V ": I$(1)="K ": I$(2)="Na ": I$(3)="Ca ": I$(4)="Cl "
E(1)=1 : E(2)=1 : E(3)=2 : E(4)=-1 : 'charges
C(1)=1.35 : C(2)=.05 : C(3)=.0002 : C(4)=.52 : 'concentrations
G(1)=1 : G(2)=8.5 : G(3)=11 : G(4)=14 : 'resistances
TS=10 : XL=0 : XG=20 : YL=-6 : YG=6 : 'min., max. X, Y(K)
P(1)=10.75 : P(2)=8.25 : 'assumed P(K)'s
GOSUB 60 : 'find values of Q(I),T(L),U(L),V(L)
FOR K=0 TO 4 : READ YI(K) : NEXT K : 'initial values of Y(K)
DATA 3.74, .26, -.73, .70, -.64
DQ=0 : 'gives repetitive but attenuated firing
'DQ=.006#: 'gives graded potential
'DQ=-.0005#: 'gives enhanced double firing
FOR I=1 TO 4 : Q(I)=Q(I)+DQ : C(I)=C(I)/E(I) : NEXT I
TS=10 : S3=8 : S2=32 : 'scaling factors for X, Y(3), Y(2)
X=XL : XS=SW/(XG-XL) : YS=SL/(YG-YL) : HI=.5/XS : N=4
10 LINE(0,0)-(SW-1,SL-1),15,B : FOR I=-1 TO 1
J=INT((YG-4*I+.6)*YS) : IF I=0 THEN K=15 ELSE K=7
LINE(0,J)-(639,J),K : LOCATE 15-8*I : PRINT 100*I : NEXT I
LOCATE 2,2 : FOR I=0 TO 4 : COLOR 10+I : PRINT I$ (I);
```

```
   NEXT I : PRINT " time (ms):"; : FOR K=0 TO 4
   COLOR 10+K : J=YS*(YG-YI(K)) : PSET(0,J) : NEXT K
20 H=HI : XT=X : DXT=DX : CK=1 : C=CK*HI : ND=1
30 IF C<.0625 THEN 40 ELSE H=H/2 : C=C/2 : ND=2*ND
   IF H>.0025*HI THEN 30 ELSE CK=0
40 XT=X : FOR I=0 TO N : YA(I)=YI(I) : R(I)=0 : NEXT I
   FOR J=1 TO 4 : YP=INT(J/2) : YP=YP*H : X=XT+YP
   FOR I=0 TO N : Y(I)=YA(I)+YP*R(I) : NEXT I
   YP=(J*(5-J)-2)*H : GOSUB 50
   FOR I=0 TO N : CR=ABS(R(I)) : IF CR>CK THEN CK=CR
   YI(I)=YI(I)+YP*R(I)/6 : NEXT I : NEXT J : LOCATE 2,26
   PRINT INT(X); : I=XS*X : FOR K=0 TO 4 : COLOR 10+K
   PRINT INT(100*Z(K)); : J=YS*(YG-Z(K)) : PSET(I,J)
   NEXT K : ND=ND-1 : IF ND>0 THEN 40
   IF INKEY$ <>"" THEN COLOR 15 : END
   IF X<XG THEN 20 ELSE CLS : X=0 : GOTO 10
50 FOR I=1 TO 4 : A(I)=0 : Z(I)=0 : NEXT I
   FOR K=1 TO 2 : S(K)=0 : NEXT K : FOR K=1 TO 2
   FOR I=1 TO 4 : L=5*(K-1)+I : CA=U(L)*Y(2*K-1)+V(L)*Y(2*K)
   Z(I)=Z(I)-CA : A(I)=(1+A(I))*(EXP(-E(I)*CA)-1)
   S(K)=S(K)+C(I)*A(I) : NEXT I : NEXT K : FOR I=1 TO 4
   K=INT((I+1)/2) : R(I)=T(I)*(Q(K)*Y(I)+S(K)) : NEXT I
   R(0)=-TS*(R(1)+Q(1)*Y(0))/P(1)
   R(5)=-TS*(R(3)+Q(2)*Y(5))/P(2)
   Z(0)=-(Y(0)+Y(1)+Y(3)) : Z(2)=Z(2)/S2 : Z(3)=Z(3)/S3
   RETURN
60 RT=.5*SQR(3) : FOR K=1 TO 2 : 'solve dispersion eqn.
   FOR I=0 TO 4 : C=P(K)-G(I) : V(I)=C*C : U(I)=C(I)*C
   NEXT I : FOR I=1 TO 4 : A(I)=0 : W(I)=0 : NEXT I
   W(0)=1 : FOR J=1 TO 4 : FOR I=J TO 1 STEP -1
   A(I)=A(I)+A(I-1)*V(J)+W(I-1)*U(J)
   W(I)=W(I)+W(I-1)*V(J) : NEXT I : NEXT J : C=A(1)
   FOR I=1 TO 3 : A(I)=A(I+1)/C : NEXT I : 'If F = frequency,
   'cubic for X = (Q/F)^2 is now X^3 + A(1) * X^2 + A(2) * X + A(3) = 0
   C=A(1)/3 : CB=C*C : CA=CB-A(2)/3 : CB=C*(CB-3*CA)-A(3)
   'cubic for Y = X + C is now Y^3 = 3 * CA * Y + CB
   CC=4*CA*CA*CA : CD=CB*CB : IF CD<CC THEN 70
```

```
    CB=.5*(CB+SQR(CD-CC)) : CB=SGN(CB)*(ABS(CB))^ (1/3)
    CD=CB+CA/CB : X=CD-C : GOTO 80
70 CC=SQR(CC-CD)/CB : CD=2*SGN(CB)*SQR(CA)
    CC=ATN(CC)/3 : X1=CD*COS(CC)-C : X=RT*CD*SIN(CC)
    IF X+1.5*C<0 THEN X=-X
    X=-.5*(X1+3*C)+X : IF X1<X AND X1>=0 THEN X=X1
80 CA=0 : FOR I=0 TO 4 : J=I+5*(K-1) : YA(J)=X+V(I)
    CA=CA+C(I)/YA(J) : NEXT I : Q(K)=CA*X : R(K)=Q(K)*CA
    PRINT "K,P,Q,R =";K;P(K);Q(K);R(K) : 'values of P, Q, R = F^2
    NEXT K : CB=1/(G(4)-G(1)) : FOR K=1 TO 2 : J=5*(K-1)
    L=2*K-1 : T(L)=TS/(G(1)-P(K)) : T(L+1)=TS/(G(4)-P(K))
    FOR I=0 TO 4 : L=I+J : U(L)=CB*(G(4)-G(I))*YA(J+1)/YA(L)
    V(L)=CB*(G(I)-G(1))*YA(J+4)/YA(L) : NEXT I : NEXT K
    PRINT "Touch any key to start: "
90 IF INKEY$ ="" THEN 90 ELSE CLS : RETURN
```

A5.1 Uses of the Hodgkin-Huxley Equations

The program listed below gives a choice of computing *either* the potentials that Hodgkin and Huxley fitted to the data obtained from their voltage clamp equations, *or* an action potential assuming the voltage dependence of the membrane conductances obtained from the same data. The computed potentials are shown as a function of time in graphical form on screen. To obtain the initial impulse for the action potential, the conductances are all given a zero initial value, and their subsequent variation is indicated below the potential curve.

```
KEY OFF : SCREEN 9 : CLS : SW=640 : SL=350 : XL=0 : XG=16
YL=-120 : YG=30 : XS=SW/(XG-XL) : YS=SL/(YG-YL) : H=.5/XS
GNA=120 : GK=36 : GL=.3 : VNA=-115 : VK=12 : VL=-10.5989
LINE INPUT"Enter 'c' for clamp, 'a' for action potential: ",A$
NE=4 : CLS : FOR K=1 TO 9 : READ XA(K),YA(K),XB(K),YB(K)
LINE (XA(K),YA(K))-(XB(K),YB(K)) : NEXT K : YP=SL-YS*YG
DATA 0,0,639,0, 639,0,639,349, 0,349,639,349, 0,0,0,349, 0,70,639,70
DATA 0,280,639,280, 200,280,200,284, 400,280,400,284, 600,280,600,284
IF A$="c" THEN 60 ELSE YI(1)=5 : YI(2)=0 : YI(3)=0 : YI(4)=0
FOR K=1 TO NE : Y(K)=YI(K) : GOSUB 20 : NEXT K
```

```
10 XT=X : FOR I=1 TO NE : YT(I)=YI(I) : R(I)=0 : NEXT I
   FOR J=1 TO 4 : YP=INT(J/2) : YP=YP*H : X=XT+YP
   FOR I=1 TO NE : Y(I)=YT(I)+YP*R(I) : NEXT I : YP=(J*(5-J)-2)*H
   GOSUB 30 : R(1)=-Y : R(2)=(1-Y(2))*AM-Y(2)*BM
   R(3)=(1-Y(3))*AH-Y(3)*BH : R(4)=(1-Y(4))*AN-Y(4)*BN
   FOR I=1 TO NE : YI(I)=YI(I)+YP*R(I)/6 : NEXT I : NEXT J : F=1
   I=CINT((X-XL)*XS) : FOR K=1 TO NE : COLOR 9+K
   GOSUB 20 : PSET(I,J) : NEXT K : NP=NP+1
   LOCATE 2,4 : PRINT "V =";Y(1);" " : IF I¡640 THEN 10
   FOR K=1 TO 7 : READ X(K),Y(K),N$(K) : I=1+X(K)/8
   J=Y(K)/14 : LOCATE J,I : PRINT N$(K); : NEXT K : GOTO 80
   DATA 200,266,"5", 392,266,"10", 592,266,"15", 504,308,"time (msec)"
   DATA 4,266,"0", 4,56,"100", 4,28,"V"
20 F=5+4*SGN(2*K-3) : J=CINT(8*YS*(YG-F*Y(K)))/8
   IF J<0 OR J>350 THEN J=SL : RETURN ELSE J=SL-J : RETURN
30 V=Y(1) : M=Y(2) : HH=Y(3) : N=Y(4)
40 AM=1 : IF V<>-25 THEN AM=.1*(V+25)/(EXP(.1*V+2.5)-1)
   AN=.1 : IF V<>-10 THEN AN=.01*(V+10)/(EXP(.1*V+1)-1)
   BM=4*EXP(V/18) : BN=.125*EXP(V/80) : AH=.07*EXP(V/20)
   BH=1/(EXP(.1*V+3)+1) : N4=N*N*N*N : M3=M*M*M
   Y=GK*N4*(V-VK)+GNA*M3*HH*(V-VNA)+GL*(V-VL): RETURN
50 M=AM*(1-EXP(-CM*X))/CM : N=AN*(1-EXP(-CN*X))/CN
   HH=AH*(1-EXP(-CH*X))/CH : N4=N*N*N*N : M3=M*M*M
   Y=GK*N4*(V-VK)+GNA*M3*HH*(V-VNA)+GL*(V-VL)
   RETURN
60 LOCATE 2,2 : PRINT"current:"; : FOR K=0 TO 10 : V=10*K
   COLOR 9+(K MOD 7) : GOSUB 40 : X=0 : CM=AM+BM
   CH=AH+BH : CN=AN+BN : LOCATE K+2,70 : PRINT "V =";V
70 X=X+H : I=XS*X : GOSUB 50 : J=YS*(YG-Y) : PSET(I,SL-J)
   LOCATE 2,11 : PRINT -INT(10*Y)/10;" " : IF X<XG THEN 70
   NEXT K
80 IF INKEY$="" THEN 80 ELSE END
```

A5.4 Artificial Insects

In this Appendix, two programs in the usual format will be listed for the simulation of the behaviour of two artificial insects. A computer with a colour monitor is important for the operation of both programs.

The first program is simply to generate a data file for the representation of the insects on the computer screen. An insect is created in a sequence of 48 different positions, and data is stored in the file 'idata' concerning the position and color of the pixels in the area of the screen occupied by the insect. In the subroutine beginning at statement number 10, the separate sections indicated create the body, the tibia (stumps) and fibula (ends of legs), the nose and eyes of the insect in all the required positions. The angle TH determines the orientation of the body. Some comments concerning the main program will be found below.

```
   'This program, called "idata.bas", generates data for "insects.bas"
   SCREEN 9 : R=3/4 : CLS : DEFINT I : DIM IA(1001),IB(1001)
   PI=3.1416 : COLOR 12 : OPEN "o",1,"idata" : PRINT #1,0; 0;
   SN=2 : SC=-1.5 : SS=1.1 : A=18 : B=10 : IC=320 : JC=140
   FOR L=0 TO 23 : TH=L*PI/12 : CA=COS(TH) : SA=SIN(TH)
   IA=5*CA : JA=5*R*SA : XC=A*CA : XS=-B*SA : YC=R*A*SA
   YS=R*B*CA : GOSUB 10 : GET (IC-40,JC-25)-(IC+39,JC+24),IA
   FOR K=2 TO 1001 : IF IA(K) <> 0 THEN PRINT #1,K; IA(K);
   NEXT K : PRINT #1,0; 0;
   GOSUB 10 : GET (IC-40,JC-25)-(IC+39,JC+24),IB
   FOR K=2 TO 1001 : IF IB(K) <> 0 THEN PRINT #1,K; IB(K);
   NEXT K : PRINT #1,0; 0; : NEXT L : CLOSE : END
10 CLS : FOR K=0 TO 255 : TH=K*PI/256 : 'body
   C=COS(TH) : S=SIN(TH) : I=IC+XC*C+XS*S : J=JC+YC*C+YS*S
   LINE (I,J)-(639-I,279-J) : NEXT K : 'stumps follow
   FOR K=0 TO 3 : ST=SC : SC=SS : SS=-ST
   I(K)=IC+SC*XC+SS*XS : J(K)=JC+SC*YC+SS*YS
   LINE (IC,JC)-(I(K),J(K)) : LINE (IC+1,JC)-(I(K)+1,J(K))
   NEXT K : 'legs follow
   FOR K=0 TO 3 : IT(N)=I(N) : JT(N)=J(N) : I(N)=I(N)+SN*IA
```

```
J(N)=J(N)+SN*JA : SN=-SN : LINE (IT(N)+1,JT(N))-(I(N)+1,J(N))
LINE (IT(N),JT(N))-(I(N),J(N)) : N=(N+1) MOD 4
IF N=2 THEN SN=-SN
NEXT K : LINE (IC+XC,JC+YC)-(IC+1.3*XC,JC+1.3*YC) : 'nose
LINE (IC+XC+1,JC+YC)-(IC+1.3*XC+1,JC+1.3*YC) : 'eyes
FOR K=1 TO 3
CIRCLE (IC+.8*XC+.6*XS,JC+.8*YC+.6*YS),K,10
CIRCLE (IC+.8*XC-.6*XS,JC+.8*YC-.6*YS),K,10 : NEXT K
RETURN
```

The main program for the simulation of insect behaviour follows. Instructions for the operation of the program appear on screen, and the early part of the program, up to statement 90, is concerned with screen instructions, reading in of data, and provision for the easy creation of an environment for the insects on the screen. Around statement 100 the simulated neural processing begins; it incorporates a learning program similar to that given for the animal cerebellum in the next Chapter. A set of synaptic weights is read from data at the end of the program, in which $W(K) = w_{ij}$ is the weight of the connection of the $I(K) = i$-th neuron with the $J(K) = j$-th neuron. The weights initially have minimum values insufficient for the motion of the insects, but increase as a result of sensitization of the synapse by repeated efforts of the insects to move.

There is provision for the repeated feeding of the insects, and for the movement of the food tray as well as blocks of the environment by a temporary interruption of the program. The food tray may be left under one of the blocks, with interesting results simulating the frustration of the insect's periodic attempts, with occasional success, to reach the food.

```
SCREEN 9 : SW=640 : SL=350 : CLS : RANDOMIZE TIMER
DEFINT A-B,I-N : NI=2 : 'NI=# of insects
'NN=# of neurons/unit NC=# of units/insect NW=# of weights
NI=2 : NN=6 : NC=2 : NW=16 : S=-2 : V=-4 : T=2 : LR=2
NU=NI*NC : H=NN*NU : PI=3.141593 : E$=CHR$(27)
DIM A(H),O(H),F(H),I(NW),J(NW),W(NU*NW)
```

```
   DIM AR(1001),AL(1001),BR(1001),BL(1001),I1(8814),I2(8814)
   DIM N(49),K(49),M(49),L(251),C(23),S(23)
   I=15 : J=11 : LINE (0,0)-(I,J),14,B : GET (0,0)-(I,J),K
   LINE (0,0)-(I,J),14,BF : GET (0,0)-(I,J),M :
   LINE (0,0)-(SW,SL),3,BF
   LINE (0,0)-(39,24),3,BF : GET (0,0)-(39,24),L
   P$(1)="This program, 'AINS', uses data in file IDATA to run."
   P$(2)="A cursor, which is also a food tray, appears on screen,"
   P$(3)="is moved by the arrow keys. An environment of blocks"
   P$(4)="is created by moving the cursor to any position, then "
   P$(5)="touching the 'Insert' or 'Delete' key to place a block. "
   P$(6)="When ready, use the 'Esc' key to begin. The insect is"
   P$(7)="fed by touching the 'f' key when the program is running."
   P$(8)="Touch 'a' to speed, 'd' to slow the insects. To move the"
   P$(9)="blocks or food tray later, touch 'm', and 'Esc' when done."
   P$(10)="'Esc' also stops the program. Touch any key to start ... "
   FOR K=1 TO 10 : LOCATE 6+K,8 : PRINT P$(K) : NEXT K
   FOR K=0 TO 23 : C=K*PI/12 : C(K)=CINT(4*COS(C))
   S(K)=CINT(3*SIN(C)) : NEXT : NS=2 : SS=2 : I=0 : J=0
   AR(0)=80 : AR(1)=50 : AL(0)=80 : AL(1)=50 : BR(0)=80
   BR(1)=50 : BL(0)=80 : BL(1)=50 : I=0 : OPEN "i",1,"idata"
10 IF EOF(1)=-1 THEN CLOSE : GOTO 20
   INPUT #1,I1(I),I2(I) : IF I1(I)<>0 THEN I=I+1 : GOTO 10
   N(J)=I : J=J+1 : GOTO 10
20 IF INKEY$="" THEN 20
   LINE (40,25)-(600,324),0,BF : IM=60 : JM=37
30 PUT (IM,JM),K,XOR : A$=INKEY$ : PUT (IM,JM),K,XOR
   IF A$=E$ THEN PUT (IM,JM),K,XOR : ON IN+1 GOTO 90,100
   IF LEN(A$)=2 THEN A$=RIGHT$(A$,1) ELSE 30
   ON INSTR("HMPKRS",A$) GOTO 40,50,60,70,80,80
40 IF JM>37 THEN JM=JM-25 : GOTO 30 ELSE 30
50 IF IM<580 THEN IM=IM+40 : GOTO 30 ELSE 30
60 IF JM<312 THEN JM=JM+25 : GOTO 30 ELSE 30
70 IF IM>69 THEN IM=IM-40 : GOTO 30 ELSE 30
80 PUT (IM-20,JM-12),L,XOR : GOTO 30
90 MA=1 : NA=INT(24*RND) : XA=210 : YA=110 : GOSUB 250
   PUT (XA,YA),AR,XOR : GOSUB 270 : MB=M : NB=N
```

```
    XB=X-39 : YB=Y-25 : MD=-1 : ND=INT(24*RND)
    XD=420 : YD=220 : GOSUB 240 : PUT (XD,YD),BL,XOR
    GOSUB 270 : MC=M : NC=N : XC=X-39 : YC=Y-25
    'Main Program for neural processing
    'Read default data for connections:
    FOR K=1 TO NW : READ J(K),I(K),W(K)
    FOR L=1 TO NU-1 : W(K+L*NW)=W(K) : NEXT L : NEXT K
    FOR I=1 TO H : A(I)=S : O(I)=-1 : NEXT I : 'Initialization
    ' Neural processing begins
100 FOR I=1 TO H : J=CINT(.52*RND+.01*NS*F(I))
    IF (I-1) MOD NN<2 THEN A(I)=A(I)+J
    NEXT I : 'Unit processing follows
    FOR I=1 TO H : IF A(I) <= S THEN A(I)=A(I)+1 : O(I)=-1
    IF A(I) >= T THEN O(I)=1
    NEXT I : FOR L=0 TO NU-1 : FOR K=1 TO NW
    I=I(K)+L*NN : J=J(K)+L*NN
    NK=K+L*NW : W=W(NK) : IF O(I)<0 THEN 120
    IF A(J) <= S THEN 120 ELSE A=A(J)+W
    IF A<T THEN A(J)=A : O(J)=-1 : GOTO 110
    A(J)=(A-V) MOD (T-V)+V : O(J)=1
110 IF A(J)<S+2 THEN 120 : 'Learning rule follows
    IF RND*100>(A-S-1)*LR THEN 120 ELSE W=W(NK)
    IF F(J)>63 THEN 120
    F(J)=F(J)+1 : IF ABS(W)<4 THEN W(NK)=W+SGN(W)
120 NEXT K : NEXT L
    IF O(6)=1 AND KA=0 THEN 130 : 'insect A(Rightswing)
    IF O(12)=1 AND KA=1 THEN 140 : 'insect A(Leftswing)
    IF O(18)=1 AND KB=0 THEN 150 : 'insect B(Leftswing)
    IF O(24)=1 AND KB=1 THEN 160 ELSE 100 : 'insect B(Rightswing)
130 GOSUB 230 : PUT (XA,YA),AR,XOR : PUT (XB,YB),AL,XOR
    GOSUB 270 : MA=M : NA=N : XA=X-39 : YA=Y-25 : KA=1
    GOTO 170
140 GOSUB 250 : PUT (XB,YB),AL,XOR : PUT (XA,YA),AR,XOR
    GOSUB 270 : MB=M : NB=N : XB=X-39 : YB=Y-25 : KA=0
    GOTO 170
150 GOSUB 260 : PUT (XD,YD),BL,XOR : PUT (XC,YC),BR,XOR
    GOSUB 270 : MD=M : ND=N : XD=X-39 : YD=Y-25 : KB=1
```

```
   GOTO 170
160 GOSUB 240 : PUT (XC,YC),BR,XOR : PUT (XD,YD),BL,XOR
   GOSUB 270 : MC=M : NC=N : XC=X-39 : YC=Y-25 : KB=0
170 A$=INKEY$ : IF A$="" THEN 100
   ON INSTR(E$+"fmad",A$) GOTO 180,190,200,210,220 : GOTO 100
180 COLOR 15 : END
190 NF=14-NF : PUT (IM,JM),M,XOR : GOTO 100
200 IN=1 : PUT (IM,JM),K,XOR : IF NF=0 THEN 90
   PUT (IM,JM),M,XOR : NF=0 : GOTO 30
210 IF NS<16 THEN NS=NS+1 : GOTO 100 ELSE 100
220 IF NS>0 THEN NS=NS-1 : GOTO 100 ELSE 100
230 'Prepare for insect A(Leftswing)
   M=MB : N=NB : X=XB+39 : Y=YB+25 : K=2*N+1 : M1=N(K)
   M2=N(K+1) : FOR K=2 TO 1001 : AL(K)=0 : NEXT K
   FOR K=M1 TO M2-1 : AL(I1(K))=I2(K) : NEXT K : RETURN
240 'Prepare for insect B(Leftswing)
   M=MD : N=ND : X=XD+39 : Y=YD+25 : K=2*N+1 : M1=N(K)
   M2=N(K+1) : FOR K=2 TO 1001 : BL(K)=0 : NEXT K
   FOR K=M1 TO M2-1 : BL(I1(K))=I2(K) : NEXT K : RETURN
250 'Prepare for insect A(Rightswing)
   M=MA : N=NA : X=XA+39 : Y=YA+25 : K=2*N : M1=N(K)
   M2=N(K+1) : FOR K=2 TO 1001 : AR(K)=0 : NEXT K
   FOR K=M1 TO M2-1 : AR(I1(K))=I2(K) : NEXT K : RETURN
260 'Prepare for insect B(Rightswing)
   M=MC : N=NC : X=XC+39 : Y=YC+25 : K=2*N : M1=N(K)
   M2=N(K+1) : FOR K=2 TO 1001 : BR(K)=0 : NEXT K
   FOR K=M1 TO M2-1 : BR(I1(K))=I2(K) : NEXT K : RETURN
270 'Sensory input, parameters (X,Y, M, N)
   IF RND<.05 THEN N=N+SGN(RND-.5) : GOSUB 290
   XI=C(N) : YI=S(N)
   IF POINT(X+10*XI,Y+10*YI)=3 THEN 280
   X=X+SS*XI : Y=Y+SS*YI
   IF RND<.01 THEN M=-M : RETURN
   IF NF=0 THEN RETURN ELSE XE=X+4*XI-IM
   YE=Y+4*YI-JM : R=SQR(XE*XE+YE*YE) : SI=SGN(RND-.5)
   IF R<8 THEN NF=0 : M=SI : PUT (IM,JM),M,XOR : RETURN
   FOR K=1 TO INT(RE/16)
```

```
    IF POINT(X-16*K*XE/RE,Y-16*K*YE/RE)=3 THEN RETURN
    NEXT K : M=SGN(XE*YI-XI*YE) : IF M=0 THEN M=SI
280 N=N+M : GOSUB 290 : RETURN : 'change direction
290 N=(N+24) MOD 24 : RETURN : 'initial weights follow
    'Data j(k),i(k),w(k) (k=1,2) for synaptic input to system
    DATA 1,1,1, 2,2,1
    'Data j(k),i(k),w(k) (k=3,...NW) for unit intraconnections
    DATA 3,1,1, 5,1,1, 6,1,1, 4,2,1, 5,2,1, 6,2,1, 4,3,-1, 6,3,-1
    DATA 2,4,-1, 3,4,-1, 6,4,-1, 1,5,-1, 2,5,-1, 5,6,-1
```

A6.4 Cortical Unit Cicuits

There are three rather similar programs listed in this Section that allow a demonstration of the learning capacity of typical units in different parts of the animal cortex.

The first program models the action of a unit of the cerebellum, where the input comes from the climbing fibers (CF) and the mossy fibres (MF), which activate the granule cells (Gr1 and Gr2). There are three types of (inhibitory) interneurons: the basket (B), stellate (St) and Golgi (Go) cells. The output of the unit is from the Purkinje (P) cells. Initially, all cells are in the resting state (green), and the synapses are unsensitized. Periodic input from the extracellular fluid is represented on screen by a blue flash. The colour of a neuron and its processes indicate its activation level. There are two potentiated levels (pale blue and red, respectively) and a sequence of refractory levels through which a neuron progresses after firing. The program shows the effect on the unit of training, in which synapses onto neurons left in a potentiated state are gradually sensitized, so that eventually the Purkinje cells fires with each new input.

The DATA statements within the program include values of the extracellular input and synaptic weights for each cell, together with its screen coordinates; the name of the cell is shown on the right and read in with the other data. The weights are progressively modified, in accordance with our statistical formulation of Hebb's Rule (three lines below statement 40), during the operation of the program. The effect on the activation of each cell can be seen in modifications to the sequence of colours on screen.

Initially all cells are in their lowest resting state (green), but when first excited, they are left in potentiated states (pale blue or red). As will be seen from the table of synaptic weights, there is a fine balance between excitatory and inhibitory synaptic input to within the unit; however, as the result of repeated extracellular activation, cells will eventually fire. The occurrence of a firing can be recognized on screen by the following automatic progression through the refractory states (purple, white, yellow, etc.) until the lowest resting state is regained. As the result of long-term potentiation, synaptic weights gradually increase in magnitude, though their sign is unchanged, so that the firings gradually become more frequent. Eventually there are no further changes in the weights, the Purkinje cells fire and return to their lowest resting state after every activation, and the unit continues to repeat the learned 'program'. The program can be stopped by touching any key. The sole purpose of statement 30 is to produce a short pause!

```
   '"PURK" models untrained neurons CF,MF,Gr1,Gr2,B,St,Go,P of
   'cerebellum with synaptic input to CF and MF, and extracellular
   'input to G1, G2, St and P. A(J)=actual level; R(J)=resting level.
   SCREEN 9 : CLS : DEFINT A-X : M=8 : R=-2 : XI=7
   RANDOMIZE TIMER : DIM W(8,8),A(8),O(8),E(8),C$(8),Z$(24)
   COLOR 10 : FOR J=1 TO M : FOR I=0 TO M : READ W(J,I)
   NEXT I : READ X(J),Y(J),C$(J) : A(J)=R : NEXT J
   COLOR 10 : FOR J=1 TO M : GOSUB 70 : NEXT J
   FOR A=1 TO 11 : X=52*A : GOSUB 20 : LINE(X,10)-(X+32,30),,BF
   NEXT A
10 X=X+5 : XI=XI+1 : IF XI<10 THEN O(0)=0 : GOTO 40
   XI=0 : O(0)=1 : COLOR 15,11 : GOSUB 30 : COLOR 15,8 :
   GOTO 40
20 C=4+((A+18) MOD 11) : IF C>7 THEN C=C+1
   COLOR C : RETURN : 'Pause for blue flash follows
30 FOR I=1 TO 1000 : Z=Z+COS(RND) : NEXT I : RETURN
40 FOR J=1 TO M : IF A(J)<R THEN A(J)=A(J)+1 : GOTO 60
   FOR I=0 TO M : IF O(I)=0 THEN 50
   W=W(J,I) : A=A(J) : A(J)=A+W
```

```
   IF A>R THEN IF 3-ABS(W)>7*RND THEN W(J,I)=W+SGN(W)
50 NEXT I
60 IF A(J)>0 THEN O(J)=1 : A(J)=A(J)-11 ELSE O(J)=0
   A=A(J) : GOSUB 20 : GOSUB 70 : NEXT J
   IF NT>0 THEN FOR I=1 TO 256*NT : Z=COS(RND) : NEXT I
   IF INKEY$="" THEN 10 ELSE COLOR 15 : END
   C$=" EX,CP,PP,Gr,B1,B2,B3,P1,P2"
   DATA 1, 0, 0, 0, 0, 0, 0, 0, 0, 40, 315, "CF"
   DATA 1, 0, 0, 0, 0, 0, 0, 0, 0, 620, 335, "MF"
   DATA 1, 1, 1, 0, 0, 0, 0,-1, 0, 200, 280, "G1"
   DATA 1, 0, 1, 0, 0, 0,-1,-1, 0, 400, 290, "G2"
   DATA 0, 1, 0, 1, 0, 0,-1, 0, 0, 240, 70, " B"
   DATA 1, 1, 0, 0, 1,-1, 0, 0, 0, 360, 105, "St"
   DATA 0, 0, 1, 1, 1, 0, 0, 0,-1, 280, 210, "Go"
   DATA 1, 1, 0, 1, 1,-1,-1, 0, 0, 320, 140, " P"
70 X=X(J) : Y=Y(J)
   ON J GOTO 80,80,90,90,100,100,110,120 : GOTO 130
80 FOR K=8 TO 10 : CIRCLE(X,Y),K : NEXT K : GOTO 130
90 FOR K=1 TO 10 : CIRCLE(X,Y),K : NEXT K : GOTO 130
   FOR K=1 TO 10: LINE(X-K,Y+K)-(X+K,Y+K)
   NEXT K : GOTO 130
100 FOR K=1 TO 10 : LINE(X-K,Y+K)-(X+K,Y+K)
   NEXT K : GOTO 130
110 FOR K=1 TO 16 : EY=Y+K-16 : LINE(X-K,EY)-(X+K,EY)
   NEXT K : GOTO 130
120 FOR K=8 TO 24 : EY=Y+24-K : LINE(X-K,EY)-(X+K,EY)
   NEXT K : FOR K=-5 TO 5 : LINE(X+K,Y)-(600+K,349) : NEXT
130 FOR K=1 TO 8: IF W(J,K)=0 THEN 150
   IF J<3 THEN LINE(X,Y-1)-(X(K),Y+1),,BF : GOTO 140
   LINE(X-1,Y)-(X+1,Y(K)),,BF
140 LINE-(X(K),Y(K))
150 NEXT K : RETURN
```

The next program models the action of a unit consisting of 12 cells of the cerebral cortex, as described in Section 6.4. The activation levels and corresponding screen colours are the same as for the previous program, and, in spite of the difference in the number of neurons, the DATA statements have the same format, and again the extracellular input is represented on screen by a blue flash.

```
'"BETZ" models action of initially untrained neurons CC,TC,S1,S2,
'M1,M2,A1,A2,B1,B2,C,P of the cerebrum, with synaptic input to
'CC and/or TC, and extracellular input to S1 or S2.
'CC=corticocortical; TC=thalmocortical; S=spiny stellate;
'M1=Martinotti; M2=neuroglialform; A=axonal tuft; B=basket;
'C=double bouquet; P=pyramid
SCREEN 9 : CLS : DEFINT A-X : R=-2 : T=45
DIM W(12,12),A(12),E(12),O(12),R(12),X(12),Y(12),N$(12)
FOR I=1 TO 12 : FOR J=0 TO 11 : READ W(I,J) : NEXT J
READ X(I),Y(I),N$(I) : A(I)=R : NEXT I : COLOR 10
FOR I=1 TO 12 : GOSUB 50 : NEXT I : FOR A=1 TO 11
X=52*A : GOSUB 150 : LINE(X,0)-(X+32,20),,BF : NEXT A
10 T=T+5 : IF T MOD 60>0 THEN O(0)=0 : GOTO 20
O(0)=1 : COLOR 15,11 : FOR I=1 TO 200 : Z=Z+COS(RND)
NEXT I : COLOR 15,0 : 'input each 60 msec.
20 FOR J=1 TO 12 : IF A(J)<R THEN A(J)=A(J)+1 : GOTO 40
FOR I=0 TO 12 : IF O(I)=0 THEN 30
W=W(J,I) : A=A(J) : A(J)=A+W : IF A(J)>4 THEN A(J)=4
IF A>R THEN IF 3-ABS(W)>7*RND THEN W(J,I)=W+SGN(W)
30 NEXT I
40 IF A(J)>0 THEN O(J)=1 : A(J)=A(J)+1 ELSE O(J)=0
IF A(J)>2 THEN A(J)=A(J)-10
NEXT J
FOR I=1 TO 12 : A=A(I) : GOSUB 150 : GOSUB 50 : NEXT I
IF NT>0 THEN FOR I=1 TO 250*NT : Z=COS(RND) : NEXT I
IF INKEY$="" THEN 10 ELSE COLOR 15 : END
'C$=" EX CC TC S1 S2 M1 M2 A1 A2 B1 B2 C X Y"
DATA 0, 0, 0, 0, 0, 0, 0, 0, 0, 0, 0, 0, 40, 315, "CC"
DATA 1, 0, 0, 0, 0, 0, 0, 0, 0, 0, 0, 0, 600, 325, "TC"
DATA 1, 1, 1, 0, 0, 0, 0, 0, 0, 0, 0, 0, 160, 280, "S1"
DATA 1, 1, 1, 0, 0, 0, 0, 0, 0, 0, 0, 0, 320, 290, "S2"
DATA 0, 1, 0, 0, 0, 0, 1, 0, 0, 0, 0, 0, 400, 315, "M1"
DATA 0, 1, 1, 0, 1, 0, 0, 0, 0, 0, 0, 0, 480, 245, "M2"
```

```
    DATA 1, 1, 0, 0, 1, 0, 0, 0, 0, 0, 0,-1, 360, 210, "A1"
    DATA 1, 0, 0, 0, 1, 0, 0, 0, 0, 0, 0,-1, 480, 70, "A2"
    DATA 0, 1, 0, 0, 1, 0, 0, 0, 0, 0, 0,-1, 200, 35, "B1"
    DATA 0, 0, 1, 0, 1, 0, 0, 0, 0, 0, 0,-1, 80, 80, "B2"
    DATA 0, 1, 0, 1, 0, 0, 0, 0, 0, 0, 0, 0, 360, 90, " C"
    DATA 1, 1, 1, 1, 1, 1, 0,-1,-1,-1,-1, 0, 240, 175, " P"
50 X=X(I) : Y=Y(I)
    ON I GOTO 60,60,70,70,80,80,90,90,100,100,110,120
60 FOR K=8 TO 10 : CIRCLE(X,Y),K : NEXT K : GOTO 130
70 FOR K=1 TO 10 : CIRCLE(X,Y),K : NEXT K : GOTO 130
80 FOR K=5 TO 15 : EY=Y+K-15 : LINE(X-K,EY)-(X+K,EY)
    NEXT K : GOTO 130
90 LINE(X-8,Y-6)-(X+8,Y+6),,BF : GOTO 130
100 FOR K=0 TO 12 : EY=Y+K : LINE(X-K,EY)-(X+K,EY)
    NEXT K : GOTO 130
110 FOR K=0 TO 20 : DX=10-ABS(K-10): EY=Y+K-8
    LINE(X-DX,EY)-(X+DX,EY) : NEXT : GOTO 130
120 FOR K=6 TO 20 : Z=Y-K+10 : LINE(X-K,Z)-(X+K,Z)
    NEXT K : FOR K=-5 TO 5 : LINE(X+K,Y)-(600+K,349) : NEXT
130 FOR K=1 TO 12 : IF W(I,K)=0 THEN 140
    IF I<3 THEN LINE(X,Y-1)-(X(K),Y+1),,BF : GOTO 140
    LINE(X-1,Y)-(X+1,Y(K)),,BF : LINE-(X(K),Y(K))
140 NEXT K : RETURN
150 C=4+((A+18) MOD 11) : IF C>7 THEN C=C+1
    COLOR C : RETURN
```

The final program is similar, but models a unit of the hippocampus. The input to the unit comes from the commissural pathway (CP) or the perforant pathway (PP), which activate the granule cell (Gr). There are three inhibitory basket cells (B1, B2 and B3), and two pyramidal cells (P1 and P2); the latter provides the output from the unit.

```
'"ALLO" models an initially untrained allocortical unit with synaptic
'input from CP and PP to Gr and extracellular input to Gr, B1,
'B3 and P2. Colour represents activation level. PP=perforant
'pathway, from entorhinal cortex; CP=commissural pathway
'from the septum and contralateral hippocampus.
```

```
SCREEN 9 : CLS : DEFINT A-X : M=8 : R=-2 : XI=7
RANDOMIZE TIMER : DIM W(8,8),A(8),O(8),E(8),C$(8),Z$(24)
COLOR 10 : FOR J=1 TO M : FOR I=0 TO M : READ W(J,I)
NEXT I : READ X(J),Y(J),C$(J) : A(J)=R : NEXT J
COLOR 10 : FOR J=1 TO M : GOSUB 70 : NEXT J
FOR A=1 TO 11 : X=52*A : GOSUB 20
LINE(X,10)-(X+32,30),,BF : NEXT A
10 X=X+5 : XI=XI+1 : IF XI<10 THEN O(0)=0 : GOTO 40
XI=0 : O(0)=1 : COLOR 15,11 : GOSUB 30 : COLOR 15,8
GOTO 40
20 C=4+((A+18) MOD 11) : IF C>7 THEN C=C+1
COLOR C : RETURN
30 FOR I=1 TO 1000 : Z=Z+COS(RND) : NEXT I : RETURN
40 FOR J=1 TO M : IF A(J)<R THEN A(J)=A(J)+1 : GOTO 60
FOR I=0 TO M : IF O(I)=0 THEN 50
W=W(J,I) : A=A(J) : A(J)=A+W
IF A>R THEN IF 3-ABS(W)>7*RND THEN W(J,I)=W+SGN(W)
50 NEXT I
60 IF A(J)>0 THEN O(J)=1 : A(J)=A(J)-11 ELSE O(J)=0
A=A(J) : GOSUB 20 : GOSUB 70 : NEXT J
IF NT>0 THEN FOR I=1 TO 256*NT : Z=COS(RND) : NEXT I
IF INKEY$="" THEN 10 ELSE COLOR 15 : END
'C$=" EX,CP,PP,Gr,B1,B2,B3,P1,P2"
DATA 1, 0, 0, 0, 0, 0, 0, 0, 0, 40, 315, "CP"
DATA 1, 0, 0, 0, 0, 0, 0, 0, 0, 620, 335, "PP"
DATA 1, 1, 1, 0,-1, 0, 0, 0, 0, 80, 140, "Gr"
DATA 1, 0, 1, 0, 0, 0, 0, 1, 0, 120, 70, "B1"
DATA 0, 0, 0, 1, 0, 0, 0, 0, 1, 320, 70, "B2"
DATA 1, 1, 0, 0, 0, 0, 0, 0, 0, 520, 70, "B3"
DATA 0, 0, 1, 1, 0,-1, 0, 0, 0, 200, 105, "P1"
DATA 1, 1, 0, 0, 0, 0,-1, 1, 0, 400, 210, "P2"
70 X=X(J) : Y=Y(J) : ON J GOTO 80,80,90,100,100,100,120,110
80 FOR K=8 TO 10 : CIRCLE(X,Y),K : NEXT K : GOTO 130
90 FOR K=1 TO 10 : CIRCLE(X,Y),K : NEXT K : GOTO 130
100 FOR K=1 TO 10 : LINE(X-K,Y+K)-(X+K,Y+K)
NEXT K : GOTO 130
110 FOR K=-5 TO 5 : LINE(X+K,Y)-(600+K,349) : NEXT K
```

```
120 FOR K=6 TO 20 : EY=Y+20-K : LINE(X-K,EY)-(X+K,EY)
    NEXT K
130 FOR K=1 TO 8: IF W(J,K)=0 THEN 150
    IF J<3 THEN LINE(X,Y-1)-(X(K),Y+1),,BF : GOTO 140
    LINE(X-1,Y)-(X+1,Y(K)),,BF
140 LINE-(X(K),Y(K))
150 NEXT K : RETURN
```

A6.5 Cortical Pattern Recognition

The following program models the activity of a set of interconnected units of the cortex, including 4 sensory association units each containing 12 neurons, 4 hippocampal units each containing 8 neurons, 4 motor association units each containing 12 neurons, and 16 cerebellar units each containing 8 neurons. The units are similar to those described in the previous Appendix, but are given synaptic weights that result from a long course of training. Synaptic input is given to one sensory neuron at the top left of the screen, and the firing of this neuron activates one neuron after another so that eventually the cerebellar Purkinje cells are activated and fire. The assumed synchronization of the output of the hippocampal cells with that of the sensory association cells is very important for the efficient activation of the cerebellar cells; without this, some cells would not regain their lowest resting states. After a single cycle, all neurons are in their lowest resting states except the last, which if left in a potentiated state. The full 'program' is executed by the system in three cycles, after which all neurons are in their lowest resting states. The activation levels of all cells are again indicated on screen by their colours.

```
'"CORT" models trained activity of 256 neurons named A$(I) in the
'cerebrum, B$(I) in the allocortex and C$(I) in the cerebellum.
'Synaptic input is to a single cell in the sensory cerebrum; activation
'levels are represented by colors and extracellular input by a blue
'flash. A(J)=actual level; the lowest resting level is -2. Connections
'between different units shown on screen. This is a graphical version
'of the program listed in the published paper.
SCREEN 9 : CLS : DEFINT A-X : NA=4 : NC=16 : M=256
```

```
    DIM N(12),WA(12,12),WB(8,8),WC(8,8),EA(12),EB(8),EC(8)
    DIM A$(12),Z$(64),I(100),J(100),EX(100),X(256),Y(256),A(M),O(M)
    M1=48 : M2=80 : M3=128 : XM=32 : R=-2
    N=1 : FOR J=1 TO 12 : N(J)= N : N=2*N : NEXT
    FOR I=1 TO 12 : FOR J=1 TO 12 : READ WA(I,J) : NEXT J
    READ EA(I),A$(I) : NEXT I
    FOR I=1 TO 8 : FOR J=1 TO 8 : READ WB(I,J) : NEXT J
    READ EB(I),B$(I) : NEXT I
    FOR I=1 TO 8 : FOR J=1 TO 8 : READ WC(I,J) : NEXT J
    READ EC(I),C$(I) : NEXT I
    FOR I=1 TO M : A(I)=R : NEXT I
    L=0 : S=1 : K=0 : XI=XM-1 : GOSUB 100
10 X=X+4 : XI=XI+1 : IF XI=XM THEN XI=0 ELSE 30
    T=4 : GOSUB 20 : COLOR 15,11 : T=1 : GOSUB 20
    COLOR 15,8 : GOTO 40
20 FOR I=1 TO 500*T : Z=COS(RND) : NEXT I : RETURN
30 FOR J=1 TO M : IF O(J)=1 THEN 40
    NEXT J : X=X+4*(XM-XI-1) : XI=XM-1 :
    FOR J=1 TO M : IF A(J)<R THEN A(J)=R
    NEXT J
40 L=1 : FOR J=1 TO M : IF J>M2 THEN Y=1
    IF A(J)<R THEN A(J)=A(J)+1 : GOTO 90
    IF J>M3 THEN P=INT((J-M3-1)/8) : IN=M3+8*P : GOTO 70
    IF J>M2 THEN P=INT((J-M2-1)/12) : IN=M2+12*P : GOTO 50
    IF J>M1 THEN P=INT((J-M1-1)/8) : IN=M1+8*P : GOTO 60
    P=INT((J-1)/12) : IN=12*P : Y=0
    IF (XI=0 AND J=2) THEN A(J)=A(J)+3
50 JI=J-IN : FOR I=1 TO 12
    IF O(IN+I)=1 THEN A(J)=A(J)+WA(JI,I)
    NEXT I : IF XI=Y+2*P THEN A(J)=A(J)+EA(JI)
    GOTO 80
60 JI=J-IN : FOR I=1 TO 8
    IF O(IN+I)=1 THEN A(J)=A(J)+WB(JI,I)
    NEXT I : IF XI=1+2*P THEN A(J)=A(J)+EB(JI)
    GOTO 80
70 JI=J-IN : Q=INT(P/4) : FOR I=1 TO 8
    IF O(IN+I)=1 THEN A(J)=A(J)+WC(JI,I)
```

```
    NEXT I : IF XI=2+2*Q THEN A(J)=A(J)+EC(JI)
80 IF J<J(L) THEN 90
    IF J>J(L) THEN L=L+1 : GOTO 80
    IC=I(L) : IF O(IC)=1 THEN A(J)=A(J)+EX(L)
    L=L+1 : GOTO 80
90 IF A(J)<1 THEN O(J)=0 ELSE O(J)=1 : A(J)=A(J)-11
    COLOR 5+((A(J)+18) MOD 11)
    FOR I=1 TO 4 : CIRCLE(X(J),Y(J)),I : NEXT I
    NEXT J : IF INKEY$="" THEN 10 ELSE COLOR 15 : END
    ' CC,TC,S1,S2, M, N,A1,A2,B1,B2, C,Py EX
    DATA 0, 0, 0, 0, 0, 0, 0, 0, 0, 0, 0, 0, "CC"
    DATA 0, 0, 0, 0, 0, 0, 0, 0, 0, 0, 0, 0, "TC"
    DATA 3, 3, 0, 0, 0, 0, 0, 0, 0, 0, 0, 3, "S1"
    DATA 3, 3, 0, 0, 0, 0, 0, 0, 0, 0, 0, 3, "S2"
    DATA 3, 0, 0, 0, 3, 0, 0, 0, 0, 0, 0, 0, " M"
    DATA 3, 3, 0, 3, 0, 0, 0, 0, 0, 0, 0, 0, " N"
    DATA 2, 0, 0, 1, 0, 0, 0, 0, 0,-4, 0, 3, "A1"
    DATA 0, 0, 0, 1, 0, 0, 0, 0, 0,-1, 0, 3, "A2"
    DATA 3, 0, 0, 1, 0, 0, 0, 0, 0,-1, 0, 0, "B1"
    DATA 0, 3, 0, 3, 0, 0, 0, 0, 0,-3, 0, 0, "B2"
    DATA 3, 0, 3, 0, 0, 0, 0, 0, 0, 0, 0, 0, " C"
    DATA 7, 4, 6, 1, 3, 0,-7,-3,-3,-4, 0, 0, 3, "Py"
    ' CP,PP,Gr,B1,B2,B3,P1,P2
    DATA 0, 0, 0, 0, 0, 0, 0, 0, "CP"
    DATA 0, 0, 0, 0, 0, 0, 0, 0, "PP"
    DATA 3, 3, 0,-1, 0, 0, 0, 0, 3, "Gr"
    DATA 0, 3, 0, 0, 0, 0, 3, 0, 3, "B1"
    DATA 0, 0, 3, 0, 0, 0, 0, 3, 0, "B2"
    DATA 3, 0, 0, 0, 0, 0, 0, 0, 3, "B3"
    DATA 0, 3, 3, 0,-3, 0, 0, 0, 0, "P1"
    DATA 3, 0, 0, 0, 0,-3, 3, 0, 3, "P2"
    ' CF,MF,G1,G2, B,St,Go, P, EX
    DATA 0, 0, 0, 0, 0, 0, 0, 0, 0, "CF"
    DATA 0, 0, 0, 0, 0, 0, 0, 0, 0, "MF"
    DATA 5, 2, 0, 0, 0, 0,-3, 0, 2, "G1"
    DATA 0, 2, 0, 0, 0,-1,-3, 0, 2, "G2"
    DATA 1, 0, 3, 0, 0,-1, 0, 0, 0, " B"
```

```
   DATA 4, 0, 0, 1,-1, 0, 0, 0, 3, "St"
   DATA 0, 3, 3, 1, 0, 0, 0,-2, 3, "Go"
   DATA 5, 0, 4, 4,-5,-4, 0, 0, 4, " P"
100 COLOR 15 : FOR J=1 TO 256 : K=J-1 : U=11 : V=16
   IF J>M3 THEN Y(J)=2*V*(INT(K/8) MOD 4)+13*V ELSE 110
   X(J)=U*(K MOD 8)+14*U*INT((K-128)/32)+3*U : GOTO 140
110 IF J>M2 THEN Y(J)=9*V ELSE 120
   X(J)=U*((K+4) MOD 12)+14*U*INT((K-80)/12)+U : GOTO 140
120 IF J>M1 THEN Y(J)=5*V ELSE 130
   X(J)=U*(K MOD 8)+14*U*INT((K-48)/8)+3*U : GOTO 140
130 Y(J)=V : X(J)=U*(K MOD 12)+14*U*INT(K/12)+U
140 FOR K=1 TO 4 : CIRCLE(X(J),Y(J)),K,10 : NEXT K
   CIRCLE(X(J),Y(J)),5 : NEXT J : FOR IC=1 TO NA
   L=L+1 : EX(L)=3 : I(L)=12*IC : J(L)=M1+8*IC-6 : NEXT IC
   FOR IC=1 TO NA : L=L+1 : EX(L)=3 : I(L)=M1+8*IC
   J(L)=M2+12*IC-10 : NEXT IC
   FOR IC=1 TO NA : FOR JC=0 TO 3 : L=L+1 : EX(L)=3
   I(L)=M2+12*IC : J(L)=M3+32*IC+8*JC-30 : NEXT JC
   NEXT IC : FOR IC=1 TO 3 : L=L+1 : I(L)=M1+8*IC
   J(L)=2+12*IC : EX(L)=3 : NEXT IC : FOR J=M3+1 TO M
   IC=INT((J-M3-1)/8)+1 : KC=8*IC-8 : JC=J-M3-KC
   IF JC<8 THEN 150 ELSE L=L+1 : J(L)=J : EX(L)=-5
   IF (IC AND 1)=1 THEN I(L)=J+5 ELSE I(L)=J-11
   IF IC<NC-1 THEN L=L+1 : I(L)=J+12 : J(L)=J : EX(L)=3
   IF IC>2 THEN L=L+1 : I(L)=J-20 : J(L)=J : EX(L)=3
150 NEXT J
   FOR J=2 TO L : I=J-1 : IC=I(J) : JC=J(J) : XC=EX(J)
160 IF J(I)>J(J) THEN I=I-1 : GOTO 160
   FOR P=J TO I+2 STEP -1 : I(P)=I(P-1) : J(P)=J(P-1)
   EX(P)=EX(P-1) : NEXT P : I(I+1)=IC : J(I+1)=JC : EX(I+1)=XC
   NEXT J : J(L+1)=M+1 : FOR J=1 TO L : FOR IC=-1 TO 1
   X=X(I(J))+IC : Y=Y(I(J)) : PSET(X,Y) : X=X(J(J))+IC
   Y=Y(J(J)) : LINE-(X,Y) : NEXT IC : NEXT J : RETURN
```

In the following program, numbered patterns may be created in the upper right portion of the screen by moving from point to point with the help of the arrows. Elements of a pattern may be created or erased at a particular point by touching any key. The patterns may be thought of as patterns of refined motor activity, to be learned by the sensitization of a set of unit circuits of the cerebellum. The program simulates the action of a zone in the cerebellum made up of C interconnected minizones (columns), each of which consists of R interconnected unit circuits (rows). The output of the zone is the firing pattern of the Purkinje cells of the unit circuits, which is progressively modified by a learning process.

The patterns are learned by trial and error, with a randomly chosen initial 'guess'. Climbing Fiber and/or Mossy Fiber input to the minizones is initially randomized but is changed in processing if the output pattern does not match a pattern pre-recorded in a 'zRC' file. Minimum weights for specified synapses are progressively modified during learning, and are stored for automatic recall as sparse matrices in sequentially numbered 'wRC' files, when learning is complete. When the pattern has been learned, not always perfectly, a new attempt may be made to learn the same or some other pattern created on screen. Since synaptic weights are stored for all learned patterns, if a previously learned pattern is created, it will be recognized and will be put immediately onto the screen with its correct number.

```
   CLS : SCREEN 9 : DEFINT A-Z : RANDOMIZE TIMER
   COLOR 15 : PRINT "Welcome to the Zonal Cerebellum Model"
   PRINT "" : PRINT "Press any key to start ..."
   ' ...............................................Definitions
   'NI=number of iterations following input
   'N=number of neurons in each unit circuit
   'R=number of unit circuits in each minizone
   'C=number of minizones in macrozone
   'T=neuron firing threshold
   'S=highest neuron refractory level
   'V=lowest neuron refractory level
   'LR=frequency of memory reinforcement (1-100)
   'W(K)=interconnection sparse matrix elements
15 IF INKEY$="" THEN 15
   SW=640: SL=200 '............Screen width and length in pixels
```

```
  CW=8: CL=8 '...............Character width and length in pixels
  RM=INT(SL/16): CM=INT(SW/38)
  LL=-1+SL/CL: LC=32*CM/CW
  '.......................................................Initialization
21 PRINT "Enter number of rows (up to";RM;"): ";
  LINE INPUT R$ : R=VAL(R$) : IF R=0 OR R > RM THEN 21
  R1=INT((R-1)/8)+1 : R2=8*R1-R
  IF LEN(R$)=1 THEN R$="0"+R$
24 PRINT "Enter number of columns (up to";CM;"): ";
  LINE INPUT C$ : C=VAL(C$): IF C=0 OR C > CM THEN 24
  NU=C*R: MM=C*R1: C1=MM-1
  IF LEN(C$)=1 THEN C$="0"+C$
  E$=SPACE$(LC): F$="Z"+R$+C$
  DIM N(MM), P(NU), F(NU): GOSUB 97
  N=6: T=1: S=-4: V=-9: NI=11: Q=4: G=R*N: H=G*C
  LR=30: NV=2: NW=22: NY=16
  DIM A(H), O(H), I(NW), J(NW), W(NU*NW)
32 S$="W"+R$+C$+P$: IF FL=1 THEN GOSUB 90: GOTO 46
  FOR I=1 TO H: A(I)=S: O(I)=-1: NEXT
  ' ...............................................Random Input Pattern
  FOR I=1 TO NU: F(I)=INT(3*RND)-1: NEXT
  '...................................Read default data for connections
  RESTORE: FOR K=1 TO NW: READ J(K), I(K), W(K)
  '..........................................Standard interconnections
  IF K <= NY THEN 44
  ON K-NY GOTO 40, 40, 41, 42, 42, 43
40 I(K)=I(K)-G: GOTO 44
41 I(K)=I(K)+G: GOTO 44
42 I(K)=I(K)-N: GOTO 44
43 I(K)=I(K)+N
44 FOR L=1 TO NU-1: W(L*NW+K)=W(K): NEXT: NEXT
  ' ......................................................Processing
46 P1=0: FOR I=1 TO LL: LOCATE I, 1: PRINT E$; : NEXT I
  ' ....................................Transfer Function
  '.........extracellular input processing
  FOR CN=0 TO C-1: FOR RN=0 TO R-1: FOR K=1 TO NV
  L=R*CN+RN : J=J(K)+N*L: A=A(J)+F(L+1)
```

```
   IF A < T THEN A(J)=A: O(J)=0: GOTO 55
   A(J)=(A-V) MOD (T-V)+V: O(J)=1: JM=(J+5) MOD 6
   L=JM+1: COLOR L+9: CIRCLE (32*CN+4*L-2, 16*RN+4), 2
   IF JM=5 THEN L=J/6: IF P(L)=0 THEN F(L)=-1 ELSE F(L)=1
55 NEXT K: NEXT RN: NEXT CN
56 '..........refractory processing
   FOR I=1 TO H: IF A(I) <= S THEN A(I)=A(I)+1: O(I)=O(I)-1
   NEXT
   '...........unit processing
   FOR CN=0 TO C-1: FOR RN=0 TO R-1: L=CN*R+RN: NN=N*L
   NK=NW*L: FOR K=1 TO NW: I=NN+I(K)
   IF K <= NY THEN 65
   '.......................................... Edge exceptions
   IF K > NY THEN IF I < 1 OR I > H THEN 75
   '......................... Synaptic input and unit intraconnections
65 IF O(I) < 0 THEN 75
   J=NN+J(K): IF A(J) <= S THEN 75 ELSE A=A(J)+W(NK+K)
   IF A < T THEN A(J)=A: O(J)=-1: GOTO 71
   A(J)=(A-V) MOD (T-V)+V: O(J)=1: JM=(J+5) MOD 6
   L=JM+1: COLOR L+9: CIRCLE (32*CN+4*L-2, 16*RN+4), 2
   IF JM=5 THEN L=J/6: IF P(L)=0 THEN F(L)=-1 ELSE F(L)=1
71 IF A(J) < S+2 THEN 75
   ' .........................Learning Rule
   FL=0: IF RND*100 > (A-S-1)*LR THEN 75
   W=W(NK+K): IF ABS(W) < 4 THEN W(NK+K)=W+SGN(W)
75 NEXT K: NEXT RN: NEXT CN
   ' .......................................................Iteration
   P1=P1+1: IF P1 < NI THEN 56
   IF INKEY$ <> "" THEN 81 ELSE LOCATE LL-1, LC+1
   IF FL=0 THEN PRINT "Learning .."; : FL=FL+1 ELSE 81
   IF FL < 8 THEN 46
   ' .......................................................Save Weights
81 OPEN "O", #1, S$
   FOR K=1 TO H: PRINT #1, A(K); O(K); : NEXT K
   FOR K=1 TO NW: PRINT #1, J(K); I(K);
   FOR L=0 TO NU-1: PRINT #1, W(L*NW+K); : NEXT: NEXT
   FOR L=1 TO NU: PRINT #1, F(L); : NEXT L
```

```
   CLOSE #1: LOCATE LL, 1
   LINE INPUT ; "Enter 'a' for another pattern, or 'e' to end: ", A$
   IF A$="a" THEN GOSUB 97: GOTO 32 ELSE CLOSE : END
   '..................................................Load Weights
90 OPEN "I", #1, S$
   FOR K=1 TO H: INPUT #1, A(K), O(K): NEXT
   FOR K=1 TO NW: INPUT #1, J(K), I(K)
   FOR L=0 TO NU-1: INPUT #1, W(L*NW+K): NEXT: NEXT
   FOR L=1 TO NU: INPUT #1, F(L): NEXT
   CLOSE #1: RETURN
   '..................................................Pattern input
97 Z$="": FOR I=1 TO MM: Z$=Z$+CHR$(0): NEXT I
   DIM CU(28), M(7): FOR I=1 TO 5: FOR J=1 TO 3
   PSET (I, J),15 : NEXT: NEXT: GET (1, 1)-(5, 3), CU
   I=256: FOR L=0 TO 7: I=I/2: M(L)=I: NEXT L : CLS
   COLOR 15: OPEN "r", 1, F$, MM: FIELD 1, MM AS Y$: LP=0
102 LP=LP+1: GET 1, LP: IF Y$ <> Z$ THEN 102
   COLOR 15 : PRINT "Next pattern #"; LP;
   LINE INPUT ; "; enter # of pattern to edit: ", P$: P=VAL(P$)
   CLS : LOCATE LL, 1: PRINT "Press 'r' to relearn, or ";
   PRINT "use arrows, 'Insert' and 'Delete', then 'e' to exit";
   FOR I=1 TO NU: P(I)=0: NEXT I
   LOCATE LL, 1: GET 1, P: W$=Y$: LM=SW-6*C-6
   LINE (LM, 0)-(SW-1, 4*R+4), , B: FOR I=1 TO R
   FOR J=1 TO C :PSET (LM+6*J, 4*I): NEXT J: NEXT I
   FL=0: L=C1: FOR IA=0 TO C1 : A$=LEFT$(W$,1)
   W$=RIGHT$(W$, L): L=L-1: N(IA)=ASC(A$): NEXT IA
   FOR IA=0 TO C1: NN=N(IA)
   J1=INT(IA/R1): J2=IA-R1*J1: J=J1+1 : I=8*J2
   FOR JB=0 TO 7: L=NN AND M(JB): IF L=0 THEN 117
   NP=R*J-R+I+1: CIRCLE (LM+6*J, 4*I+4),2,10: P(NP)=1
117 I=I+1: NEXT JB: NEXT IA
   I=1: J=1
119 JA=LM+6*J: JB=4*I: PUT (JA-2, JB), CU, XOR
   A$=INKEY$ : PUT (JA-2, JB), CU, XOR: IF A$="" THEN 119
   IF LEN(A$)=2 THEN A$=RIGHT$(A$, 1)
   FL=INSTR(CHR$(8)+CHR$(13)+"reKMPHRS ", A$)
```

```
    IF FL=0 THEN 128
    ON FL GOTO 124, 126, 134, 134, 124, 125, 126, 127, 128, 131, 125
124 IF J > 1 THEN J=J-1: GOTO 119 ELSE 119
125 IF J < C THEN J=J+1: GOTO 119 ELSE 119
126 IF I < R THEN I=I+1: GOTO 119 ELSE 119
127 IF I > 1 THEN I=I-1: GOTO 119 ELSE 119
128 CIRCLE (JA, JB), 2: JA=INT((I-1)/8): JB=I-1-8*JA
    M=R1*J+JA-R1: L=M(JB) AND N(M)
    IF L=0 THEN N(M)=N(M)+M(JB)
    NP=R*(J-1)+I: P(NP)=1: GOTO 119
131 CIRCLE (JA, JB), 2, 0: JA=INT((I-1)/8): JB=I-1-8*JA
    M=R1*J+JA-R1: L=M(JB) AND N(M)
    IF L=M(JB) THEN N(M)=N(M)-L
    NP=R*(J-1)+I: P(NP)=0: GOTO 119
134 W$="": FOR JA=0 TO C1: W$=W$+CHR$(N(JA)): NEXT
    OP=P: I=0: IF Y$=W$ THEN FL=FL-3: GOTO 139
136 I=I+1: GET 1, I: IF Y$=W$ OR I=OP THEN P=I ELSE 136
    P$=STR$(P): L=LEN(P$): P$=RIGHT$(P$, L-1)
    IF P < OP THEN FL=1: OP=P : GOTO 139
    LSET Y$=W$: PUT 1, OP: FL=0
139 LOCATE LL, 1: PRINT E$; "Pattern #"; OP; : CLOSE
    RETURN
    ' ..................................................Matrix elements
    ' ...........J(K),I(K),W(K) (K=1,2) for synaptic input to system
    DATA 1,1,1, 2,2,1
    ' ...........J(K),I(K),W(K) (K=3,...NY) for unit intraconnections
    DATA 3,1,1, 5,1,1, 6,1,1, 4,2,1, 5,2,1, 6,2,1, 4,3,-1, 6,3,-1
    DATA 2,4,-1, 3,4,-1, 6,4,-1, 1,5,-1, 2,5,-1, 5,6,-1
    ' ...........J(K),I(K),W(K) (K=NY+1,.NW) for unit interconnections
    DATA 6,3,-1, 6,2,1, 6,3,-1, 6,3,-1, 6,2,1, 6,3,-1
```

A8.3 Model of a Quantal Turing Machine

This program allows some insight into the effect of 'scanning' of quantal bits, regarded as components of the potential in channels in the membranes of a sequential set of neurons. The latter are numbered so that proximity in the sequence implies also physical proximity. The existing parameters allow the representation of set of 64 neurons, arranged in rows. The components of the potentials are given random initial values, but as a result of interaction with the neurons they soon become correlated and develop the form of a wave that can be seen on screen. Initially the neurons fire at random, but most of the firings gradually become synchronized with the maxima of the potential.

```
   P$(1)="'QWAVE' models components of the potential in the "
   P$(2)="extracellular fluid and their interaction with cells,"
   P$(3)="represented by coloured rings. Colours indicate the "
   P$(4)="phase of the extracellular potential. When the "
   P$(5)="potential is near its maximum there is a chance that "
   P$(6)="it will provide activation to a cell. A thick white "
   P$(7)="ring indicates that the cell has been activated. All"
   P$(8)="processes are in real time. Touch a key to start ..."
   CLS : SCREEN 9 : LINE(0,0)-(639,349),9,BF : DEFINT I-N
   FOR I=1 TO 8 : LOCATE I+5,12 : PRINT P$(I) : NEXT I
   N=64 : DIM X(N),Y(N),P(N),T(N),TL(N),TR(N),BL(N),BR(N)
10 IF INKEY$="" THEN 10 ELSE CLS : 'N=number of neurons
   FOR J=0 TO N-1 : T(J)=J*RND : ' determines phase angles of bits
   NEXT J : GOSUB 40 : PI=3.141593 : T0=T : PT=.95
   'begin iteration, put neurons on screen; colour shows phase
20 GOSUB 40 : DT=T-T0 : FOR J=0 TO N-1 : X=(32*J MOD 512)+32
   Y=28*INT(J/16)+28 : T=T(J)+DT : K=CINT(T) MOD 16
   'Next line uses matrix elements .5*(1+cos(T)) of bits
   FOR I=10 TO 12 : CIRCLE(X,Y),I-2,8 : CIRCLE(X,Y),I,K
   NEXT I : IF .5*(1+COS(T))<(1-.0025*RND) THEN 30
   T(J)=-DT+2*PI : FOR I=8 TO 12 : CIRCLE(X,Y),I,15
   NEXT I : IF J>0 THEN T(J-1)=(1-PT)*T(J-1)+PT*PI
   IF J<N-1 THEN T(J+1)=(1-PT)*T(J+1)+PT*PI
30 NEXT J : IF INKEY$="" THEN 20 ELSE END
40 T$=TIME$ : L=LEN(T$) : M$=MID$(T$,L-4,2)
   S$=RIGHT$(T$,2) : T=60*VAL(M$)+INT(VAL(S$)) : RETURN
```

Bibliography

1. G. L. Stebbins (1982), *Darwin to DNA: Molecules to Humanity,* W. H. Freeman: San Francisco.
2. G. J. Vermeij (1987), *Evolution and Escalation,* Princeton Univ. Press: Princeton, NJ.
3. J. von Neumann (1966), Theory of Self-Reproducing Automata (A. W. Burks, Ed.) Univ. of Illinois Press, Urbana, Ill.
4. S. Levy (1992), *Artificial Life,* Pantheon: New York.
5. H. S. Green and T. Triffet (1993), *J. Intelligent Material Systems and Structures* **4**, 35-42.
6. H. S. Green and T. Triffet (1993), *Mathl. Comput. Modelling* **18**, 1-18.
7. S. Grossberg (1976), *Biological Cybernetics***23**, 121-134.
8. S. Grossberg (1989), *Neural Networks and Natural Intelligence,* M. I. T. Press, Cambridge MA.
9. D. E. Rumelhart and J. L. McClelland (1986), *Parallel Distributed Processing,* **1,2**, M. I. T. Press: Cambridge MA.
10. J. L. McClelland and D. E. Rumelhart (1988), *Explorations in Parallel Distributed Processing,* M. I. T. Press, Cambridge MA.)
11. T. Kohonen (1988), *Self-Organization and Associative Memory,* Springer, Berlin.
12. R. Penrose (1994), *Shadows of the Mind: The Missing Science of Consciousness,* Oxford Univ. Press, Oxford.
13. D. Hodgson (1991), *The Mind Matters,* Clarendon, Oxford.
14. H. P. Stapp (1993). *Mind, Matter and Quantum Mechanics,* Springer, Berlin.
15. J. C. Eccles (1994), *How the Mind Controls its Brain,* Springer, Berlin.
16. D. Bohm (1952), *Phys. Rev.* **85**, 166-179; 180-193.
17. P. N. Kaloyerou (1994), *Physics Reports* **244**, 287-358.
18. J. S. Bell (1990), *Sixty-two Years of Uncertainty* (A. I. Miller, Ed.), 17-31, Plenum Press, New York.
19. W. H. Zurek (1982), *Phys. Rev.*D **26**, 1862-1880.
20. H. Everett III (1957), *Rev. Mod. Phys.***29**, 454-462.
21. B. S. De Witt and N. Graham, Eds. (1973), *The Many-Worlds Interpretation of Quantum Mechanics,* Princeton Univ. Press., Princeton NJ.
22. M. Born (1926), *Z. f. Phys.* **37**, 863-867; *ibid.* **38**, 803-827.
23. N. Bohr (1928), *Nature* **121**, 580-590.

24. F. Lopez da Silva (1992), *Induced Rhythms in the Brain* (E. Başar and T. H. Bullock, Eds.), 83-102, Birkhäuser, Boston.
25. N. Bohr (1933), *Nature*, **131**, 421-423; 457-459.
26. S. Hecht, S. Schlaer and M. H. Pirenne (1941), *J. of Gen. Physiol.*, **25**, 891-940
27. D. A. Baylor, T. D. Lamb and K. -W. Yau (1979), *J. Phsiol.*, **288**, 613-634.
28. E. Başar (1991), *Chaos in Brain Function*, Birkhäuser, Boston.
29. P. Jordan (1941), *Die Physik und das Geheimnis des organischen Lebens*, F. Vieweg, Braunschweig.
30. A. O. Gomez (1966), *Brain and Conscious Experience* (J. C. Eccles; Ed.), 446-468, Springer, New York.
31. H. Margenau (1984), *The Miracle of Existence*, Ox Bow, Woodbridge, CT.)f
32. P. A. M. Dirac (1930), *The Principles of Quantum Mechanics*, Oxford Univ. Press., Oxford.
33. J. von Neumann (1932), *Mathematische Grundlagen der Quantenmechanik*, Springer-Verlag, Berlin.
34. M. Born and P. Jordan (1925) *Z. F. Phys.***34**, 858-888.
35. M. Born, W. Heisenberg and P. Jordan (1926), *Z. f. Phys.* **35**, 557-615.
36. G. Tarozzi and A. van der Merwe, Eds. (1988), *The Nature of the Quantum Paradoxes*, Kluwe, Dordrecht.
37. F. Selleri (1989), *Quantum Paradoxes and Physical Reality*, Kluwe, Dordrecht.
38. E. Schrödinger (1935), *Naturwissenschaften* **23**, 807-812; 823-828; 844-849.
39. H. S. Green and T. Triffet (1991), *Aust. J. Phys.* **44**, 323-334.
40. E. P. Wigner (1962), pp. 284-301 in *The Scientist Speculates* (I. J. Good, Ed.) Heinemann, London.
41. M. Born and H. S. Green (1947), *Proc. Roy. Soc.* A **191**, 168-181.
42. H. Mori (1956), *J. Phys. Soc. Japan*, **11**, 1029-1044.
43. R. Kubo, M. Yokota, and S. Nakajima (1957), *J. Phys. Soc. Japan* **12**, 1203-1211.
44. L. Brillouin (1964), *Scientific Uncertainty and Information*, Academic Press, New York.
45. T. Triffet and H. S. Green (1975), *J. Biol. Phys.* **3**, 53-76; 77-93.
46. C. E. Shannon and W. Weaver (1949), *The Mathematical Theory of Communication*, Univ. of Illinois Press: Urbana IL.
47. P. T. de Chardin (1959), *The Phenomenon of Man*, Harper, New York.

48. J. C. Eccles (1979), pp. 1-18 in *Cerebro-Cerebellar Interactions,* (J. Massion and K. Kasaki, Eds.), Elsevier, Amsterdam.
49. T. Triffet, P. Calvert and T. W. Huntoon (1991), in *System Sciences: Architecture and Emerging Technologies* (V. Milutinovic and B. D. Shriver, Eds.) IEEE Computer Soc. Press).
50. T. Triffet and H. S. Green (1980), *J. Theor. Biol.* **86**, 3-44.
51. H. S. Green and T. Triffet (1980), *Mathematical Modelling* **1**, 41-61.
52. J. E. Le Doux (1992), *Current Opinion in Neurobiol.* **2**, 191-197.
53. B. L. Jacobs (1991), *J. Clin. Psych.* **52**, 17-23.
54. M. C. Nowycky and D. J. Triggle, Eds. (1991), *Annals of the New York Academy of Sciences*, **635**, New York.
55. N. J. Cohen and H. Eichenbaum (1993), *Memory, Amnesia and the Hippocampal System*, M. I. T. Press, Cambridge MA.
56. A. Trehub (1991), *The Cognitive Brain*, M. I. T. Press, Cambridge MA
57. L. A. Coward (1990), *Pattern Thinking*, Praeger, New York.
58. V. B. Mountcastle (1978), in *The Mindful Brain* (G. M. Edelman and V. B. Mountcastle, Eds.); M. I. T. Press, Cambridge MA.)
59. J. Szentagothai (1978), *Proc. Roy. Soc. Lond.* B **201**, 219-248.
60. M. Ito (1984), *The Cerebellum and Neural Control,* Raven Press, New York.
61. S. Haykin (1994), *Neural Networks*, Macmillan Co., New York.
62. R. Lorente de No (1981), *The Primary Acoustic Nuclei,* Raven Press, New York.
63. Ramon y Cajal (1911), *Histologie du Systeme Nerveux de l'Homme et des Vertebres*, **I, II**, Maloine, Paris.
64. S. Palay and V. Chan-Palay (1974), *Cerebellar Cortex,* Springer-Verlag, Berlin.
65. S. Palay and V. Chan-Palay, Eds. (1982), *The Cerebellum - New Vistas,* Springer-Verlag, Berlin.
66. A. Peters and E. G. Jones (1984), *Cerebral Cortex,* Plenum Press, New York.
67. W. Seifert (1983), *Neurobiology of the Hipppocampus,* Academic Press, New York.
68. R. L. Isaacson and K. H. Pribham, Eds. (1986), *The Hippocampus,* **3,4**; Plenum Press, New York.
69. G. M. Shepherd (1974), *The Synaptic Organization of the Brain,* Academic Press, New York.
70. M. L. Barr and J. A. Kiernan (1983), *The Human Nervous System,* Harper and Row, Philadelphia.

71. C. C. Wood, G. McCarthy, N. K. Squires, H. C. Vaughan, D. L. Woods and W. C. McCallum (1984), *Ann. New York Acad. of Sci.***425**, 681-721.
72. L. Kaufman, Y. Okada, J. Tripp and H. Weinberg (1984), *Ann. New York Acad. Sci.* **425**, 722-742.
73. J. M. Osepchuk, Ed. (1983), *The Biological Effects of Electromagnetic Radiation,* IEEE Press, New York.
74. H. Malitz and H. A. Sackheim, Eds. (1986), *Electroconvulsive Therapy* (Ann. N. Y. Acad. Sci., **462**.
75. R. Lorente de No (1947), *A Study in Nerve Physiology,* Studies of the Rockefeller Institute for Medical Research, **131-132**, New York.
76. S. Marrazzi and R. Lorente de No (1944), *J. Neurophysiol.* **7**, 83-102.
77. W. R. Adey (1967), *Prog. Brain Res.* **27**, 228-245.
78. W. Rall (1962), *Biophys. J.* **2**, 145-167.
79. W. Rall and G. M. Shepherd (1978), *J. Neurophysiol.* **31**, 884-915.
80. H. H. Jasper (1983), pp. 375-393 in *The Organization of the Cerebral Cortex,* (F. O. Schmitt, 1st Ed), 375-393, M. I. T. Press: Cambridge, MA.)
81. S. R. Shaw (1984), *J. exp. Biol.* **112**, 225-251.
82. T. Inouye, K. Shinosaki, A. Iyama, Y. Matsumoto and S. Toi (1994), *Cognitive Brain Res.* **2**, 87-92.
83. T. Triffet and H. S. Green (1988), *J. theor. Biol.* **131**, 199-221.
84. G. E. Hinton and J. A. Anderson, Eds. (1981), *Parallel Modes of Associative Memory,* Erlbaum, Hillside NJ.
85. J. J. Hopfield and D. Tank (1986), *Science, N. Y.* **233**, 625-633.
86. T. A. Pedley, R. Traub and I. Goldensohn (1982), pp. 255-269 in *Cellular Pacemakers,* (D. O. Carpenter, Ed.), **1**, John Wiley & Sons, New York.
87. R. K. Wong and P. A. Schwartzkroin (1982), *Cellular Pacemakers,* (D. O. Carpenter, Ed.), 1, 238-254, John Wiley & Sons, New York.
88. R. J. M. Cotterill (1988), *Computer Simulation in Brain Science* (Camb. Univ. Press: Cambridge, England)
89. H. S. Green and T. Triffet (1983), *J. theor. Biol.* **100**, 649-674.
90. E. R. Kandel (1979), *Behavoural Biology of Aplysia,* W. H. Freeman, San Francisco CA.
91. R. Llinas (1979), *The Neurosciences: Fourth Study Program* (F. O. Schmitt and F. G. Worden, Eds.), 555-571, M. I. T. Press, Cambridge MA.
92. T. Bliss and T. Lomo (1973), *J. Physiol.* **232**, 331-356.

93. G. Lynch, S. Halpain and M. Baudry (1983), *Neurobiology of the Hippocampus,* (W. Seifert, Ed.), 253-2654, Academic Press, New York.
94. B. L. McNaughton (1983), *Neurobiology of the Hippocampus* (W. Seifert, Ed.), 233-249, Academic Press, New York.
95. K. S. Lee (1983), pp. 265-272 *Neurobiology of the Hippocampus* (W. Seifert, Ed.), 265-272, Academic Press, New York.
96. U. Misgeld and M. R. Klee (1984), *Exp. Brain Res.* Supp. **9**, 325-332.
97. E. Fifkova and Anderson (1981), *Exp. Neurology* **74**, 621-627.
98. E. Fifkova, J. A. Markham and R. J. Delay (1983), *Brain Res. Osaka,* **266**, 163-168.
99. J. C. Eccles (1983), *Neuroscience***10**, 1071-1081.
100. J. C. Eccles (1984), *Cerebral Cortex,* (E. G. Jones and A. Peters, Eds.), **2**,1-36, Plenum Press, New York.
101. D. O. Hebb (1949), *The Organization of Behaviour,*John Wiley & Sons, New York.
102. V. B. Brooks (1984), *Exp. Brain Res.* Supp. **9**, 170-183.
103. A. M. Turing (1936), *Proc. Lond. Math. Soc.***42**, 230-265
104. K. Gödel (1962), *On Formally Undecidable Propositions*, Oliver and Boyd, London.
105. A. M. Turing (1950), *Mind***59**, 433-460
106. W. S. McCullough and W. Pitts (1943), *Bull. Math. Biophys.* **5,** 115-133
107. S. Grossberg, Ed. (1994), *Neural Networks***7**, 963-1190
108. S. Haykin (1994), pp. 65-77 in *Neural Networks,* Macmillan, New York
109. P. Benioff (1980), *J. Stat. Phys.* **22**, 563-591.
110. R. P. Feynman (1986), *Foundations of Phys.* **16,** 507-531
111. D. Deutsch (1985), *Proc. Roy. Soc. Lond.* A **400**, 97-117
112. R. Josza (1991), *Proc. Roy. Soc. Lond.* A **435**, 563-574
113. D. Deutsch and R. Josza (1992), *Proc. Roy. Soc. Lond.* A **439**, 553-558
114. J. J. Hopfield (1982), *Proc. Nat. Acad. Sci.* **79**, 2554-2558.
115. C. L. Wu and T. Y. Feng, Eds. (1984), *Interconnected Networks for Parallel and Distributed Processing,* IEEE Computer Society, Washington DC.
116. L. W. Tucker and G. C. Robertson (1988), *IEEE Computer* **21**, 26-38.
117. G. Carpenter (1989), *Neural Networks* **2**, 243-257.
118. K. A. Frenkel (1986), *ACM Communications* **29**, 752-758.
119. R. R. Rettburg, W. R. Crowther, P. P. Carvey and R. S. Tomlinson (1990), *IEEE Computer* **23**, 18-30.

120. H. P. Graf, L. D. Jackel and W. E. Hubbard (1988), *IEEE Computer* **21**, 41-49.
121. L. C. Chu and B. Wah (1990), *IJCNN Conference Proceedings,* **II**, 639-649.
122. M. Yasunaga, N. Masuda, M. Yagyu, M. Asai, M. Yamada and A. Masaki (1990), *IJCNN Conference Proceedings,*II.
123. B. Wah and G. J. Li, Eds. (1986), *Computers for Artificial Intelligence Applications,* IEEE Computer Society, Washington DC.
124. W. H. Nauta and H. J. Karten (1970), *The Neurosciences: Second Study Program* (F. O. Schmitt, Ed.), 7-26, Rockefeller Univ. Press, New York.
125. F. Crick (1984), *Proc. Nat. Acad. Sci.* **81**, 4586-4590.
126. J. Nolte (1988), *The Human Brain,* C. V. Mosby Co., Washington DC.
127. A. Sibbald, P. D. Whalley and A. K. Covington (1984), *Analytica Chemica Acta* **159**, 47-62.
128. B. Widrow (1987), *Proc. of First Int. Conf. on Neural Networks, San Diego* **1**, 145-157.
129. C. A. Mead and M. A. Mahowald (1988), *Neural Networks* **1**, 91-97.
130. J. G. Taylor (1990), *Neural Networks* **3**, 171-178.
131. H. C. Card and W. R. Moore (1990), *Neural Networks* **3**, 333-346.
132. N. Suga (1990) *Scientific American***262**, 60-68.
133. T. Triffet and H. S. Green (1975), *J. Biol. Phys.* **3**, 53-76; 77-93.
134. R. Endo (1993), *Prog. Theor. Phys.* **90**, 1121-1129
135. H. J. Freund and H. Hummelsheim (1985), *Brain* **108**, 697-733
136. M. Wiesdanger and J. S. Miles (1980), *Physiol. Rev.* **62**, 1234-1270
137. W. R. Uttal (1978), *The Psychology of Mind* (L. Erlbaum, Hillsdale N. J.)
138. H. H. Kornhuber (1973), pp 1-22 in *Memory and the Transfer of Information* (H. Zippel, Ed.; Plenum: New York)
139. W. Freeman (1986), *Methods of Analysis of Brain Electrical and Magnetic Signals: Handbook of Encephalography and Clinical Neurophysiology Vol.*3A/2 (Elsevier: Amsterdam)
140. L. Heimer (1983), *The Human Brain and Spinal Cord* (Springer: Berlin)
141. K. Brodman (1909), *Vergleichende Lokalizationslehre der Grosshirnrinde (*J. A. Barth: Leipzig)
142. W. Penfield and L. Roberts (1959), *Speech and Brain Mechanisms (*Princeton Univ. Press: Princeton, N. J.)
143. N. Butters and L. Cermak (1975), pp. 307-409 in *The Hippocampus* (Vol. 2: R. L. Isaacson and K. H. Pribham, Eds.; Plenum: New York)
144. J. C. Eccles (1982), *Arch. Psychiatr. Nervenkr.***231**, 423-441

145. J. C. Eccles, M. Ito and J. Szentagothai (1967), *The Cerebellum as a Neuronal Machine*(Springer: Berlin)
146. J. C. Eccles (1989), *Evolution of the Brain: Creation of the Self* (Routledge: London)
147. A. Vernadakis (1988), *Int. Rev. of Neurobiol.* **30**, 149-224 (1988)
148. H. Berger (1929), *Arch. Psychiatr. u. Nervenkrankh.* **87**, 527-570; (1930), *J. Psychol. Neurol.* **40**, 160-179
149. H. Caspars (1992), pp. 9-20 in *Slow Potential Changes in the Brain* (Birkhäuser: Boston)
150. W. J. Ellis (1994), *Molecular Physics* **82**, 973-988
151. A. T. Barker, K. Jalinous and I. L. Freeston (1985), *Lancet* **1**, 1106-1107
152. D. O. Carpenter (1982), *Extracellular Pacemakers* (2 Vols.; Wiley: New York)
153. B. Katz and R. Miledi (1967), *J. Physiol.* **189**, 535-544
154. W. R. Adey (1992), pp. 325-353 in *Induced Rhythms in the Brain* (E. Başar and T. H. Bullock, Eds.; Birkhäuser, Boston)
155. E. L. White (1989), pp. 83-105, 159-176, 207-215 in *Cortical Circuits* (Birkhäuser, Boston)
156. M. L. Barr and J. A. Kiernan (1983), pp. 13-31 in *The Human Nervous System* (Harper and Row: Philadelphia).
157. M. R. Rosenzweig and E. L. Bennett (1976), pp. 130-132 in *Neural Mechanisms of Learning and Memory* (M. I. T. Press: Cambridge, Mass.)
158. J. A. Anderson and E. Rosenfeld, Eds. (1988)), *Neurocomputing Foundations of Research* (M. I. T. Press: Cambridge, Mass.)
159. J. Nolte (1988), *The Human Brain* (C. V. Mosby: St. Louis)
160. G. M. Shepherd (1988), pp. 639-656 in *Neurobiology* (Oxford University Press, New York)
161. M. A. B. Brazier (1977), pp. 12-13, 41- 42, 64-65, 91-92, 123-124 in *Electrical Activity of the Nervous System* (Williams and Wilkins: Baltimore)
162. E. R. Kandel (1976), pp. 98-209 in *Cellular Basis of Behavior*(W. Freeman: San Francisco)
163. J-P. Changeux, A. Devillers-Thiery and P. Chemouilli (1985), pp. 216-238 in *Neuroscience* (P. H. Abelson, E. Butz and S. H. Snyder, Eds.; Amer. Assoc. Adv. Sci.: Washington D. C.)
164. S. W. Kuffler and J. G. Nicholls (1977), *From Neuron to Brain* (Sinauer Associates: Sunderland, Mass)
165. J. C. Eccles (1982), *Ann. Rev. Neurosci.* **5**, 325-339

166. H. H. Dale (1935), *Proc. Roy. Soc. Med.*28, 319-322
167. R. R. Llinás (1991), pp. 3-17 in *Calcium Entry at the Presynaptic Nerve Terminal*(E. F. Stanley, M. C. Nowycky and D. J. Triggle, Eds.; New York Acad. of Sci.: New York)
168. R. Jahn and T. C. Südhof (1994), *Ann. Rev. Neurosci.*17, 219-246
169. F. Hucho (1986), p. 169 in *Neurochemistry*(VCH: Weinhem)
170. B. Katz And R. Miledi (1969), *J. Physiol. (Lond.)* **195**, 481-492
171. F. A. Dodge Jr. and R. Rahamimoff (1967), *J. Physiol. (Lond.)* **193**, 419-432
172. S. B. Barton, I. Cohen and W. Van der Kloot (1983), *J. Physiol. (Lond.)* **337**, 735-752
173. H. Parnas, I. Parnas and J. Dudel (1986), pp. 215-237 in *Calcium, Neuronal Function and Transmitter Release* (R. Rahamimoff and B. Katz, Eds.; Martinus Nijhoff: Boston)
174. M. Frotscher and U. Misgeld, Eds. (1989), *Central Cholinergic Synaptic Transmission* (Birkhäuser: Boston)
175. T. V. Bliss and G. Collingridge (1993), *Nature*, **361**, 31-39
176. P. A. Colley and A. Routtenberg (1993), *Brain Res. Reviews* **18**, 115-122
177. I. Creese, D. R. Burt and S. H. Snyder (1979), *Nature*, **278**, 577-578
178. A. Scarpa, E. Carafoli and S. Papa, Eds. (1992), *Ion-motive ATPases: Structure, Function and Regulation* (N. Y. Acad. of Sci.: New York)
179. G. Biggio and E. Costa, Eds. (1988), *Chloride Channels and their Modulation by Neurotransmitters and Drugs*(Raven: New York)
180. H. C. Fibiger (1995), pp. 1-11 in *Depression and Mania* (G. L. Gessa, W. Fratta, L. Pani and G. Serra, Eds.; Lippincott-Raven: Philadelphia)
181. W. Rall (1989), pp. 1-62 in *Methods in Neuronal Modeling* (C. Koch and I Segev, Eds.; M. I. T. Press: Cambridge, Mass.)
182. H. C. Tuckwell (1987), *Introduction to Theoretical Neurobiology* (Vol. 1; Cambridge Univ. Press: Cambridge, England)
183. K. S. Cole (1968), *Membranes Ions and Impulses* (Univ. of Calif. Press, Berkeley)
184. R. Fitzhugh (1961), *Biophys. J.*1, 445-456
185. R. Plonsey (1981), pp. 177-205 in *Biomagnetism* (Eds. S. N. Erne, H. D. Hahlbohm and H. Lubbig; De Gruyter: Berlin)
186. A. L. Towe (1973), in *Bioelectric Recording Techniques* A, pp. 79-93 (Eds. R. F. Thompson and M. M. Patterson; Academic: New York)
187. O. D. Creutzfeldt, G. A. Ojemann and G. E. Chatrian (1992), pp. 21-42 in *Slow Potential Changes in the Brain* (W. Haschke, E. -J. Speckmann

and A. I. Roitbak, Eds.: Birkhäuser: Boston)

188. F. H. Lopes da Silva and W. Storm van Leeuwen (1977), *Neurosci. Lett.* **6**, 237-241
189. P. Andersen and S. A. Andersson (1968), *Physiological Basis of the Alpha Rhythm*(Appleton-Century-Crofts: New York)
190. E. Başar (1980), *EEG-Brain Dynamics* (Elsevier: Amsterdam)
191. R. Karrer, J. Cohen and P. Tueting, Eds. (1984), *Brain Information: Event Related Potentials* (New York Acad. of Sci.: New York)
192. C. H. M. Brunia, G. Mulde and M. N. Verbaten, Eds. (1991), *Event Related Brain Res.* (*EEG Suppl.* **42**; Elsevier: Amsterdam)
193. H. H. Kornhuber (1973), pp. 267-280 in *The Neurosciences: Third Study Program* (F. O. Schmitt and F. G. Worden, Eds.; M. I. T. Press: Cambridge, Mass.)
194. T. W. Picton and D. T. Stuss (1980), *Prog. Brain Res.* **54**, 17-49
195. T. H. Bullock and E. Başar (1988), Brain Res. Revs. **13**, 57-75
196. G. R. Mangun (1992), pp. 217-231 in *Induced Rhythms in the Brain* (E. Başar and T. H. Bullock, Eds.; Birkhäuser, Boston)
197. J. O'Keefe and L. Nadel (1978), *The Hippocampus as a Cognitive Map* (Clarendon Press: Oxford)
198. W. J. Freeman (1975), *Mass Action in the Nervous System* (Academic: New York)
199. E. Başar and T. Bullock (1992), *Induced Rhythms in the Brain* (Birkhäuser: Boston)
200. E. Lorenz (1963), *J. Atmos. Sci.*,**20**, 130-141; 448-464
201. J. Gleick (1989), *Chaos* (Sphere: London)
202. I. Stewart (1989), *Does God Play Dice?: the Mathematics of Chaos* (Blackwell: Oxford)
203. B. C. McNaughton, R. M. Douglas and G. V. Goddard (1978), *Brain Res.* **157**, 277-293
204. G. L. Collingridge and T. V. P. Bliss (1987), *Trends Neurosci.* **10**, 288-293
205. F. H. Lopes da Silva, J. -P. Pijn and W. J. Wadham (1994), *Prog. in Brain Res.*,**102**, 359-370
206. C. H. Vanderwolf (1988), pp. 225-340 in *Int. Rev. of Neurobiol.*,**30** (Eds. J. R. Smythies and R. J. Bradley, Academic: New York)
207. H. -H. Hinge, T. S. Jensen, M. Kjaer, J. Marquardsen and B. de F. Olivarius (1986), *Arch. Neurol.*, **43**, 673-676
208. J. W. Miller, R. C. Petersen, E. J. Metter, C. H. Millikan and T. Yanagihara (1987), *Neurology*, **37**, 733-737

209. H. S. Green and T. Triffet (1975), *Int. J. Quantum Chem: Quantum Biol. Symp.* **2**, 289-296
210. J. Jaynes (1976), *The Origin of Consciousness in the Breakdown of the Bicameral Mind*, (Houghton Mifflin: Boston)
211. J. A. Rogas-Ramiras and R. R. Drucker-Colin (1977), pp 57- in *Neurobiology of Sleep and Memory* (R. R. Drucker-Colin and J. L. McGaugh, Eds.; Academic: New York)
212. F. Beck and J. C. Eccles (1992), *Proc. Nat. Acad. Sci.***89**, 11357-11361
213. G. M. Edelman (1989), *The Remembered Present. A Biological theory of Consciousness (*Basic Books: New York)
214. R. Penrose (1989), *The Emperor's New Mind: Concerning Computers, Minds and the Laws of Physics* (Oxford Univ. Press: Oxford)
215. D. C. Dennett (1991), *Consciousness Explained (*Allen Lane/Penguin: London)
216. F. Crick and C. Koch (1992), *The Problem of Consciousness* in *Scientific American*, 111-117
217. J. R. Searle (1992), *The Rediscovery of Mind*(MIT Press: Cambridge Mass.)
218. E. R. John, Ed. (1990), *Machinery of the Mind* (Birkhäuser Boston)
219. G. A. Martynov and R. R. Salem (1983), *The Electric Double Layer at a Metal-Dilute Electrolyte Interface* (*Lecture Notes in Chemistry***33**; Springer: Berlin)
220. L. Brillouin (1963), *Science and Information Theory* (Academic: New York)
221. H. S. Green and R. B. Leipnik (1970), *Sources of Plasma Physics* (Nordhoff: Amsterdam)
222. L. Szilard (1923), *Zeits. f. Physik* **53**, 840-856
223. P. Debye and E. Hückel (1923), *Phys. Zeits.* **24**, 185-206
224. J. W. Gibbs (1902), *Elementary Principles of Statistical Mechanics* (Yale Univ. Press: New Haven)
225. J. F. Zemaitis *et al.* (1986), *Handbook of Aqueous Electrolyte Thermodynamics* (Amer. Inst. of Chem. Eng.: New York)
226. B. E. Conway (1981), *Ionic Hydration in Chemistry and Biophysics* (Elsevier: Amsterdam)
227. S. Vaccaro and H. S. Green, *J. theor. Biol.* **81**, 771-788
228. N. W. McLachlan (1951), *Mathieu Functions* (Oxford Univ. Press: Oxford)
229. A. L. Hodgkin and A. F. Huxley (1952), *J. Physiol.* **117**, 500-544
230. K. S. Cole (1960), *Biophys. J.* **1**, 1-14

231. K. S. Cole (1968), *Membranes Ions and Impulses* (Univ. of Calif. Press: Berkeley)
232. J. Cronin (1987), *Mathematical Aspects of Hodgkin-Huxley Neural Theory* (Cambridge Univ. Press: Cambridge, England)
233. B. Frankenhaeuser and A. L. Hodgkin (1957), *J. Physiol.* **137**, 218-294
234. L. J. Mullins (1962), *Nature* **196**, 986-987
235. R. A. Sjodin and L. J. Mullins (1958), *J. Gen. Physiol.* **48**, 49-53
236. R. Fitzhugh (1981), pp. 25-35 in *The Biological Approach to Excitable Systems* (W. J. Adelman and D. E. Goldman, Eds.; Plenum: New York)
237. B. C. Abbott, A. V. Hill and J. V. Howarth (1958), *Proc. Roy. Soc. Lond.* B **148**, 149-187
238. A. Rabinovitch, R. Thieberger and M. Friedman (1994), *Phys. Rev.* E **50**, 1572-1578
239. S. R. Vaccaro (1993), *Mathl. Comput. Modelling* **18**, 49-61
240. B. Sakmann and E. Neher, Eds. (1983), *Single Channel Recording* (Plenum: New York)
241. J. F. Sherwood and T. Triffet (1977), *First Int. Conf. on Mathematical Modelling,* **2**, 19
242. S. R. Vaccaro and H. S. Green (1979), J. theor. Biol., **81**, 777-802
243. S. W. Kuffler and D. D. Potter (1964), *J. Neurophysiol.* **27**, 290-320
244. R. E. Coggeshall and D. W. Fawcett (1964), *J. Neurophysiol.* **27**, 229
245. J. G. Nicholls and S. W. Kuffler (1964), *J. Neurophysiol.***27**, 645-673
246. J. G. Nicholls and D. A. Baylor (1968), *J. Neeurophysiol.***31**, 740-756
247. A. E. Stuart (1970), *J. Physiol.***209**, 627-646
248. J. G. Nicholls and D. Purves (1970), *J. Physiol.* **209**, 647-667
249. J. G. Nicholls and D. Purves (1972), *J. Physiol.* **225**, 637-656
250. D. C. van Essen (1973), *J. Physiol.* **230**, 509-534
251. K. J. Muller and J. G. Nicholls (1974), *J. Physiol.* **238**, 357-369
252. J. K. S. Jansen, K. J. Muller and J. G. Nicholls (1974), *J. Physiol.***242**, 289-305
253. K. W. Yau (1976), *J. Physiol.* **263**, 489-512
254. S. Miyazaki and J. G. Nicholls (1976), *Proc. Roy. Soc. Lond.* B **194**, 295-311
255. K. J. Muller and V. J. McMahan (1976), *Proc. Roy. Soc. Lond.* B **194**, 481-499
256. W. B. Kristan, Jr. and G. S. Stent (1976), *Cold Spring Harbor Symp. Quantum Biol.***40**, 663
257. P. B. Sargent, K. W. Yau and J. G. Nicholls (1977), *J. Neurophysiol.***40**, 446-452

258. P. B. Sargent (1977), *J. Neurophysiol.***40**, 453-460
259. J. G. Nicholls and B. G. Wallace (1978), *J. Physiol.***281**, 157-170
260. D. Bowling, J. G. Nicholls and I. Parnas (1978), *J. Physiol.* **282**, 169-180
261. E. R. Kandel (1979), *The Harvey Lecture Series* **73**
262. C. R. Gallistel (1980), *Amer. Sci.* **68**, 398-409
263. N. Lakshminarayanaiah (1969), *Transport Phenomena in Membranes* (Academic: New York)
264. E. E. Bitter, Ed. (1970), Chs. 6-7 in *Membranes and Ion Transport* **2**, (Wiley: New York)
265. D. Geduldig and R. Gruener (1970), *J. Physiol. Lond.* **211**, 217-244
266. M. V. Thomas and A. L. F. Gorman (1977), *Science* **196**, 531-533
267. N. Akaike, K. S. Lee and A. M. Brown (1978), *J. Gen. Physiol.* **71**, 509-531
268. Z. Ahmed and J. A. Connor (1979), *J. Physiol.* **286**, 61-82
269. I. Kupfermann and E. R. Kandel (1969), *Science***164**, 847-850
270. I. Kupfermann and H. Pinsker (1969), p. 356 in *Reinforcement and Behavior* (J. Tapp, Ed.; Academic Press: New York)
271. V. Castellucci, H. Pinsker, I. Kupfermann and E. R. Kandel (1970), *Science* **167**, 1745-1748
272. E. R. Kandel, T. J. Carew and J. Koester (1976), *Electrobiology of Nerve, Synapse and Muscle* (J. B. Reubens, D. P. Purpura, M. V. L. Bennett and E. R. Kandel, Eds.; Raven Press: New York)
273. E. R. Kandel, M. Brunelli, J. Byrne and V. Castellucci (1976), *Cold Spring Harbor Symp. Quantum Biol.***40**, 465
274. E. R. Kandel (1979), *Sci. Amer.***241** (9), 60-70
275. I. Kupfermann, H. Pinsker, V. Castellucci and E. R. Kandel (1971), *Science***174**, 1252-1255
276. M. Klein and E. R. Kandel (1978), *Proc. Nat. Acad. Sci. USA* **75**, 3512-3516
277. R. Rahaminoff (1974), p. 943 in *The Neurosciences: Third Study Program* (F. O. Schmitt and F. G. Wordon, Eds.; M. I. T. Press: Cambridge, Mass.)
278. T. Shimara and L. Shimara (1977), *Brain Res.* **127**, 168-172
279. T. Triffet and H. S. Green (1983), *J. Theor. Biol.***100**, 645-674
280. A. L. Hodgkin and A. F. Huxley (1957), *Proc. Roy. Soc. Lond.* B **148**, 1-37
281. P. Skorupski (1992), *J. Neurophysiol.* **67**, 664-679
282. S. I. Head and B. M. H. Bush (1992) *J. exp. biol.* **163**, 187-208

283. U. Bässler, T. Hoffman and U. Schuch (1986), *Physiol. Entomol.* **11**, 359-356
284. U. Bässler (1993), *Brain Res. Rev.* **18**, 207-226
285. M. Burrows (1992) *TINS* **15**, 226-232
286. U. Bässler (1986), *Biol. Cyber.***54**, 65-69
287. K. G. Pearson (1985), pp. 307-315 in *Feedback Control in Invertebrates and Vertebrates* (W. J. P. Barnes and M. H. Gladden, Eds.; Dover: London)
288. R. D. Beer (1990), *Intelligence as Adaptive Behavior* (Academic: Boston, Mass.)
289. R. D. Beer, H. J. Chiel and L. S. Sterling (1991), *Amer. Scientist* **79**, 444-452
290. K. von Frisch (1967) *The Dance Language and Orientation of Bees*Harvard Univ. Press: Cambridge, Mass.)
291. J. S. Albus (1981), *Brains, Behavior, and Robotics*(BYTE Books-McGraw-Hill: Peterborough, N. H.)
292. A. M. Turing (1963), *Computers and Thought (*E. A. Feigenbaum and J. Feldman, Eds.; McGraw-Hill, New York)
293. J. von Neumann (1959),*The Computer and the Brain* (Yale Univ. Press: New Haven, Conn.)
294. W. S. McCullough and W. Pitts (1943), *Bull. Math. Biophys.* **5**,115-133
295. F. Rosenblatt (1958), *Psych. Rev.* **65**, 386-408
296. N. Wiener (1948), *Cybernetics: Control and Communication in the Animal and the Machine* (Wiley: New York)
297. W. R. Uttal (1978), *The Psychobiology of Mind* (Lawrence Erlbaum: Hillsdale, N. J.)
298. C. Hampden-Turner (1981), *Maps of the Mind* (Collier Books-Macmillan: New York)
299. K. Parsaye, M. Chignell, S. Khoshafian and H. Wong (1989), pp. 161-22 in *Intelligent Databases: Object-Oriented, Deductive Hypermedia Technologies*(Wiley: New York)
300. J. C. Bezdek and S. K. Pal (1992), *Fuzzy Models for Pattern Recognition* (IEEE Press: Piscataway, N. J.)
301. R. K. Lindsay, B. G. Buchanan, E. A. Feigenbaum and J. Lederberg (1980), *Applications of Artificial Intelligence for Organic Chemistry: The DENDRAL Project* (McGraw-Hill: New York)
302. W. A. Martin and R. J. Fateman (1971), pp. 59-75 in *Proc. Second Symposium on Symbolic and Algebraic Manipulation* (Los Angeles, Cal.)

303. F. Hayes-Roth, D. A. Waterman and D. B. Lenat (1983), *Building Expert Systems* (Addison-Wesley: Reading, Mass.)

304. G. M. Edelman and V. B. Mountcastle (1982), *The Mindful Brain: Cortical Organization and the Group-Selective Theory of Higher Brain Function* (M. I. T. Press: Cambridge, Mass.)

305. P. J. Werbos (1989), pp. 209-216 in *Proc. Int. Joint Conference on Neural Networks*, **1**(Washington, D. C)

306. C. C. Klimasauskas and J. P. Guiver (1988), *NeuralWorks*, (NeuralWare, Inc., Sewickley, Penn.)

307. J. J. Hopfield (1982), *Proc. Nat. Acad. Sci. USA* **81**, 3088-3092

308. D. E. Goldberg (1989), *Genetic Algorithms: in Search, Optimization & Machine Learning* (Addison-Wesley: Reading, Mass.)

309. J. A. Anderson (1993), pp. 77-103 in *Associative Neural Memories* (M. Hassoun, Ed.; Oxford Univ. Press: Oxford, England)

310. T. Triffet and H. S. Green (1989), *Mathl. Comp. Modelling***12**, 673-694

311. H. S. Green and T. Triffet (1989), *J. theor. Biol.***136**, 87-116

312. B. Widrow (1990), *30 Years of Adaptive Neural Networks: Perceptron*30 Years of Adaptive Neural Networks: Perceptron, Madaline and Backpropagation", *Proceedings of the IEEE*, 78, 1415-1442

313. P. M. Morse and H. Feshbach (1953), *Methods of Theoretical Physics*, **1**,434-443, McGraw-Hill, Inc., New York

314. S. Kirkpatrick, C. D. Gelatt, Jr. and M. P. Vecchi (1983), *Science* **220**, 671-680

315. G. A. Carpenter and S. Grossberg (1991), *Pattern Recognition by Self-Organizing Neural Networks* (M. I. T. Press: Cambridge, Mass.).

316. R. Hecht-Nielsen (1990), *Neurocomputing* (Addison-Wesley: Reading, Mass.).

317. J. A. Freeman (1991), *Neural Networks* (Addison-Wesley: Reading, Mass.)

318. D. H. Hubel and T. N. Wiesel (1977) *Proc. Roy. Soc. Lond.* B **198**, 1-59

319. K. Fukushima, S. Miyake and T. Ito (1983), IEEE Trans.: Systems, Man and Cybernetics **13**, 826-834

320. N. H. Farhat, D. Psaltis, A. Prata and E. Paek (1985), *Applied Optics* **24**, 1469-1475

321. G. L. Sewell (1986), *Quantum Theory of Collective Phenomena* (Oxford Univ. Press: Oxford, England)

322. W. J. Freeman (1992), *Int. J. of Bifurcation and Chaos in Appl. Sci. and Eng.* **2**, 451-482

323. J. H. Holland (1992), *Adaptation in Natural and Artificial Systems* (M. I. T. Press: Cambridge, Mass.)
324. G. Nicolis and I. Prigogine (1989), *Exploring Complexity* (W. H. Freeman: New York)
325. V. Milutinovic and B. D. Shriver, Eds. (1991), *Proceedings of the Twenty-Fourth International Conference on Systems Science: Architecture and Emerging Technologies*, **1** (IEEE Computer Soc. Press: New York)
326. M. Minsky (1985), *The Society of Mind* (Simon and Schuster: New York)
327. R. C. Schank and P. G. Childers, *The Cognitive Computer* (Addison-Wesley: Reading, Mass.).
328. W. Hubbard, D. Schwartz, J. S. Denker, H. P. Graf, R. E. Howard, L. D. Jackel, B. Straughn and D. M. Tennant (1986), pp. 151, 227-234, 182-187 in *A. I. P. Conference Proceedings*, (R. G. Lerner, Ed.; American Institute of Physics)
329. C. A. Mead and M. Ismail (1989), *Analog VLSI Implementation of Neural Systems*, (Kluwer-Academic: Boston, Mass.)
330. T. Triffet and H. S. Green (1993), *Mathl. Comput. Modelling* **17**, 75-88
331. T. Triffet and H. S. Green (1992), pp. 51-60 in *Intelligent Engineering Systems Through Artificial Neural Networks*, **2** (C. H. Dagli, L. I. Burke and Y. C. Shin, Eds.)
332. T. Triffet and H. S. Green (1993), pp. 195-205 in *Third International Conference on Microelectronics for Neural Networks* (UnivEd Technologies: IEEE, Edinburgh)
333. F. M. Gray (1991), Ch. 2 in *Solid Polymer Electrolytes* (VCM Publishers)
334. A. J. Bard and L. R. Faulkner (1980), *Electrochemical Methods* (Wiley: New York)
335. T. Gambke and B. Metz (1989), *Glastech. Ber.* **62**, 38-45.
336. E. Fifkova and A. van Harreveld (1975), *J. Neurocytol.* **6**, 211-230
337. S. E. Fox, S. Wolfson and J. B. Rank, Jr. (1983), pp. 303-317 in *Neurobiology of the Hippocampus*, (W. Seifert, Ed.; Academic: New York)
338. J. Szentagothai (1984), *Exp. Brain Res.* Supp. **9**, 347-358
339. T. Bliss and A. Gardner-Medwin (1973), *J. Physiol.***232**, 357-374
340. T. J. Teyler and P. D. Scenna (1987), *Ann. Rev. Neurosci.* **10**, 131-161
341. R. Karner, J. Cohen and P. Tueting (Eds.,1984), *Brain and Information* (Ann. New York Acad. Sci. **425**)

342. H. H. Kronhuber (1984), *Exp. Brain Res.* Supp. **9**, 315-323
343. K. Sasaki (1984), *Exp. Brain Res.* Supp. **9**, 347-358
344. G. Lynch, (1986), *Synapses, Circuits, and the Beginnings of Memory* (M. I. T. Press: Cambridge Mass.)
345. M. P. Witter, H. J. Groenewegen, F. H. Lopes de Silva and A. H. M. Loman (1989), *Prog. in Neurobiol.* **33**, 161-253
346. L. Nadel, L. Cooper, P. Culicover and R. M. Harnish, Eds. (1988), *Neural Connections, Mental Computations* (M. I. T. Press: Cambridge MA)
347. L. Weiskrantz (1978), pp. 373-387 in *Functions of the Septo-Hippocampal System (*CIBA Foundation Symposium **58**; Elsevier: Amsterdam)
348. B. van der Waerden (1967), *Sources of Quantum Mechanics* (North Holland : Amsterdam)
349. W. Heisenberg (1925), *Zeits. d. Physik* **33**, 879-893
350. W. Heisenberg (1927), *Zeits. d. Physik* **43**, 172-198
351. F. J. Dyson (1949), *Phys. Rev.* **75**, 486-502; 1736-1755
352. P. Busch, P. J. Lahti and P. Mittelstaedt (1991), *The Quantum Theory of Measurement,* (Springer: Berlin)
353. J. F. Cornwell (1984), *Group Theory in Physics* (2 Vols.) (Academic: London)
354. H. S. Green (1995), *Aust. J. Phys.* **148**, 613-633
355. P. Ghose, D. Home and G. S. Agarwal (1992), *Phys. Lett.* **A168**, 95-99
356. Y. Mizobuchi and Y. Ohtaké (1991), *Phys. Lett.* **A168**, 1-5
357. A. Einstein, B. Podolsky and N. Rosen (1935), *Phys. Rev.* **47**, 777-780
358. L. Janossy (1952), *Acta Phys. Hungar.* **1**, 423-468 (1952), also (1953) as *Ann. d. Physik,* **11**, 323-361
359. H. S. Green and T. Triffet (1969), *J. Math. Phys.* **10**, 1069-1089
360. H. S. Green (1958), *Nuovo Cimento***9**, 880-889
361. L. de Broglie (1959), *J. Phys. Radium* **20**, 963-979
362. R. Landauer (1995) *Phil. Trans. Roy. Soc. London A* **353**, 367-376
363. D. P. DiVincenzo (1995) *Phys. Rev. A* **51**, 1015-1022
364. T. Triffet and H. S. Green (1996), *Mathl. Comput. Modelling* **24**, 37-56
365. H. S. Green and T. Triffet (1996), *Math. Scientist* **21**, 73-84
366. A. Scott (1995) *Stairway to the Mind* 80-94 (Springer: New York)
367. D. Chalmers (1995) *Journal of Consciousness Studies* **2**, 200-219
368. S. Mithen (1996) *The Prehistory of the Mind* (Thames and Hudson Ltd.: London)

Index